The Neurology of Thinking

The Neurology of Thinking

D. FRANK BENSON, M.D.
The Augustus S. Rose Professor of Neurology
UCLA School of Medicine
Los Angeles, California

New York   Oxford
OXFORD UNIVERSITY PRESS
1994

Oxford University Press

Oxford New York Toronto
Delhi Bombay Calcutta Madras Karachi
Kuala Lumpur Singapore Hong Kong Tokyo
Nairobi Dar es Salaam Cape Town
Melbourne Auckland Madrid

and associated companies in
Berlin Ibadan

Copyright © 1994 by Oxford University Press, Inc.

Published by Oxford University Press, Inc.,
200 Madison Avenue, New York, New York 10016

Oxford is a registered trademark of Oxford University Press

All rights reserved. No part of this publication may be reproduced,
stored in a retrieval system, or transmitted, in any form or by any means,
electronic, mechanical, photocopying, recording, or otherwise,
without the prior permission of Oxford University Press.

Library of Congress Cataloging-in-Publication Data
Benson, D. Frank (David Frank), 1928–
The neurology of thinking / D. Frank Benson.
p. cm. Includes bibliographical references and index.
ISBN 0-19-505882-8
1. Cognition disorders. 2. Cognitive neuroscience.
3. Cognition. I. Title.
[DNLM: 1. Thinking—physiology. 2. Nervous System Diseases—
complications. 3. Cognition Disorders—complications.
4. Neuropsychology. WL 103 B474n 1994]
RC394.C64B45 1994
616.8—dc20 DNLM/DLC
for Library of Congress 93-6521

9 8 7 6 5 4 3 2 1
Printed in the United States of America
on acid-free paper

Preface

> No brain . . . no mind, no intellect, no nothing.
>
> J. Z. YOUNG, 1987

The fundamental approach used in this volume, basing the analysis of mental activities on illustrative case reports, deserves comment. Despite a long and productive history, interpretation from clinical observation is not regarded highly as a technique for the study of mental activities. Anecdotes cannot be measured and, in the current technical era, are ranked closer to literature or entertainment than to science. *The Man Who Mistook His Wife for a Hat* (Sacks, 1987) is considered nonfiction literature, not a medical treatise.

Despite their limitations, descriptions of clinical cases in which thought processing is deranged do provide an avenue for approaching the mysteries of thinking. If disorders of thinking can be linked to the brain and its functions, some insight can be gained into the neural mechanisms necessary for thought. Most of the mechanisms proposed in this volume are derived directly from observations of behavioral abnormality in individuals who suffered focal brain disorders. Such observations provide a potentially powerful method for both formulating and validating theories of thinking.

A sizable body of knowledge relevant to the neurology of behavior has been collected over the past century, but relatively little of it has been applied to thinking. Most neuroscientists concentrate on individual aspects of disordered behavior; most investigators of the mind ignore the knowledge of brain function currently available. While mindless studies of the brain and brainless studies of the mind have provided valuable data, correlation remains a problem. To understand thinking as a brain process demands input from both neuroscience and cognitive science. The case study approach is a valid investigative technique that can provide valuable information for both neurobiological and cognitive approaches.

Most of the information presented in this volume comes from observations of patients whose misfortunes shed light on brain mechanisms. A few cases were taken from the literature (and are appropriately designated), but the majority were examined by the author. Many of these cases have also been published and are identified as such. Many others, however, are descriptions of individuals that were seen by the author but not previously published. These cases are identified by the designation "DFB."

An altogether too obvious difficulty for this book concerns the limitations and biases of the author. The scope of the topic is immense; any attempt to investigate the many approaches to thinking, much less to present them in an accurate though abridged form, borders on the implausible. As with all single-author volumes, the prejudices, biases, and knowledge base of the author shape the discussion. In keeping with the author's career as a practicing neurologist, thinking is viewed as a neurologic function in this book. Other important approaches are omitted or downplayed.

Over the years my study of clinical cases was highlighted, augmented, and channeled by the efforts of many teachers, colleagues, and students. Most of the patients presented in this volume were studied by groups of clinicians involved in the study of brain and behavior. While far too numerous to name, most of these colleagues are represented in the bibliography. I have learned from all of them, and, to a greater or lesser extent, all have been influential in the development of this monograph.

Acknowledgement is due to the Veterans Administration, to the UCLA School of Medicine, and to the Augustus S. Rose Chair of Neurology. In various ways each has provided the time and support needed for this project. Ms. Bonita Porch deserves major accolades for her tireless editing of the multiple manuscript drafts, construction of the tables, and careful management of the reference listings. On a different editorial level, Jeffrey House of Oxford University Press has made valiant efforts to reduce redundancy, improve the author's prose, and produce a comprehensible volume.

Finally, this monograph is dedicated to my wife, Donna, whose long-time support has made this project possible.

Los Angeles   D.F.B.
March 1993

Contents

Background Considerations

1. Toward a Neurology of Thinking, 3
2. Two Approaches to Thinking, 13

Neurological Disorders Affecting Thinking

3. The Neurology of Sensory Disorders, 29
4. The Neurology of Motor Disorders, 50
5. The Neurology of Basic Mental Control Disorders: Alertness, Attention, Mental Tone, 74
6. The Neurology of Emotional Disorders, 99
7. The Neurology of Visual Imagery, 119
8. The Neurology of Communication Disorders, 141
9. The Neurology of Memory Disorders, 177
10. The Neurology of Cognitive Disorders, 198
11. The Neurology of Higher Mental Control Disorders, 208
12. The Neurology of Thought Disorders, 227

Theoretical Considerations

13. The Neural Basis of Thinking, 247

References, 261
Index, 307

Background Considerations

Toward a Neurology of Thinking

> The most sublime intelligence will never be able to find in a closet, what only exists in the vast field of nature.
> —FRANZ JOSEPH GALL, 1838
> (VOL. V, P 317)

> Behold this ruin! Twas a skull
> Once of ethereal spirit full;
> This narrow cell was Life's retreat,
> This space was Thought's mysterious seat.
> —ANNA JANE VARDHILL (1781–1852)
> *LINES ON A SKELETON* (IN MORLEY AND EVERETT, 1953)

Thinking has always been difficult to define. All recorded attempts reflect the intellectual limitations of the day. Early definitions centered on introspectively grasped mental phenomena such as sensations, images, feelings, and ideas, while the substantial influence of external stimuli on thinking remained underappreciated. Modern approaches to thinking tend to concentrate on specific mental tasks (e.g., problem solving, categorization) or identifiable mental processes (e.g., visual–spatial imagery, language) that can be construed as the building blocks of the mind. The influence that brain functions have on thinking received relatively little attention and even less formal investigation until recent decades.

The omission of brain activity from serious considerations of thinking in the past is understandable—until the late nineteenth century almost no functions of the cortex of the brain were understood. In the past century, however, a vast body of anatomical, physiological, and, of late, biochemical data concerning higher brain functions has been gathered. The correlation of these data with selected mental processes (e.g., memory) has become a major scientific challenge, but few attempts have been made to relate the accumulating scientific knowledge of brain function to the overall process called *thinking*. For many serious students of mental activity, the mind remains remote from the mundane functions of neural structures.

Brain and mind cannot be separated, of course. There is a growing consensus that, as Cellerier (1980) wrote, "We are slightly better off nowadays because both participants in this kind of dialogue, whatever their views may be on the Neo-Darwinian Theory of Evolution, would agree that cognition is mechanistically related to the functioning of the brain and the brain itself is a construct of biological evolution." The brain is obviously necessary for thinking or, as John Searle (1984) bluntly states, "brains cause minds." It should be possible to improve the understanding of thinking by correlating it with information on brain function. A broad diversity of approaches to individual brain functions is now available, from philosophy to psychology and neuroscience. Bringing these diverse efforts together has proved difficult, largely because we lack an approach inclusive of the many aspects of thinking.

One possible way to achieve an overview of the brain's role in thinking is through the study of clinical phenomena resulting from malfunction of the brain, the province of neurology. Among the data gathered by neurologists in their practice are observations of behavioral changes following damage to restricted areas of the brain. Specialists in this aspect of neurology (behavioral neurologists) study human behavior stripped of relatively discrete segments of the complex interrelationships making up normal brain function. Neurobehavioral observations provide an opportunity to bridge the chasm between the relatively abstract approach to mental activities practiced under the rubric of philosophy or cognitive science and the experimental work of contemporary neuroscientists. By studying the disorders of thinking that arise from damage to, or dysfunction of, discrete brain areas or systems, we can try to develop a neurology of thinking.

REQUISITE DEFINITIONS

A major hurdle in any attempt to bridge disciplines is terminology. Creative variation in language usage may produce lexically rich poetry but often fails to allow precise reporting. Ever present, the language problem becomes exacerbated when investigators must deal with terms that have acquired multiple meanings. In science, as in daily life, some agreement on the meaning of key terms is essential. Two crucial (and broadly abused) terms, *thinking* and *cognition,* deserve immediate discussion.

Thinking

Thinking has many connotations. In the most elementary definition, it is the formulation of images or concepts in one's mind (*Dorland's Illustrated Medical Dictionary,* 1974), but the accepted meaning of the term goes well beyond this definition. *New Webster's Dictionary* (1975) defines *to think* as "to form or conceive mentally as a thought, or to speculate upon or ponder; to exercise the intellectual faculties in forming ideas, judgments, etc.; to reason, meditate; to form an idea or have a mental image." This definition encompasses most higher level mental functions. More operational definitions subdivide thinking. G. Wallas (1976) proposed three stages to designate most mental functions: (1) engagement (involvement), (2) reference, and (3) preference. Others (Lezak, 1976; Pick, 1931/1973; Shallice, 1978) have proposed similar multistep operations. Many current investigations of thinking focus on a single functional approach within one of the overall operations (e.g., categorization, logical reasoning, problem solving), tending to ignore the overall process. Before presenting the definition of thinking to be used in this volume, another term widely used in discussions of thinking, *cognition,* needs consideration.

Cognition

Although of considerably more recent origin than *thinking, cognition* is defined with even less precision and encompasses a vast number of attributes. *Dorland's Illustrated Medical Dictionary* (1974) states that cognition includes all aspects of perceiving, thinking, and remembering; The *American Illustrated Medical Dictionary* (1947) emphasizes the processes of understanding and reasoning; and the *New Webster's Dictionary* (1975) defines *cognition* as the "coming to know of or knowing knowledge." The glossary of the *Comprehensive Textbook of Psychiatry* (Freedman, Kaplan, and Sadock, 1975) defines *cognition* as the mental process of knowing and becoming aware, one of the ego functions that is closely associated with judgment. Contemporary psychologists tend to study cognition by investigating individual components such as memory or selective attention, but for most, *cognition* is synonymous with *thinking.* To this group, cognition includes a variety of basic psychological functions (Ellis and Young, 1988) and can be deemed similar to, if not totally synonymous with, thinking.

Despite this background, a considerably more restricted definition of the term will be used in this book: *cognition is the process by which information is manipulated in the brain.* The information to be manipulated comes from diverse sources such as the individual's memory storage (fund of knowledge), the body of available motor responses, and the almost constant stream of newly received sensations, both external and internal. By this definition, cognition represents one step in the process of thinking.

Thinking, as the term will be used here, *represents the activities of a number of diverse, precisely interrelated nervous system functions that process thought contents.* Inherent in this definition is a rigid separation of thought content from thought process. *Thought content* represents all the data received and accumulated by the individual; it is idiosyncratic despite large bodies of standard teaching and common experience. The acts of receiving, perceiving, comprehending, storing, manipulating, monitoring, controlling, and responding to the steady stream of data can be considered *thought processing.* Thinking is a process, a biological function performed by the brain. While thought content can and does influence thought processing, the action itself, thinking, continues to operate through firmly established patterns. It is the breakdown of these patterns of thought processing, through either structural damage or chemical dysfunction, that will be the object of study in the neurological approach to thinking.

THE MIND/BRAIN DICHOTOMY

In the above discussion, two major terms, *mind* and *mental*, were downplayed, but not because they are unimportant. Both terms are, and will continue to be, commonly used by investigators of higher functions in humans. The trouble is that they suggest the age-old idea of separation of mind and body. Originally it was body and soul that were separated; now it is brain and mind.

René Descartes (1637–1955) is often credited with originating the body/soul dichotomy, because he so clearly outlined and forcefully presented it. The issue had been recognized for centuries, however. Plato (Wiener, 1973) made a sharp distinction between mind and body, and most Greek and Roman writers on the topic accepted it. As the philoso-

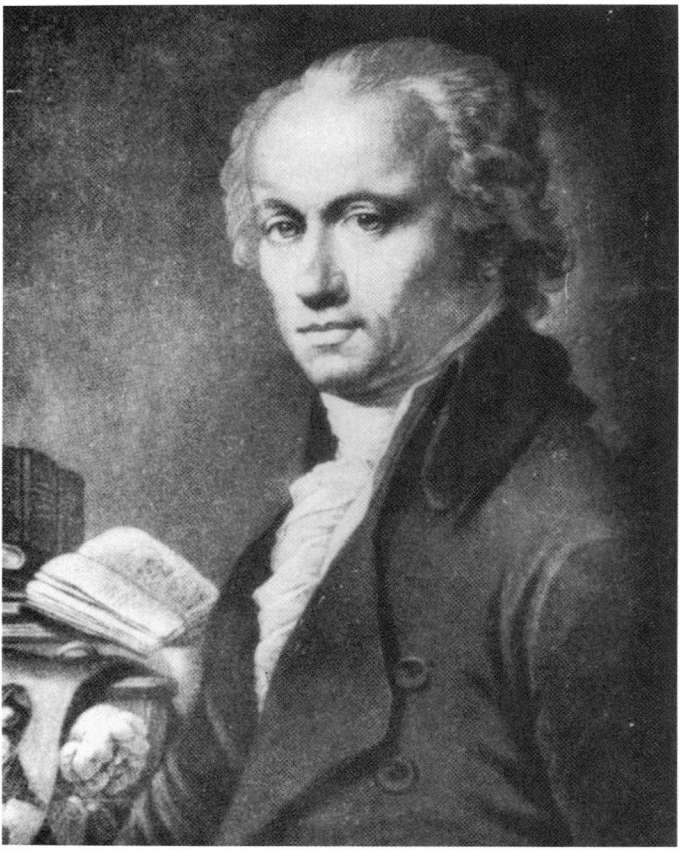

Fig. 1.1. Franz Joseph Gall (1758–1828). From Hedderly, 1970.

pher Hannah Arendt (1978) noted: "The ancient body–mind dichotomy with its strong hostility to the body was adopted, virtually intact, by the Christian creed" (p. 163). Thus, by the time of Descartes a strong tendency to separate the loftier mental (spiritual) activities from mere body functions was solidly established.

In his introspective philosophical manner, Descartes determined that the personal self ("I") existed solely in thought. "What am I then? A thing which thinks. What is a thing which thinks? It is a thing which doubts, understands, conceives, affirms, denies, wills, refuses, which also imagines and feels." Descartes himself accepted that the soul (mind) and body were united, but his writings provided strong support for their separate consideration, with emphasis on the soul (Malcolm, 1971).

With an understanding of neuroanatomy that was advanced in his day, Franz Joseph Gall molded a theory of mental activity sharply distinct from the tradition represented by Descartes. Gall (1809) assigned a number of psychological (mental) attributes to discrete areas in the cerebral

Table 1.1. Mental Faculties of Phrenology

I. Literary, Observing, Knowing Propensities (low prefrontal)

Individuality	Calculation
Form	Eventuality
Size	Locality
Weight	Time
Color	Tune
Order	Language

II. Reasoning, Reflective, Intuitive Propensities (high prefrontal)
  Causality
  Comparison
  Wit
  Intuition

III. Selfish Propensities (temporal)
  Aggressive Energy
  Acquisitiveness
  Secretiveness
  Combativeness
  Vitativeness
  Alimentiveness

IV. Domestic, Social Propensities (occipital parietal)
  Friendship
  Inhabitiveness
  Philoprogenitiveness
  Conjugality
  Amativeness

continued

Table 1.1. Mental Faculties of Phrenology (continued)
V. Self-Perfecting Propensities (lower frontal parietal)
Agreeableness
Imitation
Ideality
Sublimity
Constructiveness
VI. Egoistic, Selfish Propensities (parietal)
Firmness
Self-Esteem
Approbativeness
Cautiousness
Continuity
VII. Moral, Ethical, Spiritual Propensities (upper frontal parietal)
Benevolence
Veneration
Faith
Hope
Conscientiousness

Adapted from Hedderly, 1970.

cortex, challenging centuries of intellectual dogma. Among these attributes were wit, combativeness, and conjugality (see Table 1.1). The phrenology maps developed from this theory (Fowler and Fowler, 1849; Hollander, 1901) have proved to be mere fantasy. The correlation of cranial mensuration with psychological function (phrenology) was then and is still ridiculed, but Gall's approach eventually spawned attempts to correlate specific psychological functions with localized areas of the brain (Bouillaud, 1825; Young, 1970/1990). Phrenology provided a strong impetus to include the brain in the study of behavior.

Dualist dogma was challenged as early as the seventeenth century by John Toland (Jacobson, 1982): "thought is a function of the brain, as taste is a function of the tongue." The eighteenth century physician David Hartley (Jacobson, 1982) took a broader view: "The action of the brain on thought proves that matter and mind differ in degree but not in essence." The English physiologist David Ferrier, in his Galstonian lectures (1886), stated: "That the brain is the organ of the mind, no one doubts. And that, when mental aberrations, of whatever nature, are manifested, the brain is diseased organically or functionally, we take as an axiom. And that the physiological and psychological are but different aspects of the same anatomical substrate—these are the conclusions to which all modern research tends."

It is generally held that the content of an individual's thought is learned, not innate. The information processed in thought stems from personal (learned) experience and thus forms a body of knowledge unique to that individual. It is crucial to recognize, however, that this thought content represents only one aspect of mind.

The mental mechanisms, the brain activities that process thought content, are fundamental to any modern view of mind. Some mental processes (e.g., memory, language) are widely accepted as neurally based; others (e.g., concept formation, problem solving) are but poorly correlated with underlying neural systems. Nonetheless, an approach to thinking that highlights the brain activities involved in thought processing rather than the content of an individual's thoughts has much to offer.

THOUGHT AND LANGUAGE

That a close relationship exists between language and thought has long been recognized, but the nature of their functional interaction remains controversial (Butler, 1890/1962). In a formal discussion of this relationship, Jenkins (1969) offered three hypotheses: (1) thought is dependent on language, (2) thought is language, and (3) language is dependent on thought. He presented evidence to support each of the three postulates, accepted much of the evidence as true, and concluded that the correct answer was "all of the above." Jenkins's second hypothesis, "thought is language," however, is an absolute statement representing a powerful and circumscribed approach to thought.

Many serious students of thinking, particularly philosophers and linguists, argue that language and thought are identical. Emmanuel Kant (1781) defined thinking as "talking with oneself." The nineteenth century German linguist Max Müller included in his book *The Science of Thought: No Reason Without Language: No Language Without Reason* (1887) a section titled, "Language and Thought Inseparable." He argued that, "What we have been in the habit of calling thought is but the reverse of a coin of which the adverse is an articulate sound, while the current coin is one and indivisible, neither thought nor sound, but word." Years later the behaviorist John Watson (1930), in a chapter titled "What Is Thinking," echoed Kant: "What the psychologist has hitherto called thought is in short, nothing but talking to ourselves." He did accept word substitutes, however, so that ". . . we can say that thinking is like some vocal talking—provided we hasten to explain that it can occur without words." More recently, Arendt (1978) declared: "No speechless thought can exist. . . ." (p. 100) and further stated: "discursive thought is inconceivable without words already meaningful . . ." (p. 99). For Arendt, "Mental activities invisible themselves and occupied with the invisible, become manifest only through speech" (p. 98). Contemporary linguists tend to substitute sentences or phrases for individual words (Chomsky, 1972; Fodor, 1975) but continue to stress the crucial role of language in thinking.

Others disagree, flatly declaring that words are not the building blocks of thought processes. John Locke (1687/1934) conceived of language as having an external relationship to thinking: "Words, in their primary or immediate signification, stand for nothing but the ideas in the mind of him that uses them." Locke noted that at times words accurately expressed the individual's thoughts but that at other times they incorrectly projected this state. Jean Piaget (1926, 1950) demonstrated mental processing (thinking) in the preverbal stages of child development and concluded that thought processing appeared before language and was, therefore, an activity separate from it. In his book titled *Thinking,* the English psychologist George Humphrey (1963) took a neutral view: ". . . in general, thinking is possible without verbalization, but verbalization improves and refines it" and concluded that available experimental and clinical evidence stands against the equating of thought with language. Nevertheless, he agreed that human thinking is strongly permeated with language. In an influential treatise, Lev Vygotsky (1934/1962) noted that the relationship between a thought and a word is a living process, that the connection between them is neither preformed nor constant but is, rather, a relationship that is learned and that evolves.

Arnold Pick (1931/1973) postulated four steps between thought and verbal expression: (1) unformulated, intuitive thought; (2) structured thought; (3) sentence schema; (4) choice of words to express the thought. While Pick's schema has not been widely accepted, two of his stages are well established—(2) thought formulation and (4) language expression. For instance, Weisenburg and McBride (1933/1964) held that "The typical verbal formulation, whether expressed or not, is preceded by a process where thought becomes ordered and falls into a structure which will admit a verbal expression."

While controversy concerning the separateness of thought and language continues, both the review of pertinent arguments and well-recorded observations on the retained intelligence of individuals with acquired language loss (see Chapter 8) support the separation. In fact, recognition that language represents only a single process among the many processes that occur in thinking is a major premise of this book: *language and thought are separable brain functions.*

TOWARD A NEUROLOGY OF THINKING

If one accepts the truism that the brain is fundamental to thinking, it becomes axiomatic that alteration of a brain function involved in thought processing will alter thinking. An abnormality of the mechanism of thinking is not necessarily equivalent to abnormal thought, however. The notion that abnormal neurons generate abnormal thoughts stands discredited, and the equally simplistic idea that abnormality of thought is the direct product of social and environmental stressors appears equally inadequate. While the expressed content of abnormal thoughts may be traced to the individual's fund of learned information and investigated only through inquiry into the individual's background, the alteration of mental processing that permits the expression of abnormal thought represents an abnormality of brain function.

The use of neurological case material to investigate abnormal mental processing has a distinguished history. Early neurological studies of aphasia (the impairment of language caused by brain damage), especially those of the renowned nineteenth century investigators Paul Broca (1861, 1865) and Carl Wernicke (1874), remain crucial to the investigation of language function. Clinical observations have permitted the correlation of different memory disorders with different sites and types of brain damage or disease. Basic sensorimotor functions, from the simple registration of pain to the intricacies of visual-perceptive discrimination, have also been studied extensively in neurological cases. Observations of defects produced by damage to or malfunction of discrete parts of the brain present a substantial, albeit complicated, information base for the analysis of mental activities.

Neurology deals with abnormalities stemming from disease or damage to the nervous system (Adams and Victor, 1989). The clinical manifestations are never identical from case to case. Even patients with relatively circumscribed pathological conditions (e.g., pituitary adenoma, posterior cerebral artery occlusion) will present signs and/or symptoms not seen in others with the same disorder. This variability is significantly compounded in disorders based on variable pathology such as closed head trauma or drug intoxication (Alexander, 1982; Geschwind, 1975b). The uniqueness of a single clinical finding may be of diagnostic significance (e.g., prosopagnosia, the acquired inability to recognize familiar faces), but reliance on a single observation may misdirect the clinician (e.g., hysteria). Familiarity with the features of disease, obtained through experience, is fundamental to neurological diagnosis. Multiple observations that a combination (cluster) of clinical findings occurs when a specific neuroanatomical locus is damaged or a single disease process is present suggest a common underlying problem. Most neurologists form impressions based on the cluster of clinical findings (a syndrome) presented by the patient; the syndrome is fundamental to neurological diagnosis. While more of an art form than a science, the study of syndromes yields important insights into the working of the body, including the nervous system.

In current neurological practice, impressions from the clinical examination are supplemented by information from a variety of sources. Imaging methods—angiography, x-ray computed tomography (CT scan), positron emission tomography (PET), single-photon emission-computed tomography (SPECT), isotope brain scan, and magnetic resonance imaging (MRI) (Damasio and Damasio, 1989; Gado et al., 1982; Oldendorf, 1980)—provide valuable data concerning the "where" of brain pathology. Electroencephalography (EEG), evoked response, and tomographic EEG brain mapping (Desmedt and Noel, 1973; Engel, 1989; Harner, 1975) chart the electrophysiological patterns of brain function and dysfunction, while chemical and histological analyses of brain or other tissues can provide additional useful information. Correlation of the laboratory results with the salient clinical features has established a considerable body of knowledge concerning both the "where" and the "what" of nervous system dysfunction. Whenever available, relevant information from laboratory studies will be included in the descriptions of the case studies in this volume.

A discipline that features relatively formal testing of higher brain functions is neuropsychology. The correlation of information from neuropsychological tests with clinical, anatomical, physiological, and chemical data can provide additional insights into brain function. Neuropsychological studies will not be featured in this volume, but, for many of the case studies, neuropsychological data have provided valuable support and, where relevant, results of neuropsychological testing will be presented.

Clinical observations of the effects of lesion studies in animals have helped identify the brain processes that carry out high-level functions. The procedure is not without pitfalls, however. Well over a century ago, Hughlings Jackson (1932) noted one serious problem: the behavioral abnormalities observed in brain-damaged patients do not represent dysfunction in the finite area of the brain involved; rather, they reflect the ability of the individual's nervous system to compensate for the damage. Direct correlation of an observed behavioral abnormality with the site of central nervous system damage can lead to the erroneous conclusion that the damaged area is the locus (center) for the observed behavior. The brain, even more than most organs, is blessed with considerable ability to make alternative arrangements when something goes wrong. Neurological syndromes are the result of this compensatory ability. Nonetheless, when multiple studies demonstrate a consistent correlation between salient behavioral disturbances and a pattern of nervous system damage, a tenable hypothesis can be made concerning the neural basis of the behavior in question. This book will feature observations of the abnormal behavior that accompanies neurological disorders and, as much as possible, will correlate these observations with neuroanatomical data. On this basis an outline of the neural basis of thinking will be proposed.

2

Two Approaches to Thinking

> The knowledge that thinking has conquered for humanity is vast, yet our knowledge of thinking is scant. It might seem that thinking eludes its own searching eye.
> —DAVID RAPPAPORT, 1951

> Everyone agrees that all knowledge and thought are somehow related to the brain, but many thinkers pay little attention to this fact: the word "brain" is not mentioned in the index to Gilbert Ryle's *Concept of Mind* (1949). When philosophers think about thinking, they mostly examine their own thoughts. When scientists think about brains they refer not to their own brains but to observations made by neuroscientists.
> —J. Z. YOUNG, 1987

Thinking about thinking has a long, illustrious history that has led to the development of a wide variety of theoretical frameworks. The original theological and philosophical views were supplemented by clinical and scientific observations and more recently by experimental work. None has proved powerful enough to eclipse all others. Early in this century reflexology (Sechenov, 1963; Pavlov, 1927; Bekhterev, 1913), behaviorism (Skinner, 1957; Watson, 1930), and psychoanalysis (Freud, 1966; Jung, 1906) attempted to offer broad syntheses of mental activities. More limited approaches have explored verbal learning (Ebbinghaus, 1885/1964; Bourne, 1966; Bourne, Ekstrand, and Dominowski, 1971), concept formation (Bruner, Goodnow, and Austin, 1956; Osgood, 1953; Piaget, 1950; Vygotsky, 1934/1962), problem solving (Bolton, 1972; Johnson-Laird and Wason, 1977; Gilhooly, 1982), and language (Chomsky, 1957, 1965, 1980; Lenneberg, 1967; Miller, 1965; Vygotsky, 1934/1962).

An outgrowth of World War II, information processing (Cherry, 1953; Broadbent, 1954, 1971) became a cornerstone for computer-based data manipulation and spawned artificial intelligence (AI). Figure 2.1 presents D. E. Broadbent's diagrammatic illustration of information processing. Debate on the question "Can computers think?" has flourished since the

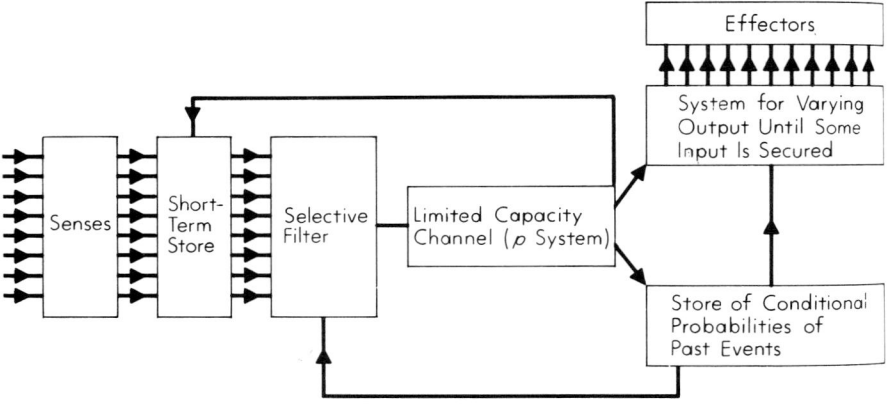

Fig. 2.1. Broadbent's (1958) flowchart illustrating the processing of information.

concept was originally proposed (Gardner, 1985; McCullough and Pitts, 1943; von Neumann, 1958), with the most intense argument revolving around the definition of thinking. If thinking is defined simply as the manipulation of symbols (weak AI), as suggested by Newell and Simon (1972), computers are seen to excel at the task (Hofstadter, 1983). If more is demanded, i.e., an ability to initiate original thoughts (strong AI), the analogy becomes controversial (Searle, 1980, 1984). While computers have fabulous memory systems, they are weak at categorization and lack the emotional tone, monitoring skills, capacity for future anticipation, and response planning of human brains. Most significantly, contemporary computers are serial processors, whereas it is now recognized that the brain operates multiple, parallel, and simultaneous channels of thought (Hinton and Anderson, 1981; James, 1890; Neisser, 1963). The field of AI has provided useful engineering concepts (e.g., servomechanisms, feedback-feedforward, holograms), but not an accurate description of human thought processing. In fact, most of the approaches to thinking listed here appear inadequate as explanations of the complex processes that occur during human thinking.

Despite similar limitations, two other broad approaches are crucial to a neurology of thinking and will be discussed at more length in this chapter. One, termed *associationism*, charts the influence that sensations and ideas have on each other; the second, *functionalism*, deals with the neural basis of individual brain functions.

ASSOCIATIONISM

The nature of thought has been extensively explored by philosophers: one of their earliest theories, associationism, refers to the process that make it "possible for one experience to be reproduced by another" (Watt, 1905/1906). Aristotle took an interest in the manipulation of images and noted that mental associations are strengthened by the mechanics of similarities, contrasts, and contiguity (Aristotle, 1931). Thomas Hobbes (1650/1840) proposed that sensation was the major element of thought. Locke (1687/1934) coined the term *associationism* (Mandler and Mandler, 1964), and proposed that "idea is the object of thinking" and "all ideas come from sensation or reflection." Locke's theories were developed, challenged, and modified by a series of British philosophers, including David Hume, David Hartley, George Berkeley (1710/1942), Alexander Bain (1868), and James and John Stuart Mill, father and son. Called *British empiricists,* they treated thought as a product of sensations and/or recollected images that formed ideas, strengthened by repetition, contrast, and contiguity.

The prime intellectual tool of the British empiricists was introspection; Locke (1687/1934) stated: "I can speak but of what I find in myself." The cornerstones of associationism, as proposed by the British empiricists, were introspection, the denial of a spiritual basis for thought, and the mechanical processing of sensation into thought. All three premises came under steady attack, and by the early twentieth century a variety of new psychological theories had undermined the simple associationist explanation of thought (Reeves, 1965). British empiricism ceased to be a major influence in the philosophy of mental functions.

Nonetheless, the importance of association in thought processing remains widely acknowledged. Arthur Koestler (1967) noted that "Associationism is dead, but association remains one of the fundamental facts of mental life." Examples of mental association abound and deserve illustration as a cornerstone for the neurology of thinking. One remarkable use of introspection and association appears in the early papers of Sir Francis Galton (1879a), who recorded his own mental activities during a period of high visual stimulation:

> On several occasions, but notably one when I felt myself unusually capable of the kind of effort required, I walked leisurely along Pall Mall, a distance of 450 yards, during which time I scrutinized with attention every successive object which caught my eyes, and I allowed my attention to rest on it until one or two thoughts had arisen through direct association with that object; then I took a very brief mental note of them, and passed onto the next object. . . . The number of objects viewed, was, I think, about three hundred, for I have subsequently repeated the same walk under similar conditions and endeavoring to estimate their number, with that result. It was impossible to recall in other than the vaguest way the numerous ideas that had passed through my mind; but of this, at least, I was sure, that samples of my whole life had passed before me, that many bygone incidents, which I never suspected to have formed part of my stock of thoughts, had been glanced at as objects too familiar to awaken the attention. I saw at once that the brain was vastly more active than I had previously believed it to be, and I was perfectly amazed at the unexpected width of the field of its everyday operations.

Galton repeated the walk after several days and was again struck by the variety of mental associations and the frequent occurrence of thoughts that had not consciously occupied his mind for many years. Admiration of his own mental capacity was diminished, however, as he noted a considerable repetition of ideas produced in the two walks. Galton had made important observations about mental association—the rapid, transient nature and broad diversity of freely formed associations—and about the tendency for a given stimulus to reproduce the same association on repeated exposure.

In a second experiment (1879b) Galton devised a system for exposing words in a random fashion. He then recorded the first few thoughts that followed viewing the written word, timing and recording each response. Although he never allowed more than a few seconds for the response, Galton noted that from one to four thoughts were produced by each stimulus word. A surprising number of the associations stemmed from experiences that had occurred many years earlier. In fact, almost 40 percent of the responses dated from his boyhood and youth, 45 percent from subsequent early manhood, and only 15 percent reflected recent experiences. Through this well-described series of observations of his own thought processes, Galton demonstrated that multiple associations can and do occur after a single stimulation, that the response is likely to be the same or very similar when a sensory stimulus is repeated, and that many of the associations had been formed early in life.

Experimentation in Russia at the beginning of the twentieth century provided further insight into the process of association. Accepting the original premise of I. M. Sechenov (1863) that the reflex act was a key element of behavior, Ivan Pavlov (1927) manipulated external sensory stimuli and produced a conditioned reflex (e.g., ringing a bell with each offering of food until the sound of the bell alone could promote gastric secretion). Pavlov stated: "All learning can, in the final analysis, probably be reduced to conditioning. . . ." (Mowrer, 1976). V. M. Bekhterev (1913) produced an entire system of psychology, reflexology (1917/1926), based on the conditioned reflex.

In the United States, John Watson (1930) adopted the ideas of association psychology and Pavlovian conditioned reflex to develop a mechanistic account of mental activity that came to be known as behaviorism. Watson claimed that all mental activities were responses to a stimulus and that stimulus ⟶ response epitomized all behavior: "When a complicated habit is completely analyzed, each unit of the habit is a conditioned reflex" (Watson, 1930). Language was included among the complex reflex acts, and Watson proposed that thinking was a subvocal language activity; thus, silent thinking would be accompanied by occult movements of the tongue, lips, pharynx, and so forth. Numerous tests have been constructed to confirm the presence of ongoing subvocal language during thought processing, but to date they have failed either to prove or to repudiate the subvocal activation theory (Sokolov, 1972).

The associationism of Watson, Skinner, and other behaviorists has

THE FAR SIDE By GARY LARSON

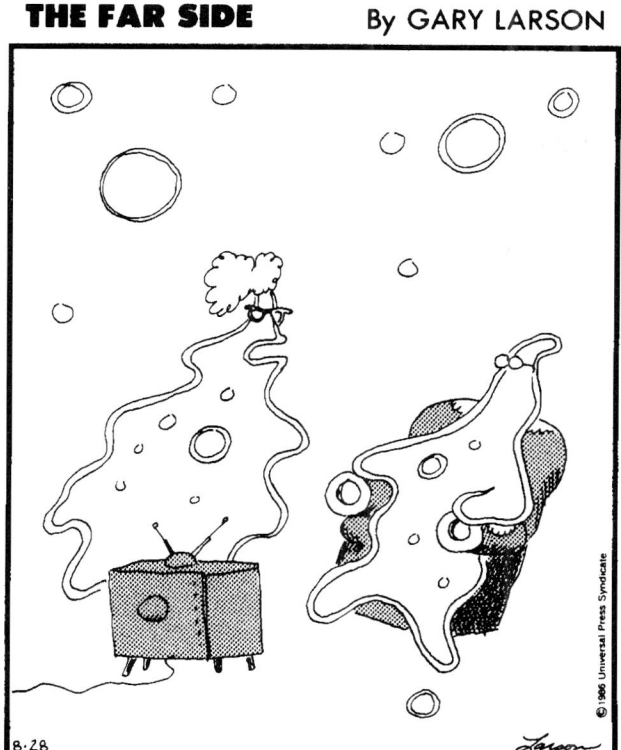

Fig. 2.2. THE FAR SIDE Copyright 1986 Universal Press Syndicate. Reprinted with permission. All rights reserved.

come under severe criticism. From a linguistic viewpoint, Noam Chomsky (1957) denied that mechanically constant associations would be capable of producing the vast richness of sentence construction available to humans. Similar criticisms were noted for many realms of psychology (Miller, 1965), and current activities in cognitive science recognize that the vast complexity of mental activity cannot possibly be encompassed in the simple principles of behavioral associationism. Despite the apparent truth of these challenges, the underlying principle of association remains an integral, indeed essential, element in the understanding of thought processing (Voss, 1969). Humphrey (1963) clearly affirmed this status: "It may be said that the history of the psychology of thinking consists largely of an unsuccessful revolt against the doctrine of association."

Crucial to the concept of association in human thought processing is the ability to link information from one modality (e.g., sensation, memory) with that from other modalities. Termed *intermodal*, *cross-modal*, or *transmodal* association, this process is so fundamental to human thought that it is difficult to realize that most animal species possess little or no ability to transfer information from one sensory modality to another.

To illustrate the importance of cross-modal associations, a single study can be cited. A British psychologist, George Ettlinger (1967), trained monkeys to push a lever when a cross (food reward) was flashed but not when a circle (shock punishment) was flashed. The animals became proficient, reaching better than 95 percent accuracy, and were able to maintain the learned response without rehearsal for several weeks. The number of trials needed to reach this proficiency was recorded. Ettlinger then repeated the experiment with the same animals but substituted a tactile presentation, a three-dimensional cut-out of a circle and cross presented in a darkened, nonvisual environment. He again recorded the number of trials needed to attain a consistent level of accuracy and found that there was virtually no difference in the number of trials needed to attain competency in the two sensory presentations. The animals failed to correlate the visual stimulus with the tactile stimulus and, therefore, had to learn the association anew. As an imaginary continuation of Ettlinger's experiment, what would happen if a human was fully trained to respond to a visual presentation of the cross and circle figures and was then presented with a tactile cross? The correct response would be almost immediate, as the similarity of the basic figure, even across the different sensory modes, would be recognized (associated) almost automatically. Easy passage of information between sensory modes is essential for human thought processing. Human thoughts are rich multimodal constructs that combine elements of sensation (visual, auditory, tactile) with appropriately related memories, feeling tone, and visceral responses.

FUNCTIONALISM

Brains are the organs of thought, and it is axiomatic that students of thinking must know something about the brain and its operations. The effort to correlate basic mental operations with brain structure–function can be called "functionalism," and it obviously requires a knowledge of neuroscience. Only a few aspects of that vast field can be reviewed here, in severely abridged form.

Comparative Neuroanatomy

The human brain is relatively massive in size, ranking only behind those of the whale, elephant, and dolphin in actual weight and above these species in ratio of brain weight to body weight. Of even greater potential importance are the novel or considerably enlarged areas of the human brain. While the subcortical neural structures of the human brain closely resemble those of other advanced species except for size, the cortical mantle of the human brain contains several potentially important differences. Three areas of human cortex—the prefrontal cortex, the second temporal gyrus, and the angular gyrus (interparietal area) of the parietal lobe—are

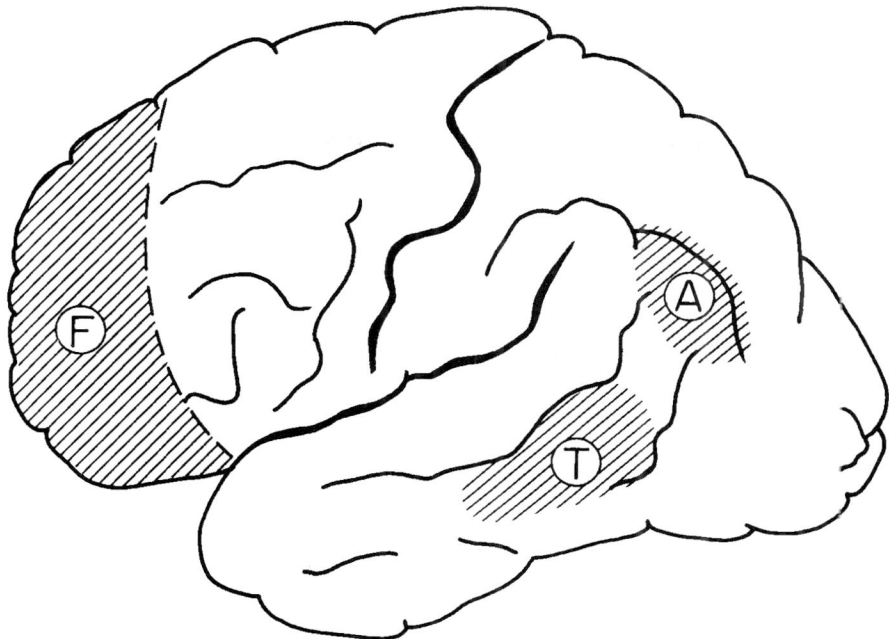

Fig. 2.3. Graphic representation of the human left hemisphere with shaded areas representing areas that are either phylogenetically novel or of greatly increased cortical dimension compared with other animal species. F = prefrontal cortex; T = 2nd temporal gyrus; A = angular gyrus.

either absent or much smaller in other animal species. Figure 2.3 graphically displays these three areas.

While prefrontal cortex is present in higher mammals, the increase in the size of this area in humans is considerable, an alteration long considered fundamental to man's superior mental function (Teuber, 1964; Tilney, 1928). The demonstration of specific frontal lobe functions, however, has proved difficult; this will be discussed in Chapter 11. The second temporal gyrus appears novel to the human brain, and its location would be consonant with a role in the interpretation of discrete, sequential auditory signals, particularly those of language. This aspect of the second temporal gyrus will be discussed in Chapter 8. Finally, the angular gyrus of the parietal lobe, a prominent structure in the human brain, is present in apes, relatively small in monkeys, and virtually absent in lower species; its location, abutting each of the three major sensory cortices, implies a key role in communication between sensory modalities. The major task proposed for the angular gyrus is cross-modal association. It can be postulated that each of these three primarily human neuroanatomical areas carries out important functions in the processing of thought.

Hemispheric Specialization

The human brain consists of two almost symmetrical hemispheres—right and left. The corpus callosum, the largest individual neural pathway in the central nervous system (more than 200 million fibers), connects the cerebral aggregates of the two hemispheres, and smaller but significant interhemispheric pathways augment this sizable connection. That the cerebral hemispheres might represent two independent sources of mental activity is a relatively recent idea. A convincing body of evidence (Bogen, 1986; Kruper, Palton, and Koskoff, 1971; Wenzel, Tschirgi, and Taylor, 1962) demonstrates that either hemisphere alone can sustain mental life. An entire hemisphere, either right or left, may be removed in children or in adults (Dennis, 1980; Smith, 1966), and, while significant neurological and psychological deficits will occur, the behavior (personality, thinking) of posthemispherectomy patients appears to remain remarkably intact. They learn, communicate, have emotions, and freely present their own thoughts, demonstrating that a single cerebral hemisphere can operate as an independent mental unit (Bogen, 1977).

From a different perspective, the study of patients who have had the two hemispheres separated by surgical section of the corpus callosum reveals that each hemisphere can carry out behaviors independent of the other (Gazzaniga and Sperry, 1967). In fact, the two separated hemispheres may present different responses to the same stimulus (Critchley, 1970a,b; Sperry, 1968; Trevarthen, 1984). Each hemisphere, when allowed to act separately, is capable of independent response.

These observations have led to the notion of a "dual mind" (Bogen, 1969b, 1986; Wigan, 1844), which has obvious implications for mind/brain relations (LeDoux, Wilson, and Gazzaniga, 1977; Lishman, 1969, 1971b; Puccetti, 1981). Some (Orenstein, 1972; Wigan, 1844) have even suggested that the two separate mental units of the human brain, constantly vying with each other, represent a major source of psychiatric disorder. Table 2.1 presents a synopsis of potential implications derived from the study of independent hemispheric functioning.

One striking demonstration of brain asymmetry is the ability of one hemisphere to carry out a significant mental function better than the other, so-called hemispheric specialization. The obvious example is lan-

Table 2.1. Postulated Brain/Mind Combinations

Hemisphere	Brain	Mind	Clinical State
One hemisphere	One half brain	One mind	Hemispherectomy
Two hemispheres	Two half brains	Two minds	Split brain
Two hemispheres connected—synchronous	One brain	Two minds—collaborative	Hemispheric specialization (e.g., language)
Two hemispheres connected—dyssynchronous	One brain	Two minds—disjunctive	Psychosis

Adapted and altered from a presentation by Joseph E. Bogen to the UCLA Neurobehavior Seminar, January, 1990.

guage, a high-level cognitive function performed almost exclusively by the left hemisphere of most adults (Benson, 1985; Broca, 1865; Roberts, 1969). Several functions such as melody (McFarland and Fortin, 1982) and visual–spatial discrimination (Sergent and Corballis, 1990) are better performed by the right hemisphere. Hypotheses as to how information is processed differently by the two hemispheres have been presented (Bogen, 1969b; Orenstein, 1972; Semmes, 1968) but have proved difficult to substantiate. Each hemisphere appears to have an equal potential to learn the performance of most mental functions (Zangwill, 1960). There is little doubt that hemispheric specialization exists, but the concept has been overused and oversimplified (Efron, 1990).

Consciousness, an obvious but unexplained aspect of human mental activity, has been a popular target of right–left hemisphere speculation (Zangwill, 1974). Some suggest that the highest mental activities are the product of a single, unitary "consciousness" (Eccles, 1966; Sperry, 1985). They interpret split-brain studies as demonstration that consciousness acts in a supraordinate (unifying) capacity to control functions of both brains (hemispheres). Others, however, interpret the same observations as indicating that each hemisphere possesses an independent "consciousness" (Bogen, 1969b, 1986; Orenstein, 1972). Early observations (Rosandi and Rossi, 1967; Serafetinides, Hoare, and Driver, 1965) suggested that consciousness was a left-hemisphere function, but later studies demonstrated that removal of the left hemisphere in children (Dennis, 1980) and in adults (Smith, 1966) did not remove consciousness. It appears unlikely that either hemisphere is dominant (specialized) for consciousness.

The two hemispheres are so closely integrated that under normal circumstances little nonreflex activity occurs in one hemisphere that is not immediately reflected in the other (Efron, 1990). Each hemisphere carries out multiple activities but most are not performed without communication with the opposite hemisphere (Innocenti, 1986). While some highly specialized cognitive functions (e.g., language, construction, music appreciation) and some high-level basic response modes (analysis, synthesis) may be handled differently by the two hemispheres (Bogen, 1969a; Gordon and Bogen, 1974; Piercy and Smyth, 1962; Semmes, 1968), the similarity and close interrelationship of the two hemispheres is of far more consequence than their individuality. Although each hemisphere is capable of independent function, most higher level brain functions involve both hemispheres, although possibly not equally.

Cellular Neuroanatomy

It is a marvel of nature that nerve cells, structurally and physiologically very similar, carry out vastly different functions. This contrasts with most other biological systems in which the units (e.g., the nephron of the kidney) carry out restricted functions, interchangeable with the activities of other similar cells. Not so in the brain. One neuron may subserve visual–sensory reception, another be active in motor response, a third par-

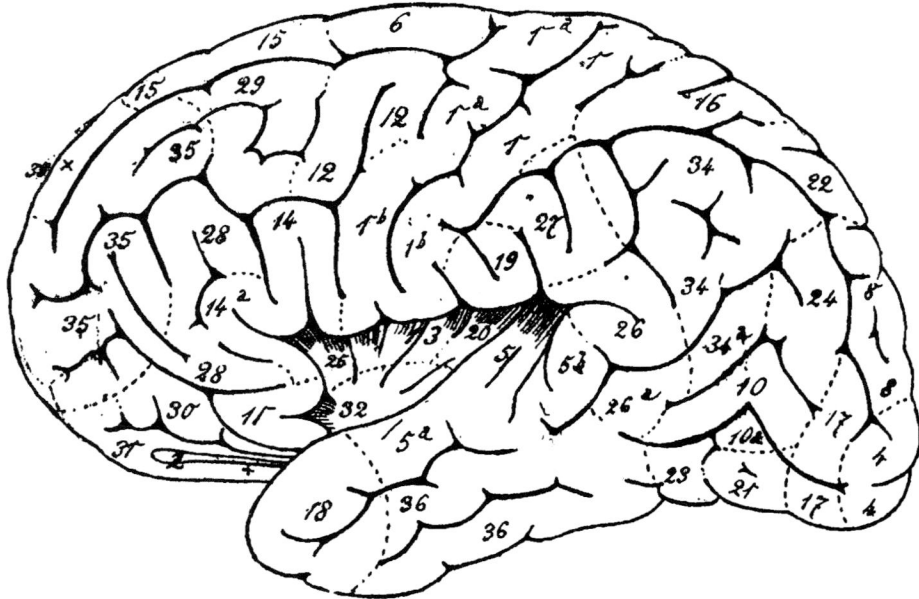

Fig. 2.4. Flechsig's (1901) representation of different cortical areas based on the temporal differences in the initiation of myelinogenesis. The numbers are sequential, the lowest numbers indicating the areas that first show myelin formation. From Flechsig, 1901.

ticipate in specific emotional response; others interact to maintain sequences of information, to communicate between and compare sensory modalities, to maintain and modulate complex motor movements, to anticipate, plan, and monitor novel mental decisions, and even to contemplate and plan future actions. The vast repertoire of mental activities subserved by neurons is not explained by structural differences in individual cells. Rather, combinations of neurons act synergistically to produce widely varied responses. Neuronal aggregates and their connections are the functional units of the central nervous system and of thought processing.

Observable differences between combinations of nerve cells in the cortex have led to numerous classifications based on gross anatomical location, cytoarchitectonics, cortical–cortical connections, cortical–subcortical connections, myelinogenesis (Fig. 2.4), and other characteristics. Despite the diversity of observations, there is basic agreement on the subdivisions of the cortex. The areas that subserve sensory reception (vision, somesthetic, auditory) and direct motor response are traditionally called *primary sensory*—or *motor*— cortex. These areas differ from the surrounding cortical areas in cytoarchitectonic patterns, in the period during development when myelin first appears, and in both long and short connecting pathways. Surrounding each of the four primary cortical areas are

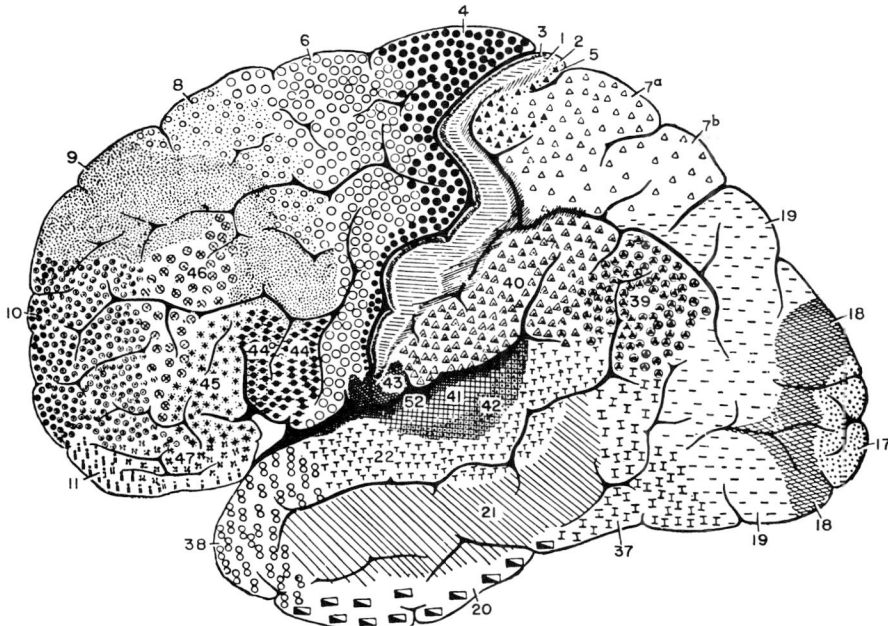

Fig. 2.5. Brodmann's (1908) psychoarchitectural map of the human brain. The numbered areas represent subtle but real differences in the neuronal distribution and organization of the cortex. From Crosby, Humphrey, and Lauer, 1962.

regions termed *sensory* or *motor* association cortex. Finally, the three relatively novel brain areas noted earlier (prefrontal cortex, second temporal gyrus, and interparietal area) have been called *tertiary* association cortex.

A number of schemes have been used to depict differences in the cortex. One distinguishes the primary sensorimotor cortex, the surrounding secondary association cortex, and the tertiary association cortex on the basis of cellular architecture, primarily the relative density of cells in different layers of the six-layered cortex. Figure 2.5 presents the Brodmann (1908) map of the human cortex based on differences in cytoarchitecture, which has been widely accepted.

The developmental stage (age) at which myelin is first laid down within the central nervous system provides another approach to the same demarcations. Flechsig (1901) demonstrated three periods in the development of cortex, depending on the period during which myelination first appears, that correspond to the primary, secondary association, and tertiary association areas defined above (Fig. 2.4). Later investigations (Yakovlev and Lecours, 1967) confirmed Flechsig's divisions and showed that the angular gyrus and the prefrontal cortex are the last areas to begin myelination (as late as three years of age). It has been suggested that full mental function (e.g., language, cognitive control) cannot be carried out until myelination is relatively well established in all areas of the cortex (Stuss and Benson, 1986; Yakovlev and Lecours, 1967).

On the basis of combined studies of cytoarchitecture and connecting pathways, Mesulam (1985b) proposed a relatively comprehensive functional classification of cortex with two divisions of autonomic and three divisions of sensorimotor cortex. In Mesulam's classification the primary sensorimotor cortex is called *idiotypic cortex,* the surrounding sensorimotor association cortex, *unimodal cortex;* and the tertiary association cortex (of Flechsig), *heteromodal cortex.* As in the earlier divisions, the idiotypic cortex is dedicated to a single sensory or motor modality. It receives (or sends) fibers subserving that one modality, and its connections are, almost entirely, limited to adjacent unimodal cortex. Unimodal (association) cortex surrounds the idiotypic cortex and performs more complex sensory or motor activities. Unimodal cortex is also dedicated to a single modality and may well be the site of much memory storage (see Chapter

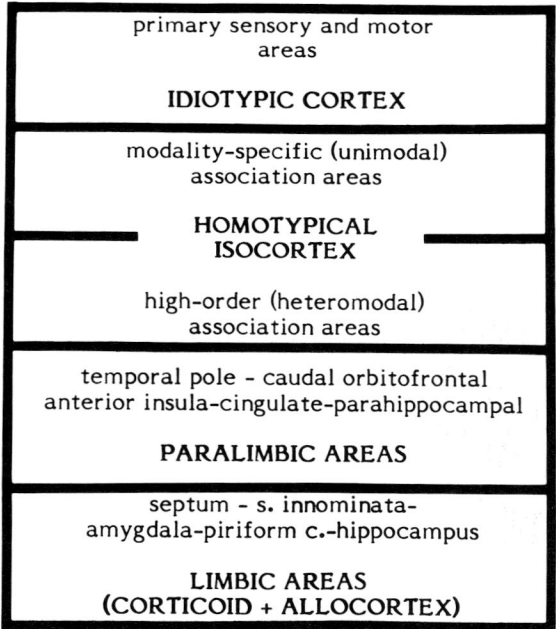

Fig. 2.6. Mesulam's diagrammatic representation of the varieties of human cerebral cortex with differentiation into idiotypic (primary), unimodal (secondary), and heteromodal (tertiary) association cortices and paralimbic and limbic cortices. From Mesulam, 1985a.

9). Heteromodal (association) cortex, as the name implies, has a considerably broader range of connections. Although the connections of the three major heteromodal cortical areas vary considerably, in general they interact with the unimodal association cortex of each major modality, with the other areas of heteromodal association cortex, and with a variety of subcortical regions. Mesulam's terminology, illustrated in Figure 2.6, will be used in this volume.

Functional Systems

Those trying to understand the intricacies of human mental activity have tended to subdivide behavior and to focus on individual mental functions. This approach was clearly represented in the faculty psychology of German and Scottish philosophy (von Wolff, 1734; Reid, 1785/1853). In recent years many labels have been applied to the individual functions. Fodor (1983) and Gazzaniga (1985) both used the term *module* to identify individual mental functions. Others have proposed such terms as *schema* (Shallice, 1982), *intelligences* (Gardner, 1983), and *functional systems* (Stuss and Benson, 1986) for different sets of mental activities. Most current investigations of brain function focus on a single aspect—memory, language, attention—with limited acknowledgement of the subtle or considerable effect that other brain operations may have on the function under investigation. Although it may appear narrow to concentrate on an isolated psychological function, this affords much more precision for investigation. The success of contemporary neuropsychology rests on this ability to subdivide complex mental activities into units that can be investigated scientifically.

Thought processing, however, demands interrelationships between these functional systems. To understand thinking, both the neuroanatomical base and the type of activity performed within the major functional systems must be studied. Subdivision into operational units, while both arbitrary and artificial, is essential if the complex of mental activities that participate in thought processing is to be investigated. For the purpose of this volume, nine functional systems will be presented as distinct units (Table 2.2).

Table 2.2. Functional Systems

Sensory (visual, auditory, tactile)
Motor
Basic mental control
Emotion/autonomic
Memory
Visual imagery
Language
Cognition
Higher mental control

Each of the nine systems, to a greater or a lesser degree, has a consistent neuroanatomical network dedicated to its operation. That is, specific neuroanatomical entities (cortical and subcortical nuclear areas and their connecting pathways) are involved, while other parts of the central nervous system have little or no influence on the behavior. The same neural entities underlie the function in all humans (and, to a considerable degree, in all higher mammals). Yet it is also clear that the function is carried out by a network; no behavior depends exclusively on a single anatomical area (center). Damage to one part of the network, however, will usually interrupt or distort only an element of the behavioral function; a characteristic behavioral impairment may be seen that indicates involvement of a specific portion of the network.

While each functional system operates through its own dedicated network, some of the neural entities (nuclear centers and their connections) are shared with other functional systems, a pattern that allows integration of brain functions but also means that damage within a single brain area almost invariably involves more than one functional system. Because the site and extent of structural damage to the brain are highly variable and more than one functional system is likely to be involved, considerable variability in behavioral symptomatology is the rule in clinical observations. Carefully discriminative study is needed for each case.

One additional consideration deserves emphasis. Within the rich matrix of integrated neural networks, multiple activities are occurring simultaneously at all times. The final product, observable behavior, results from a linking together of simultaneously operating subunits. Attempts to define the interaction of the individual subunits by simple computation fail to reflect the rich potential of human thought processing (Gibson, 1979). Current investigations include more complex analyses, at least partially encompassing multiple, concurrent brain activities required for thinking. While individual functional systems can be accepted as real entities, and their study is of unquestioned value, thinking is a distillation of these activities. The study of thinking demands that a synthesis follow the analysis of individual functional systems.

Neurological Disorders Affecting Thinking

3

The Neurology of Sensory Disorders

> . . . what perception must do is to so represent the world as to make it accessible to thought.
>
> –J. A. FODOR, 1983

> The brain scientist's working model of perception is as follows. Environmental stimuli are transduced peripherally and encoded in patterns of impulses in primary nerve fibers. These quasi-isomorphic representations of the external world are transmitted through and transformed at various levels of the sensory systems by the local microstructure, by dynamic neuronal processing mechanisms, and by the action of the central state control systems. The final distributed pattern of neural activity—an abstracted representation—is then surmised to be in a form suitable for storage in memory, and for matching with patterns previously stored there.
>
> –V. B. MOUNTCASTLE, 1986

AXIOMS/POSTULATES

Sensation conveys the information from external and internal sources that is used for ongoing thought.

Multiple, separate sensory channels are simultaneously active.

Sensation undergoes complex processing, modality specific at first but with later cross-referencing between modalities.

Cross-referenced sensations comprise essential elements for both conscious and unconscious thought.

Most received sensations remain unconscious, entering into reflex level response patterns.

Basic neurological function can be characterized as a motor response to a sensory stimulation. Sensorimotor reactions represent the procedure by which all brain and body functions, from respiration to writing, occur. The overwhelming majority of sensations are processed without conscious awareness, but sensory input and motor responses are crucial elements of thought processing. Although often overlooked, variables within sensorimotor response patterns significantly influence both thought processing and thought content.

Sensory and motor functions are traditionally considered separately. Not only do they operate in tight collaboration, however, but the sensorimotor response is fundamental to mental life. Chapters 3, 4 and 5 will deal with basic sensory, motor and control functions, while Chapters 6 through 12 will address "higher" mental functions, brain operations that influence basic sensorimotor responses.

While the relationship between sensory input and thought has long been recognized, the specifics remain controversial. Much depends on the definition of terms and the dividing line between pure sensory input and the complex mental activities of conscious thought. The subtly different definitions of perception and apperception (see below) concocted during the nineteenth century (Herbart, 1816; Wundt, 1873–74) emphasized but did not answer this question. The boundary separating sensation from thought remains undetermined. To demonstrate the position of sensation in the neurology of thought, basic definitions must be established; clinical case material will then be presented and the neuroanatomy of sensation reviewed before a neural basis of sensory processing is suggested.

VARIETIES OF SENSATION

The study of sensation is complicated by the diversity of sensory stimuli and by the complex alterations that occur during processing (Hamburger, Pribram, and Stunkard, 1970). To compensate, studies of sensory function tend to subdivide and specialize (Bridger, 1970).

It is traditionally accepted that there are five sensory modalities: vision, hearing, somesthesis, smell, and taste. The olfactory and gustatory senses are excluded in this discussion despite the probability that one or both affect thought processing, because available information is, at best, fragmentary and open to question. A third modality, vision, is so complex, has enjoyed so much meaningful investigation in recent years, and is of such pivotal importance to human thinking that higher level visual processing will be given separate consideration (Chapter 7). In this chapter only two sensory modalities—audition and somesthesis—will be discussed fully, but, as the essentials of primary visual sensory processing are similar to the other two, initial visual sensory processing will be included.

Each type of sensory input can be subdivided for evaluation. Investigations of auditory functions demand knowledge of tone, pitch, rhythm, melodic quality, sequential processing, and so forth. Subdivisions of somesthesis (also called *somatic, tactile,* or often just *sensory* function) are even more obvious. Simple somesthetic sensations include the appreciation of touch, pain, pressure, temperature, posture, and vibration, but a more complete range of somesthetic discriminations include mixtures of the individual elements such as stereognosis (the ability to identify a palpated object based on recognition of texture, size, shape, and so forth), localization of a sensory stimulus on the body, graphesthesia (appreciation of numbers or letters written on the body), ability to discriminate two separate, simultaneous stimuli, and others. Basic visual sensations include light intensity, dimension, direction of movement, color, and form. There are many complex combinations such as recognition of faces, objects and environmental landmarks, and the ability to visualize two- and three-dimensional constructions, and to read language symbols, maps and illustrations.

Basic sensory reception has been well documented in human and animal experiments, but, of necessity, the investigation of advanced sensory processing has been largely introspective, and this led to artificial subdivisions. One of the most prominent was the effort to distinguish perception from apperception. Leibniz (Dewey, 1888) contrasted "obscure perceptions" with those that were clearly apprehended or "apperceived"; the term *apperception* eventually came to designate a process that included the assimilation and interpretation of new impressions (Herbart, 1816; Kant, 1781). To Wundt (1873–74), apperception was the process by which elements of experience were appropriated and drawn into clear consciousness. While *apperception* has lost significance in this century, the intention behind the separation of perception from apperception still reflects the relationship of sensory input to thinking. Four reasonably distinct steps in sensory processing can be suggested—reception, discrimination, unimodal association, and heteromodal association. The entire process (all four steps) is often termed *perception* (Efron, 1968); Hamburger, Pribram, and Stunkard, 1970). An independent factor, selective attention, plays an important modifying role during sensory processing, and the concept will be developed further in Chapter 5. The four primary steps of sensory processing will be defined before clinical examples of discrete disturbances within this process are presented.

Reception refers to the activities of the specialized sensory tissues that receive the external (or internal) stimulus (e.g., the retina for vision, cochlea for auditory stimuli) as well as the transmission of the stimulus to cortical centers for processing in the brain. This is not a simple transmission process; the stimulus undergoes alteration, restructuring, and categorization at stages of the receiving and transmission processes (Hubel and Wiesel, 1979; Melzack and Wall, 1965). These alterations are significant, but for this discussion of thought processing the term *reception* will embrace all the neural activity that takes place from the primary receptor to the primary sensory areas of the cortex (Brodmann areas 3, 1, and 2 for somesthetic stimuli; Brodmann area 41 for audition; and Brodmann area 17 for vision). At intermediate synapses in the brain stem and thalamus, there is some processing of stimuli but the primary function of this step is the presentation of information received from the external milieu to a modality-specific area of the cortex.

Discrimination, in this discussion, will refer to the ability to compare and distinguish sensory stimuli received through the modality-specific reception chain. Discrimination of sensory variables includes both qualitative and quantitative differences in the stimuli received but represents only the comparison of simultaneous or serially received stimuli of a like nature (e.g., degree of loudness of sound, severity of pain, intensity of light)—". . . a mechanism sensitive to changes in conditional probabilities . . ." (Barlow, 1985). Most responses to this initial level of discriminated stimuli occur as a reflex, but discriminated sensory material becomes available for higher level unimodal processing.

Unimodal association, the third step in sensory processing, involves comparison of the discriminated sensory stimuli with previously processed stimuli. Both qualitative and quantitative aspects of the stimuli are analyzed and correlated with prior experience. A reflex response may be initiated, and/or limited identification may occur. With this step the sensory information (conventionally called a *percept*) becomes available for higher level brain processing that can lead to conscious (or unconscious) recognition of the sensation. Unimodal association demands memory function to associate the discriminated stimulus with prior experience (see Chapter 9). Unimodal association is an important step in the formation of memories.

Heteromodal or *cross-modal association,* the final stage in the processing of a sensation, is the ability to correlate a percept (data derived from the three unimodal steps) with information (memories) from other sensory and motor modalities. Only with this association of the unimodal percept and other modalities does a sensory stimulus reach full appreciation. Conscious recognition of a *sensation,* in the usual sense of the term, becomes possible only at the level of heteromodal association.

A simple example illustrates these proposed steps in sensory processing. A bell rings; the stimulus is received by the peripheral auditory apparatus and transmitted to the cortex (step 1, reception), where the specific auditory stimulus is distinguished from other sounds in the ambient environment (step 2, discrimination). This information is then compared and related to previously noted auditory stimuli of a similar nature (step 3, unimodal association), and the percept is then compared with a broad fund of information encompassing other modalities to give full meaning to the original stimulus (step 4, heteromodal association). Depending on information gleaned from these steps, an alarm clock may be shut off, the telephone answered, or the building evacuated because of fire danger. This simple, four-step breakdown is inadequate and open to exceptions, but it provides a basic working conception of sensory processing (Table 3.1).

Table 3.1. Sensory Processing

Step	Activity
Reception	Reception and transmission of external or internal stimuli
Discrimination	Comparison and distinguishing of the received stimuli
Unimodal association	Matching of the discriminated stimulus with previously experienced sensations of the same modality to form a percept
Heteromodal association	Comparison of the percept with previously experienced percepts from other modalities

CLINICAL EXAMPLES

The clinical disorders discussed in this chapter affect higher level sensory processing. The physiological, psychological, and neurological literature contains vast quantities of data on disorders affecting the peripheral sensory system. While dysfunction at the periphery may alter thought contents, the alterations are primarily quantitative and are recognized as such by the perceiving brain. In keeping with the above discussion of thought processing, only a few selected higher level sensory disorders relevant to the mechanics of thought processing will be presented here.

Auditory Disturbances

By far the most important disturbance of the auditory system is deafness, most often based on disorder of the receptive elements of the auditory nervous apparatus, the end organ (cochlea), the eighth nerve, or the brain stem auditory centers. Deafness based on cortical disorder is rare as a pure entity, much more often discussed than demonstrated (Bahls et al., 1988).

Case 3.1

A 64-year-old man was transferred from a Veterans Administration psychiatric hospital to a VA general hospital for neurological evaluation. History (as gathered from the chart, not from the patient) revealed that approximately two years earlier a radical change in his behavior was noted by his neighbors. While he was always considered a loner, there was an abrupt cessation of meaningful communication and an increasingly hedonistic behavior pattern that upset his neighbors. He was eventually seen medically, a diagnosis of schizophrenia was suggested, and he was placed in a mental hospital where he proved to be aggressive, assaultive, and negative, refusing to communicate with the hospital staff. This behavior and his failure to improve with standard medication regimes prompted transfer to a VA facility for long-term institutional care. Here the absence of prior psychiatric disorder and the apparently abrupt onset of the problem raised the possibility of an organic cause, warranting transfer for neurological evaluation.

During examination by the neurology service his behavior was negative; he refused to respond to verbal inquiry but occasionally produced some meaningful verbal output (e.g., "Go away!"; "Don't bother me!"; "What do you care?"). Even this was only occasionally in context. Basic neurological evaluation revealed no significant abnormality, but on physical examination atrial fibrillation and a moderately elevated blood pressure were noted. A full behavioral examination showed that he could understand and respond to written language, which led to the demonstration of competent language function but bilateral deafness.

He was totally unable to identify verbal (language) or nonverbal (e.g., telephone ring, hand-clapping, whistling) auditory stimuli. The deafness was not peripheral; he consistently showed that he could hear sounds. For instance, if a melody was sung or hummed, while neither able to name the tune nor identify it as music, he could accurately follow the beat (rhythm) with his hand. He always appeared aware when a sound was made, although he was unable to identify the sound. He insisted that he heard sounds he could not identify. When the nursing staff was instructed to communicate with him only in the written form, a notable alteration in his behavior occurred; he became friendly, tractable, and relatively happy. He was eventually discharged to his own home with a discharge diagnosis of cortical deafness, probably based on cerebrovascular infarctions affecting hemispheric auditory pathways bilaterally. (DFB)

In this case it can be suggested (no absolute anatomical proof was available) that bilateral, probably bitemporal, damage had produced a cortical deafness that precluded identification of either verbal or nonverbal auditory stimuli even though the patient insisted that he was aware of the auditory stimulus. That this was not a primary language defect (aphasia) was readily demonstrated by his ability to comprehend written material and produce normal speech. That it was not a peripheral deafness was more difficult to prove, but his excellent ability to respond to noises, even though he could not identify them, suggested that the disturbance affected a higher level of processing.

Case 3.2
A 56-year-old patient with known cardiac arrhythmia secondary to several myocardial infarctions was admitted to the hospital because of a sudden change in language use. The referring diagnosis was cerebrovascular accident that had produced aphasia. Careful examination revealed no basic neurological disability such as paralysis, sensory loss, or visual field defect. The patient's verbal output was fluent with occasional paraphasic substitutions (these disappeared after a few weeks). He could neither comprehend spoken language nor repeat what was said. In contrast, he named objects and actions on visual confrontation accurately and easily named nonlanguage noises (whistling, clapping, ringing of bells). His ability to comprehend written language was normal. A diagnosis of pure word deafness was suggested, and an isotope brain scan performed during the acute state demonstrated a single lesion deep in the posterior temporal lobe (Fig. 3.1). Over many months the patient regained some ability to comprehend spoken language, particularly when it was presented slowly; this ability was enhanced if he could look at the speaker's lips during conversation. (DFB)

A focal lesion was demonstrated in the left temporal lobe Heschl's gyrus area (the primary auditory cortex) and the pathways carrying auditory stimuli to Heschl's gyrus. It can be assumed that the vascular lesion disconnected the left temporal lobe cortex from auditory stimuli carrying verbal information to the left primary auditory cortex, as well as fibers bringing such information from the right temporal auditory area. Although the patient could hear them, he could not discriminate or analyze auditory verbal signals.

Case 3.3
A 57-year-old man, an independent and relatively successful manufacturer of leather goods, noted an acute change in hearing one afternoon. After he visited several hospital emergency rooms and a number of physicians, a cardiac arrhythmia was discovered and easily converted to normal rhythm. The patient was then transferred to the Boston VA Hospital for evaluation of "aphasia." No basic neurological disability could be demonstrated; there was no problem with visual, sensory, or motor function, and his auditory system appeared intact on bedside testing. He had a fluent verbal output contaminated with occasional semantic

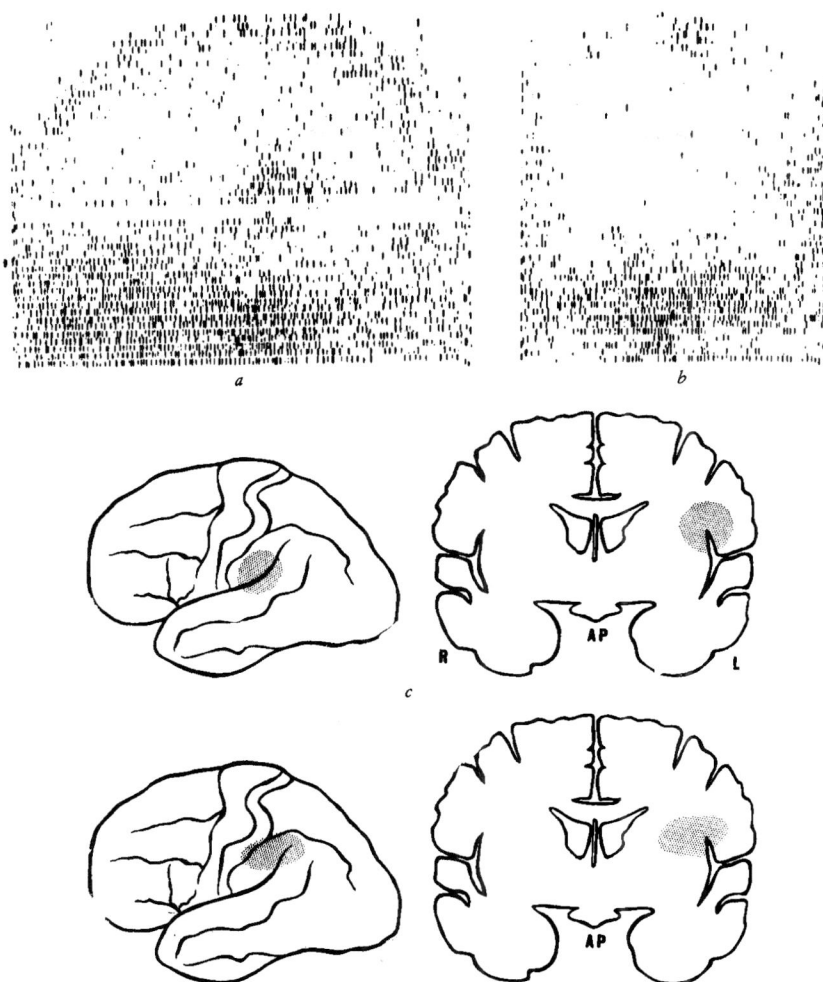

Fig. 3.1. Radionuclide brain scan (a,b) demonstrating increased uptake in the left posterior medial temporal region and an artist's conception (c,d) of the location of this lesion. From Benson and Patten, 1967.

paraphasias (word substitutions). An original difficulty comprehending spoken language improved considerably over a period of several days. Nonetheless, the patient often asked for questions to be repeated and requested that the examiner speak more slowly or use a different selection of words so that he could understand. This problem improved until his comprehension of spoken language was within normal limits on formal testing. He consistently complained, however, of hearing difficulty. Tests of peripheral hearing (audiograms) were entirely normal, but he claimed inability to recognize nonverbal sounds in the environment; when this was formally tested, his failure was almost total. Unless visualized, the difference between whistling, clapping the hands, or snapping the fingers could not be discerned, although he accurately noted whenever a sound had been made. Similarly, he could not distinguish a telephone ring, a dog bark, or the sound of horse hooves but was aware of each sound. His inability to identify nonverbal sounds remained constant for several years. He became paranoid and suspicious of his physicians, his former employees, and even his wife. He complained of failure to appreciate the meaning of spoken language, although he continued to pass formal tests of this function. It seems probable that he was unable to identify the affective quality of spoken output, probably due to his inability to discern melody (see Chapter 6). Brain imaging studies available at that time failed to define a specific focus, but it was suspected that he had sustained a small right temporal lobe embolic infarction that had produced a nonverbal auditory agnosia. (Albert et al., 1972)

The striking finding in this individual, his inability to perceive nonverbal sounds, is often called *auditory agnosia* (Vignolo, 1969). A limited literature indicates that this problem usually follows structural damage to the right temporal lobe primary auditory cortex and to the pathways feeding sensory information to it. As such, auditory agnosia is a right-hemisphere analog of the pure word deafness described in Case 3.2; some prefer to call the two disturbances *verbal auditory agnosia* and *nonverbal auditory agnosia*.

Each patient described above suffered a defect in the final stages of reception, discrimination, and/or association of auditory sensory stimuli. The demonstration of defects further along in auditory sensory processing (heteromodal association) becomes entangled with language processing and will be discussed in Chapter 8.

Each of the above cases showed significant emotional disorder, most prominently a suspicious, noncooperative attitude—paranoia. That damage to temporal lobe structures plays a direct role in this behavioral change has been suggested, but available data remain incomplete (Benson, 1973, 1992). The emotional disorder following damage to the auditory pathways may be sufficient to warrant psychiatric management, but, as Case 3.1 illustrates, it is best managed by communication through other, intact sensory input channels.

Somesthetic Disturbances

Many disturbances of the somesthetic sensory system are recognized; most represent peripheral, or at least nonhemispheric, disturbances and will not be discussed here. The six cases below illustrate varieties of higher level disturbance of sensory discrimination that have a bearing on the neural basis of thinking.

Case 3.4

A 62-year-old man was transferred to a VA hospital for rehabilitation following an acute left-brain stroke. Approximately three weeks earlier he had suffered acute right hemiparesis (arm considerably more involved than leg) and numbness and paresthesia in the right upper extremity, accompanied by a garbled, incoherent verbal output. The paresis disappeared in a few days, leaving a sensory loss involving the right upper extremity that affected higher (cortical) sensory functions such as two-point discrimination, touch localization, graphesthesia, and joint position sense, but not pain, touch, temperature, or vibration sensibilities.

The patient's cortical sensory functions improved, but several months after onset he began complaining of an uncomfortable, dull, aching sensation vaguely localized to the right upper extremity. While he accurately recognized pain over all parts of his body, including the paresthetic right arm, an indifference to deep pain could be demonstrated on the right side. Severe noxious stimulation (e.g., strong pressure on muscles, jabs with pins, venous engorgement from blood pressure cuff constriction) applied to the right arm produced only a mildly unpleasant sense of discomfort, not described as pain. Similar stimulation to the left arm produced a rapid, angry, defensive reaction and a report of sharp pain. (DFB)

The paresthetic disorder in Case 3.4 was considered a pseudothalamic pain syndrome, and the decreased response to deep pain has been termed *pain asymbolia* (Biemond, 1956). Both disorders are, at best, vague and inadequately defined in the clinical literature. They have been reported only with partial severance of pathways linking the thalamus and the primary cortical sensory areas, and it can be suggested that they represent a breakdown in the process of sensory perception. The sensation of pain is apparently appreciated at a subcortical level, but the steps of discrimination, unimodal association, and heteromodal association demand cortical activity that was disordered in Case 3.4.

Case 3.5

A 67-year-old man was hospitalized for surgical treatment of chronic pain due to prostatic carcinoma with metastasis to the pelvis. Increasingly severe bone pain had not been alleviated by either drug or x-ray treatments. The patient received one-quarter grain of morphine intramuscularly every 2 hours, and even with this analgesic regime he complained of constant discomfort and became anxious and irritated over any delay in receiving the medication. He was mentally clear with no evidence of basic neurological or mental dysfunction.

Bilateral cingulumotomy—stereotactically placed thermal lesions in the band of white matter underlying the cingulate cortex—was performed to control the pain. The postoperative state was uneventful except for an anticipated disturbance of orientation for time (Whitty and Lewin, 1960), which disappeared in 10 days. Immediately following surgery the patient no longer needed opiates and appeared considerably more comfortable and relaxed. When asked if he still had pain, he replied "yes," and if asked whether the pain was decreased he indicated that it was at least as bad as before the surgery. When asked why he no longer requested narcotics, he replied that the pain did not seem to bother him as much as before surgery. Unfortunately, this happy situation was short lived; within three months he again experienced severe pain necessitating opiate analgesia. (DFB)

The relief of intractable pain by various destructive brain operations (e.g., thalamotomy, cingulumotomy, frontal leucotomy) is well known (Ballantine et al., 1967; White and Sweet, 1955). Of particular interest in this case is the alteration of the emotional impact of the pain by a surgical lesion that did not involve the primary sensory network. Pain was accurately perceived, but at least one heteromodal association, that involving the limbic system, appears to have been altered. The neurological basis of emotion will be discussed in Chapter 6, but the alteration of pain appreciation in Case 3.5 represents a striking variation of higher sensory processing.

Case 3.6
A 48-year-old woman (same as Case 12.6) was seen because of long-standing "atypical" facial pain. Approximately eight years earlier she first noted discomfort in the right temporal region. This increased in intensity and unpleasantness despite multiple medications and many physical, psychological, and spiritual treatments by a great variety of physicians (neurologists, otolaryngologists, psychiatrists, and head and neck surgeons) and healers (naturopaths, chiropractors, acupuncturists, Chinese herb specialists, and faith healers). The patient became frustrated, irritable, depressed, and increasingly unpleasant. Both her husband and her children abandoned her, and she eventually lived as a recluse in a mountain cabin.

The most notable finding on examination was an unending stream of negative, critical, anhedonic, acerbic conversation. The patient was sharply critical of the medical profession and all others who had attempted to help her; she constantly made rude and nasty remarks about the examiner and others around her and clearly showed that she thoroughly despised everyone. No basic neurological abnormalities could be demonstrated, but on examination of her mouth the rear molars on both sides appeared abnormally shaped. Dental consultation led to a diagnosis of severe dental malocclusion. This condition was corrected through several weeks of grinding to reshape her teeth and allow better occlusion. By the end of this period the discomfort had disappeared, and she became a friendly, pleasant individual whose personality had changed remarkably. (DFB)

In Case 3.6, the diagnosis of Kosten's syndrome, painful temporomandibular joint disease, was confirmed by the dental examination. The major clinical finding, the personality disorder, proved to be a product of the chronic pain. Unimodal perception of the pain was accurate but had produced a profound alteration of interpersonal response, a condition based on heteromodal associations.

Pain is a fascinating entity, the nature of which remains under investigation. It can be defined simply as the "sensory experience evoked by stimuli that injure" (Mountcastle, 1968), but this is inadequate. In fact, pain is more accurately recognized as a psychological state that may or may not reflect a proximate physical cause (Wall, 1985). Pain is better classed with bodily sensations such as hunger or thirst than as a precise response to a peripheral stimulation. In both Cases 3.4 and 3.5 the awareness of painful stimuli was dramatically altered by damage to specific portions of the brain—the dominant hemisphere supramarginal gyrus area in Case 3.4 and the cingulum bilaterally in Case 3.5. Watson, Heilman, and colleagues have demonstrated that damage to several areas of the central nervous system including the pontine and midbrain reticular substance

(Watson et al., 1974), thalamus (Watson and Heilman, 1979; Watson, Valenstein, and Heilman, 1981), cingulate gyrus (Heilman and Valenstein, 1972; Watson, Heilman, Cauthen, 1973), and dorsolateral frontal lobe (Heilman and Valenstein, 1972) can decrease the appreciation of (response to) sensory stimuli, including pain. The experience of pain appears to represent a noxious sensory stimulus coupled with an emotional (probably limbic) response; the balance between the two can vary enormously from individual to individual, from situation to situation, and with duration of the pain.

The treatment of pain is based on one of two approaches. The first, and most successful, is removal of the source of pain. Obvious examples are treatment of tooth decay or removal of an inflamed appendix. Case 3.6, though more complicated, shows that treatment of the pain source can not only relieve the pain but also alter complex psychological responses to chronic pain. Too often, however, the source of pain is not readily correctable. The second approach, then, is to ameliorate the psychological components of the pain syndrome. Traditionally, this is achieved with analgesic and narcotic medications, apparently dulling the perception of pain by altering opioid neurotransmitter systems within the brain. While this reduces pain, a strong tendency for both physiological and psychological addiction develops. Attempts to control chronic pain with neurosurgical procedures have had limited success (White and Sweet, 1955). Peripheral nerve destruction—rhizotomy, neurectomy, and cordotomy—may separate the peripheral pain source from higher centers but too often are unsuccessful. Destruction of central nervous structures (e.g., thalamus, cingulum) is often only transiently effective. Intermittent volleys of electrical stimulation to thalamic or brain stem centers have a better chance of remaining effective but demand placement of electrodes into precise central nuclear areas, a difficult and often unsuccessful procedure. Transient electrical nerve stimulation (TENS) to peripheral nerves is simpler and safer but often only partially successful in pain relief.

Currently available data suggest that a broad neural network with multiple peripheral and hemispheric connections responds to pain; with ongoing volleys of stimulation from a chronic pain source, this network can become semiautomatous, producing the experience of pain even after the actual source of the pain is separated from higher processing areas.

Case 3.7

A 46-year-old man was rendered unconscious in a traffic accident. A boggy contusion was present over the right parietal scalp, and skull radiographs demonstrated a nondepressed skull fracture in this region. On recovery of consciousness, the patient had decreased use of the left upper limb. When his mental state cleared sufficiently, examination demonstrated that primary sensations—pain, temperature, touch, and vibration—were sensed equally on both sides, but more complex sensory functions such as two-point discrimination, touch localization, and position sense were performed poorly in the left upper extremity. Even greater disturbances were noted in graphesthesia (the ability to recognize from tactile sensation numbers written on the skin) of the left upper extremity, and the patient was almost entirely unable to name objects palpated by his left hand. When given an object such as a pencil, comb, or paper clip, in the left hand with his eyes closed, he either failed to name it or made a confabulatory response. When the same item was placed in his right hand, he immediately gave the name. Although no motor loss was noted in either hand and the sensory disorder was limited to the upper extremity, the left limb was ignored and almost never used for unimanual activities. (DFB)

In Case 3.7 damage to the parietal area of the nondominant hemisphere caused a disturbance in the ability to identify palpated objects (astereognosis) despite intact basic sensory function. Somesthetic stimuli were received and discriminated adequately but could not be associated with prior experience in that modality. That the failure to name was not based on a higher level heteromodal recognition disorder (aphasia) was readily demonstrated by the patient's ability to name the object when it was placed in his other hand.

This patient's tendency to ignore the left upper extremity deserves comment. Although mild, the decreased sensory input apparently obviated use of the left limb unless other sensory modalities such as vision or language were brought into play. Denny-Brown and colleagues (Denny-Brown, 1963; Denny-Brown and Banker, 1954; Denny-Brown, Meyer, and Horenstein, 1952) used the term *amorphosynthesis* to describe decreased utilization of a limb following damage to the sensory input system, a source of unilateral neglect (see Chapter 5). Postulating that a long-standing perceptual equivalence between the two hemispheres had been altered in favor of the undamaged hemisphere, Denny-Brown and his colleagues concluded that the limb contralateral to the side of damage would be used less. Despite fully normal motor capability, the altered processing of sensory stimuli at the unimodal association level disrupted routine sensorimotor responses.

Case 3.8

A 42-year-old man was admitted to a hospital with evidence of left hemiparesis and altered mental state. Past history revealed a neurological problem with a differential diagnosis of multiple sclerosis or cerebrovascular disease. A radioisotope brain scan at admission demonstrated increased isotope uptake in the deep white matter just to the right of the genu of the corpus callosum, considered most consistent with deep vascular lesion.

As the patient's mental state cleared, evaluation demonstrated minimal motor disturbance in the left upper extremity (slight hyperreflexia) and no disorder of primary sensory modalities. However, he was unable to name objects placed in the left hand when his eyes were closed, although he readily named the same objects placed in his right hand. If an object he had failed to name when placed in his left hand was put in a sack with several other items, his left hand unerringly chose the correct item. This selection was done with certainty even though he still failed to name the object. On occasion he would mime the use of the palpated object but rarely was this a sufficient hint to allow correct naming. In addition to the tactile naming disorder, he could not write with his left hand, producing only a stereotyped scrawl, and could not perform left limb movements to command that he readily performed with the right limbs (callosal apraxia; see Chapter 4). The minimal paresis of the left limb could not account for the motor disabilities, as he copied writing and readily performed most limb movements on imitation. He was reevaluated regularly for many years, and the left limb dysfunctions remained unchanged. (DFB)

It was assumed that the lesion demonstrated on the isotope brain scan in Case 3.8 had severed pathways that connected left-hemisphere language areas with right-hemisphere motor response areas. Not only did this keep the patient from carrying out language-based movements with the left hand, but also it did not allow him to transfer normally perceived somesthetic sensations to the language areas of the left hemisphere for naming. This case represents an anterior callosal separation syndrome featuring ideomotor apraxia, inability to write (to dictation), and inability to name objects (by palpation) with the nondominant (left) hand, a syndrome well described by Liepmann (1905), Geschwind (1965), Bogen (1979), Patel (1969), and others. These investigators surmised that information could not be transferred from the left (language dominant) hemisphere to the right hemisphere and vice versa because of the callosal separation. Thus sensory information properly appreciated in the right hemisphere is not transferred to the left hemisphere for linguistic identification. The patient's occasional inability to mime use of the object palpated by the left hand is more difficult to explain, but his failure to name the object on those few occasions when he did realize the use of the object is not; he was unable to transfer the kinesthetic image of left limb movement across the callosum to the dominant hemisphere for language response.

Case 3.9

At age 22 years, a man developed notable neurological findings, including bilateral internuclear ophthalmoplegia, right hemiplegia, right hypesthesia, and bilateral Babinski signs. Cerebrospinal fluid study revealed an elevated gammaglobulin content. A diagnosis of multiple sclerosis was suggested.

All signs and symptoms cleared rapidly but partially recurred several years later. At age 26 years, the patient noted acute onset of right hemianesthesia, weakness of both legs, and a tactile illusion of a second right arm lying across his lower chest and abdomen. The illusory arm appeared to be attached to the chest wall and extended across the midline. While the lower forearm, wrist, and palm of the illusory arm were only vague, the impression of the fingers lying on the abdominal wall was vivid (see Fig. 3.2). The illusion could persist from a few minutes to 30 minutes and was always coincident with a feeling of increased numbness, stiffness, and burning in his right arm and hand. No relationship between these episodes and either environmental or emotional changes could be noted by the patient. The episodes continued to occur frequently but irregularly for a period of almost four months, at which time they spontaneously abated. The other neurological abnormalities also improved at that time, leaving only a minimal right hemihypesthesia and slight increase in the right-sided reflexes. (Mayeux and Benson, 1979)

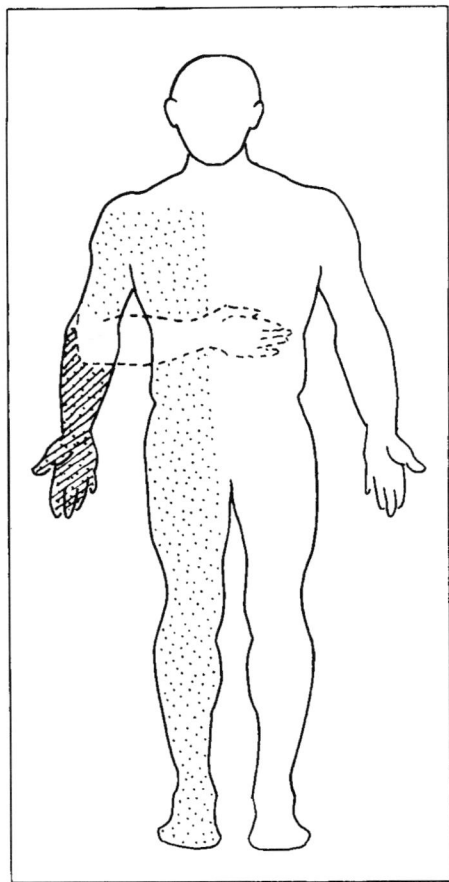

Fig. 3.2. Artist's conception of the phantom hand position described in Case 3.9. The stippled area on the right trunk and arm indicates hypesthesia, and the heavily lined area of the right forearm indicates hypalgesia. From Mayeux and Benson, 1979.

The clinical and laboratory findings in Case 3.9 supported a diagnosis of multiple sclerosis, and careful clinical analysis (this patient was seen before MRI came into use) suggested plaque formation in the ascending sensory pathways of the low brain stem or upper cervical spinal cord. In this case a discrete anatomical lesion separated sensory stimuli affecting the intact limb from higher sensory processing areas; a reception disorder allowed misperception of the (phantom) limb in space. The disorder shows that loss of sensory reception from an involved limb does not remove the mental image of the limb and is particularly illustrative because the limb involved was motorically intact. The phantom limb phenomenon was well recognized in the eighteenth and nineteenth centuries (Mitchell, 1871; Valentin, 1844) and has been carefully recorded since then (Tatlow and Oulton, 1955; Weinstein, 1969). The mental images that represent the position of the body in space are, at least to some degree, separable from the sensory input. The phantom limb phenomenon demonstrates in a dramatic way that the heteromodal aspect of somesthetic processing may operate in isolation from the modality-specific percept.

NEUROANATOMICAL SUBSTRATE

Peripheral components of the somesthetic sensory system transmit somesthetic stimuli into a series of processing channels, some of which lead to the cortex. Significant peripheral structures include the specialized sensory nerve endings, the peripheral nerves, and the pathways and synapses of the spinal cord and brain stem leading to the thalamus. From the thalamus most somesthetic data are relayed to the anterior parietal cortex. The components connecting peripheral sensors with the thalamus are fixed and rigidly organized. They are amenable to animal research and are considerably less complicated than the anatomical substrate for higher sensory interpretations.

Similar multistep programs of stimulus processing and conduction of stimuli can be outlined for the auditory and the visual systems. Details of the anatomical basis of each system are available in any textbook of neuroanatomy. Figures 3.3, 3.4, and 3.5 illustrate, in simple diagrammatic form, the peripheral aspects of the sensory systems.

Alterations in the peripheral sensory networks decrease sensory input and result in neglect and/or misrepresentation of the stimulus. The anatomical bases of such disorders are well defined in the literature and need not be discussed here. We will focus, instead, on alterations in sensory input after it reaches the brain (primarily the thalamus and the cortex).

The thalamus is a mandatory way-station for all exterosensory modalities and carries out categorizing functions (Angevine and Cotman, 1981; Nauta and Feirtag, 1986). Although all three of the sensory modalities discussed here synapse in the thalamus, no functionally significant cross-modal association occurs at this level. Each of the major sensory modalities remains separate through their thalamic processing.

At the cortical level, the three major sensory modalities have similar neuroanatomical arrangements. Each has a primary cortical reception area with a functionally significant architectural organization. The primary cortex of the somesthetic system has been characterized as a modified homunculus (Fig. 3.6); variations distinguishing sound wave frequency and tonal qualities are discretely represented in the primary auditory cortex; the receptor fields of the retina are reproduced in a crudely linear fashion in the primary visual cortex, with central (foveal) vision most posterior. The primary sensory cortices possess only limited neural

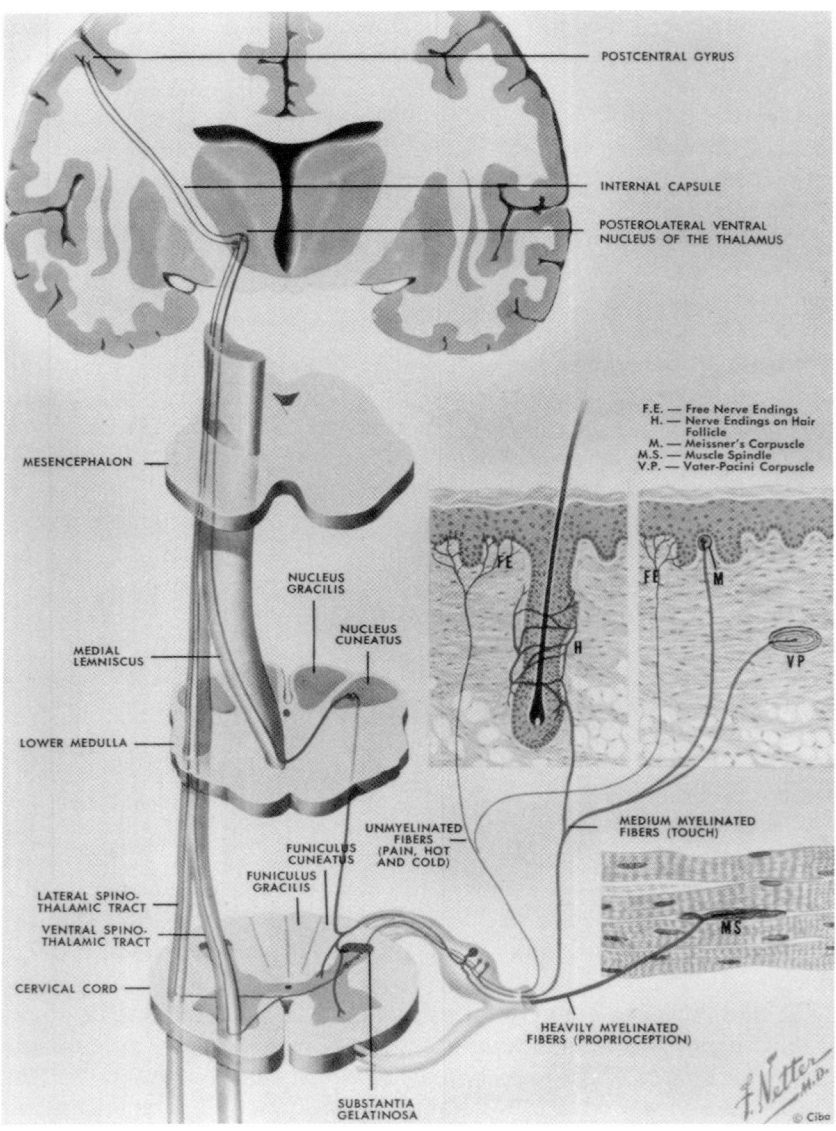

Fig. 3.3. Artist's conception of the pathways within the central nervous system for processing of somesthetic stimuli. From Netter, 1980.

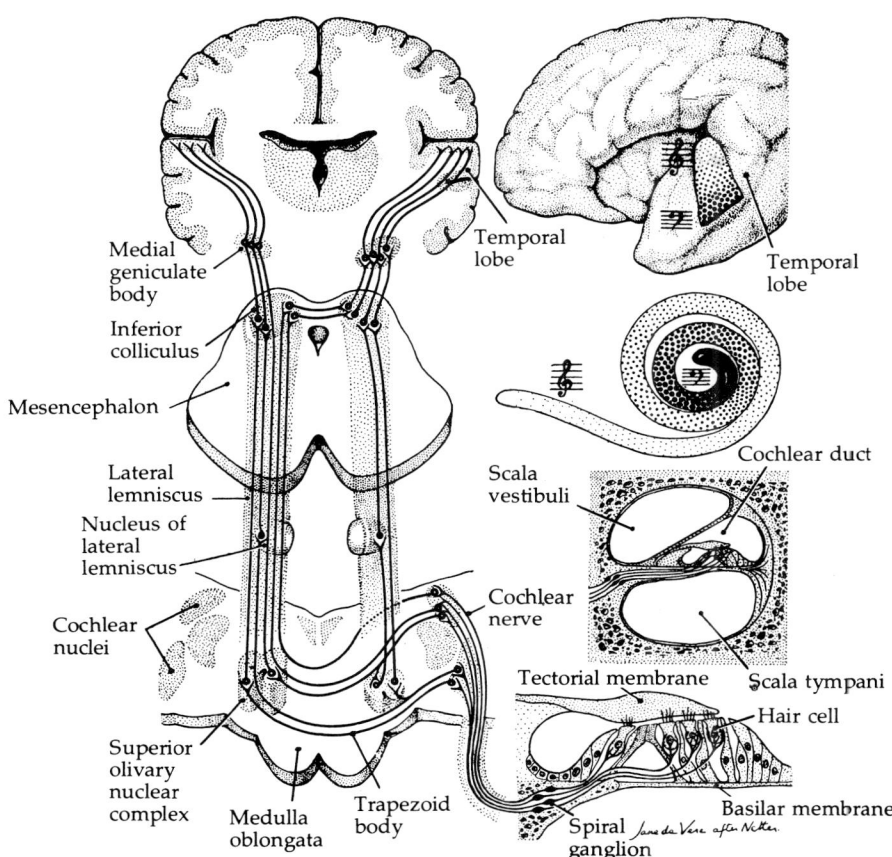

Fig. 3.4. Artist's conception of the auditory sensory system. From Angevine and Cotman, 1981.

connections; the vast majority of fibers leaving the primary sensory cortices travel only to the adjacent association cortex, while a small number of fibers connect, via the corpus callosum, to a homologous area in the opposite hemisphere to correlate midline stimuli (Pandya and Seltzer, 1986). With the exception of the callosal connections, no long cortical–cortical connections emanate from the primary sensory cortices.

The unimodal association area that surrounds each primary sensory cortical area is relatively vast and operates through functional subunits. These functional aggregations have been called *columns* (Hubel and Wiesel, 1979; Mountcastle, 1957) or *modules* (Eccles et al., 1967; Mountcastle, 1979; Szentagothai, 1975); information received from the primary cortex is transformed in the modules with increasingly complex levels of processing (Hubel and Wiesel, 1979; Mountcastle, 1968); the absence of subjective reports from the animals used for sensory experiments limits

46 Neurological Disorders Affecting Thinking

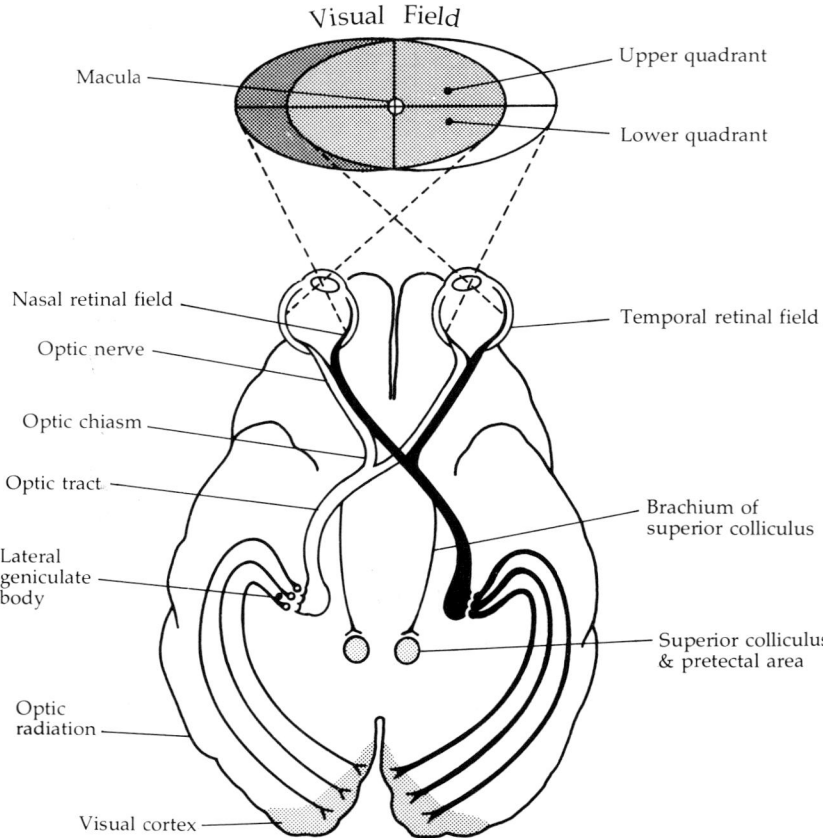

Fig. 3.5. Artist's conception of the primary visual receptive system. From Angevine and Cotman, 1981.

these studies, but it can be demonstrated that discrimination and unimodal association functions take place in the sensory association cortices. Both short and long tracts emanate from sensory association columns to carry impulses to other brain areas. Through these connections, the processed sensory input (percept) of the unimodal association areas becomes available for higher mental processing.

Multiple short nerve pathways connect the unimodal sensory complexes to contiguous cortical areas (Mesulam, 1985a), and a number of longer tracts emanate from the sensory association cortices providing connections to many brain areas (Nauta and Feirtag, 1986; Pandya, Hallet, and Mukherjee, 1969). Four major pathways deserve emphasis.

First, the association cortex of each major sensory modality produces a large body of transcallosal connections to homologous cortical areas of the opposite hemisphere and a smaller body of interhemispheric connections to a variety of other areas of the opposite cortex (Pandya and Seltzer,

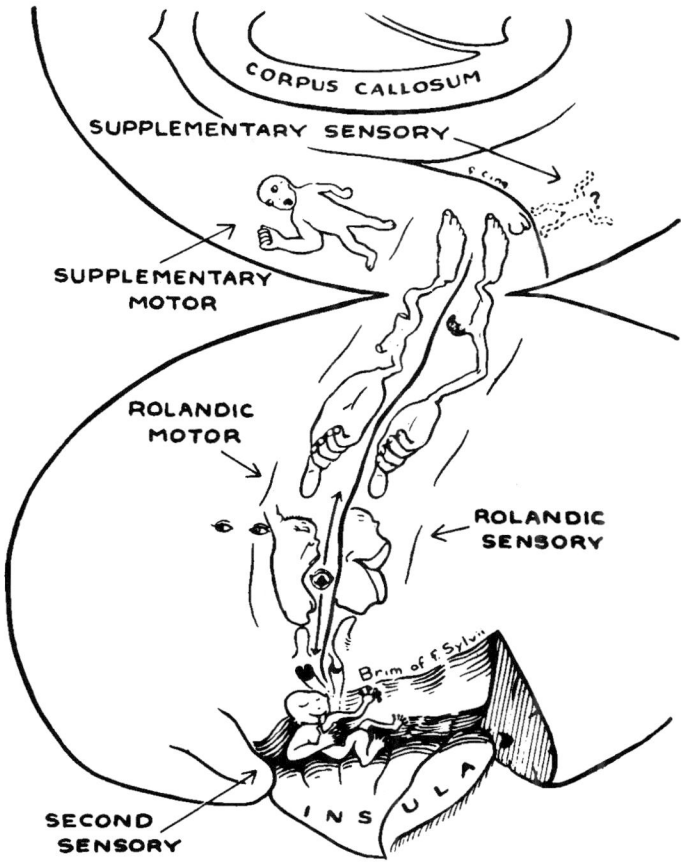

Fig. 3.6. The cortical homunculus for sensory and motor functions. From Angevine and Cotman, 1981.

1986). Through this rich transcallosal network a stimulus received in a single, primary cortical area (e.g., a tactile stimulus sensed in one hand) rapidly becomes available for processing by both hemispheres. A second major pathway from the association cortex of each sensory modality travels forward to the motor association cortex (Brodmann area 6), primarily via three white matter bundles—the superior and inferior occipital–frontal fasciculi and the superior longitudinal fasciculus (Crosby, Humphrey, and Lauer, 1962). Additional fibers travel in the same fasciculi to selected areas of the prefrontal cortex (Fuster, 1989). A third major pathway involving the visual system descends into the inferior temporal area (Crosby, Humphrey, and Lauer, 1962; Gross, 1973). This pathway and its target in the posterior, inferior temporal cortex are apparently essential for the processing of complex visual patterns (Gross, 1973; Levine, 1978), a high-level unimodal association.

In the human, a fourth major sensory connecting pathway, one considered crucial to higher mental function (Butters and Brody, 1968; Geschwind, 1965), connects the association cortex of each sensory modality to the angular gyrus of the parietal lobe, the phylogenetically recent area of cortex ideally located to act as a heteromodal association area for the three primary sensory association areas. From the angular gyrus (inferior parietal lobule in the monkey) a vast number of pathways lead to many areas of the nervous system (Pandya and Kuypers, 1969).

NEURAL BASIS OF SENSATION

All of the major pathways discussed here are bidirectional, allowing both feedforward and feedback of information. The unimodal sensory association areas not only transmit processed sensory data to a variety of cortical areas but also receive information from these and other areas. The heteromodal sensory association cortex (primarily the angular gyrus) has broad bidirectional interconnections. Sensory input, very modality-specific at the unimodal association level, becomes widely integrated with other sensory modalities at the levels of the heteromodal association areas.

The steps and connections can be further illustrated by the example used earlier. If one hears a bell ringing in a crowded and noisy room, the sensation is received by the auditory system and transmitted to the primary auditory cortex (reception). With further transmission it is distinguished from concurrent auditory stimuli (discrimination) and then compared with known auditory stimuli (unimodal association). A response may be generated (probably via long white matter tracts to the frontal motor areas), particularly if the individual was anticipating the stimulus. More often, though, additional associations with prior percepts of ringing bells occur, a process in which the percept is recognized/identified (heteromodal association) by matching with a name, with a feeling of urgency or concern, or with an unspoken verbalization such as, "That's the phone ringing." While occurring almost instantaneously, the four steps outlined in Table 3.1 are distinct functional activities.

As another illustration of sensory connections, a subject's hand is placed into a sack containing an assortment of fresh fruit. The sensation that comes from the palpation of the fruit is received through the peripheral sensory system, travels to the level of the primary somesthetic cortex in the parietal lobe (reception), and is compared with sensory stimuli coming from palpation of other fruit in the sack to provide a gauge of texture, size, firmness, and so forth (discrimination). These attributes are then matched with previous sensory experiences (unimodal association), and a percept is formed. The percept is then compared with previously learned information from other modalities such as the name of the fruit palpated, the desirability of one piece of fruit versus another, and even visual images and potential taste of the unseen fruit (heteromodal association). While much of this information is processed within the primary sensory system and its adjacent, dedicated unimodal association cortex, use for thought demands interconnection with nonsensory functional systems (such as memory, language, and executive control). Simple sensation provides essential data (percepts) for mental life, but increasingly complex steps are necessary before simple sensations can become elements of thought.

Association (with a capital A as discussed by the British empiricists) resurfaces as an obvious description for the processing of sensation. Despite the claim of the Würzburg school (Ach, 1905; Külpe, 1893) that image-less thought is possible and attempts by the Gestalt school (Köhler, 1924) to disprove association as a major mental activity, the multistep activities outlined for sensation in this chapter are best depicted as associations. While some forms of thought processing may not demand (or stimulate) sensory images, these are exceptional; most thoughts are accompanied by images involving multiple modalities; fully processed sensory percepts are essential elements in this activity.

In summary, sensations are amalgamated into thought through a fixed series of steps carried out by a similarly fixed set of neural structures. The processed information becomes increasingly sophisticated with each step until conscious awareness, recognition, and identification can be accomplished. Sensory information furnishes much of the material that becomes thought content and the processing of this information base (thinking), demands increasingly complex neural activities.

4

The Neurology of Motor Disorders

> Thought is action in rehearsal.
> —SIGMUND FREUD, 1938

> The scientific status of movement is ambiguous; as an observed fact it can be described; as a revelation of the process which produces it, it becomes an object of interrogation and experimentation beyond itself.
> —M. JEANNEROD
> THE BRAIN MACHINE, 1985

> From a control theory viewpoint, our human motor system is a multi-loop system of interminable complexity, consisting of feedback loops, all of which can be effortlessly tuned from comparatively simple regulation of the myotatic reflex gain to the most complex of cognitive work in which speech and thought are linked. We regard this multi-loop system as dependent on an anatomic substrate, but substrate used for the flexible creation and recreation of loops by various physiologic mechanisms.
> —GRIMM AND NASHNER, 1978

AXIOMS/POSTULATES

Most motor responses are overlearned and performed without conscious recognition—they are called *reflexes*.

Motor responses are the product of numerous independent neurally based functions operating synergistically to provide the final action.

Directed motor responses, particularly those devoted to novel tasks, demand cooperative participation of multiple brain activities that link the motor response system to thought processes.

Contrary to popular opinion, motor functions deserve serious consideration in the study of thought processing. Sherrington (1906) divided motor responses into two realms—reflex and integrative (higher mental) activities. Watson (1930), Thurstone (1938), and others stressed the involvement of motor function in thinking, arguing that to think was to expect to act. Oberg and Divac (1979) made a case for the involvement of the basal ganglia in a wide range of cognitive functions by demonstrating the apparent influence of neostriatal structures on the pathways of behavioral expression. A sizable literature focuses on the motor aspect of verbal expression (speech) and its relationship with thought (Ackerly and Benton, 1947; Luria and Homskaya, 1964; Sokolov, 1972; Stuss and Benson, 1986; Vygotsky, 1934/1962). Recent investigations (Botez et al., 1985; Leiner, Leiner, and Dow, 1989; Schmahmann, 1991) indicate that the cerebellum influences cognitive function. Strazalkowski (1982) goes so far as to contend that many "mental processes, especially memory, imagination, and thinking, are of motor origin."

VARIETIES OF MOTOR FUNCTION

As one of the most thoroughly studied of neural systems, motor function is described in a variety of ways. Two overlapping approaches—the first anatomical, the second combining anatomy and physiology—offer a practical base.

The most elementary clinical–anatomical approach to the motor system distinguishes upper and lower motor neuron disorders. This division presupposes an almost mythical entity, a two-neuron effector for motor activities. The first neuron arises in the cortex and runs through the deep white matter of the cerebral hemisphere to the brain stem, where it decussates (crosses to the opposite side), descending as the cortical spinal tract to end eventually in the anterior horn of the spinal cord (see Fig. 4.1). This single cell has been termed the *upper motor neuron*. Following synapse in the anterior horn, a second (lower) motor neuron traverses the anterior spinal root, enters a peripheral nerve, and eventually arrives at the effector organ (e.g., muscle, gland). Paralysis may follow damage to either of the two neuronal groups but with a strikingly different clinical picture, depending on whether the upper or lower motor tract is involved. Table 4.1 lists some of the obvious differences between upper and lower motor neuron paralysis. While a clinical differentiation clearly exists and is honored in the practice of neurology, the simplistic view of upper versus lower motor neuron is misleading. Both neurons, but particularly the upper motor neuron, fall under the influence of many additional neurons that both facilitate and inhibit neural function and therefore modulate the eventual outcome.

A second, time-honored division of motor functions separates pyramidal from extrapyramidal motor systems—the former dedicated to volitional movements, the latter to ballistic control qualities such as speed and smoothness. While useful in the clinic, this differentiation also has built-in inaccuracies and is widely criticized. First, the pyramidal system is not the only motor apparatus that controls volitional motor activities. Second, the term *extrapyramidal* is imprecise—literally, it should represent all motor

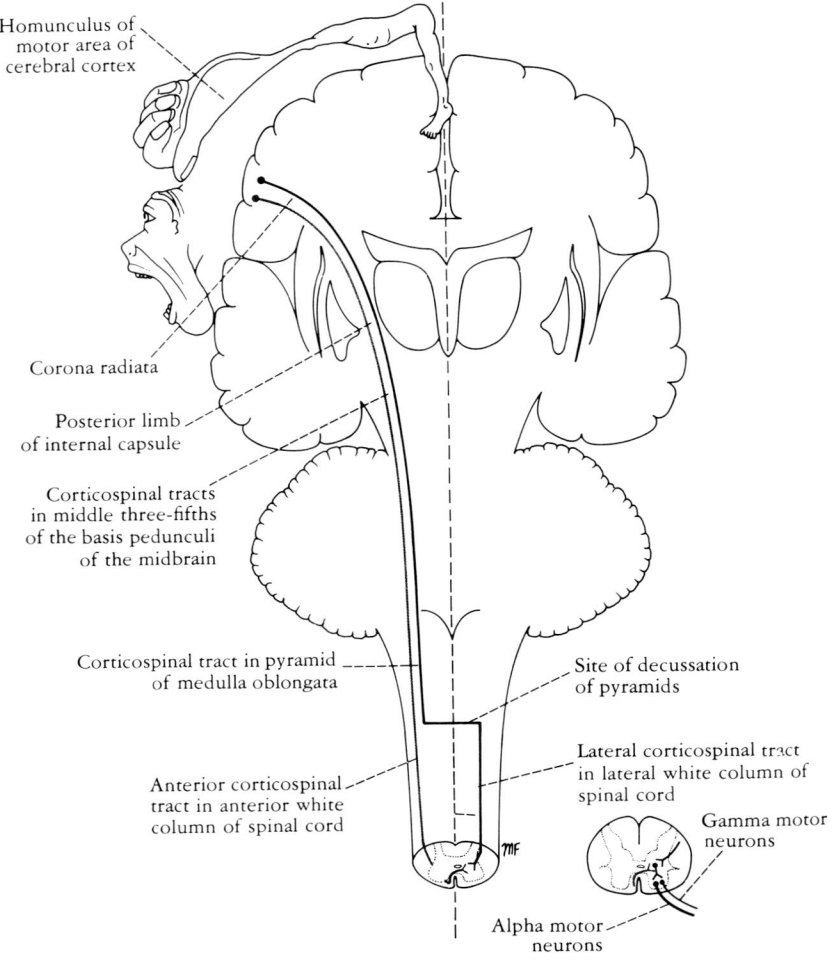

Fig. 4.1. Artist's outline of the elementary motor system depicting the upper motor neuron (cortex to spinal cord) and lower motor neuron (beyond the spinal cord). From Snell, 1980.

Table 4.1. Characteristics of Motor Paralysis

	Upper Motor Neuron	Lower Motor Neuron
Muscle units involved	Grouped	Individual
Muscle tone	Spastic	Flaccid
Muscle atrophy	Slight	Marked
Fasciculations	Absent	Present
Deep tendon reflexes	Hyperactive	Hypoactive or absent
Plantar reflexes	Extensor	Flexor or mute

systems that do not emanate from the cortical pyramidal cells or send fibers through the medullary pyramids, but in practice the term is usually reserved for the motor activities governed by the basal ganglia (striato-pallidal-nigral system). Third, the pyramidal/extrapyramidal dichotomy excludes a third major motor control system, that associated with the cerebellum. A tripartite anatomical differentiation is preferable—cerebellar, striato-pallidal-nigral, cortico–spinal. This differentiation allows relevant correlations between clinical findings and the site of functional abnormalities of the motor system. Table 4.2 presents some distinct manifestations of dysfunction in these three systems. The clinical differentiation presented in Table 4.2 is not as simple as the upper motor/lower motor separation but comes closer to categorizing motor disabilities as seen in actual practice. In many clinical situations, however, the malfunction is widespread; placement of observed dysfunctions into only one of the three types of abnormal motor function can be misleading.

While these crude anatomical divisions are helpful to the clinician, they do not do justice to the richness of the many influences that play upon the motor system. Taking different approaches, Yakovlev (1948) and MacLean (1970) described three functionally distinct motor systems, each occupying a specific area within the neural axis and each operating in a quasi-independent manner.

In Yakovlev's ontogenetic analysis (see Fig. 4.2), the innermost unit, the *motor system of visceral activities,* almost completely devoid of myelin, lies next to the hollow core of the remnant of the embryonic neural axis and deals with autonomic functions. Surrounding this inner

Table 4.2. Varieties of Cerebral Motor Dysfunction

	Cerebellar Dysfunction	Striato-Pallidal-Nigral Dysfunction	Cortico-Spinal Dysfunction
Muscle tone	Hypotonic	Rigid (cogwheel)	Hypertonic (spastic)
Distribution of abnormal tone	All muscle groups	Flexors of all four limbs	Flexors of arms, extensors of legs
Abnormal involuntary movements	Titubation, tremor	Tremor, chorea, athetosis, dystonia	Absent
Abnormal voluntary movements	Dysmetria, past pointing dysdiadochokinesis, excessive rebound	Slowness, clumsiness	Paralysis
Deep tendon reflexes	Hung (delayed response)	Hypoactive	Hyperactive
Plantar reflexes	Flexor or mute	Flexor or mute	Extensor

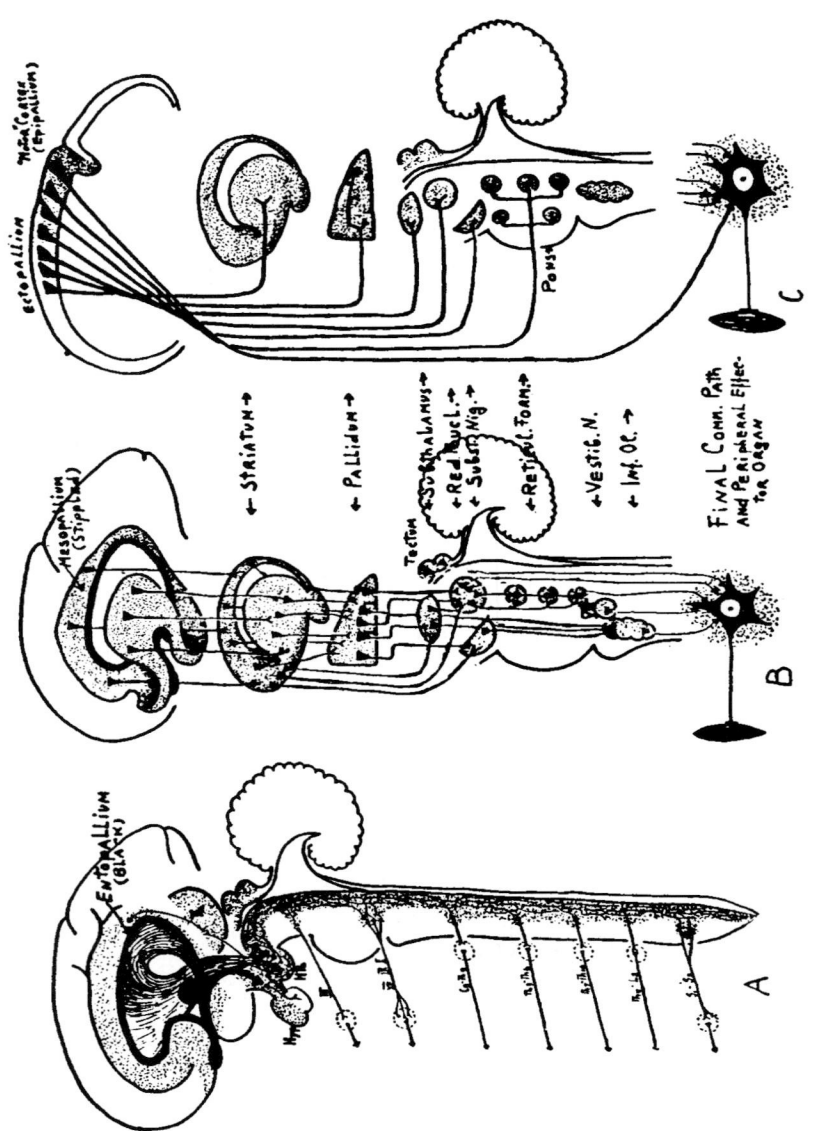

Fig. 4.2. Yakovlev's conception of three motor systems: A represents the motor system of visceral activities, B represents the motor system of behavioral expression, and C represents the motor system of effective behavior. From Yakovlev, 1948.

core is an intermediate system, a *motor system of behavioral expression*, consisting of many short neural processes organized into a reticulate network. None of the fibers is long; all apparently operate in series, producing a "huge synaptic surface of reciprocally overlapping, repeatedly recurrent synaptic relays." Yakovlev contended that the intermediate system controls outward expression, including facial emotion, vocalization, speech, gesture, body attitude, muscle tone, and posture, all of which reflect the internal state of the organism. Finally, the outermost motor system, the *motor system of effective behavior*, present only in the mammal and vastly enlarged in the human, has many well-myelinated neurons with cells of origin predominantly located in the cerebral cortex; it connects to lower brain stem and spinal motor centers in parallel. Yakovlev argued that this system controls skilled, learned movements. In higher primates it governs behaviors such as gesture, vocalization, and manual dexterity, and in humans the system has evolved to carry out behaviors such as manufacture, language, and symbolized thought.

MacLean's phylogenetic view, a tripartite scheme, is sketched in Figure 4.3. The most archaic unit, the *reptilian brain*, apparently controls basic drives (the four Fs: feeding, fleeing, fighting, and the act of procreation [MacLean, 1958]). The *paleomammalian–limbic brain* manages basic autonomic functions such as respiration, digestion, and cardiac activity. Alterations within either of these two basic systems can affect human behavior, and thought processes, but in general their actions are carried out automatically and unconsciously. Both systems are monitored by and respond to the outermost *neomammalian (effector) brain*, the neural

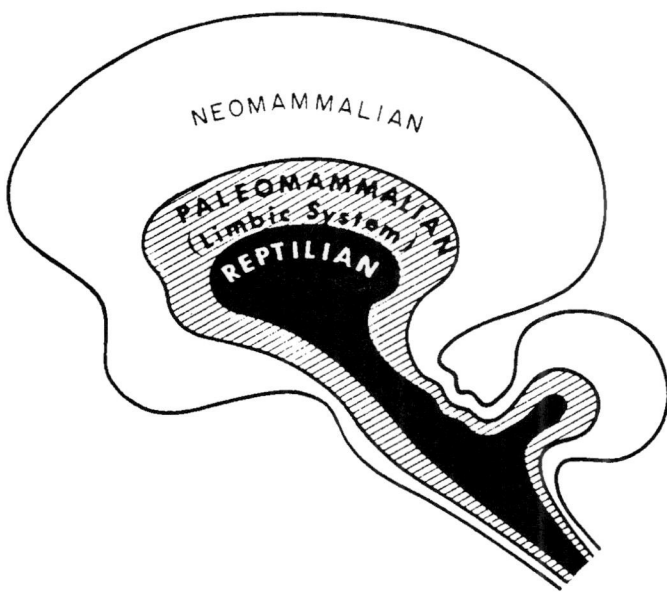

Fig. 4.3. MacLean's tripartite scheme of motor function. From MacLean, 1970.

apparatus for control of all nonautomatic motor output. In MacLean's scheme the two primitive systems have a reciprocal influence on all motor activities.

The Yakovlev and MacLean schemes outlined total motor function. More restricted categorizations have been offered. Attempting to analyze the clinical disorder called *apraxia*, Jules Dejerine (1914/1977) charted the steps that he believed necessary for the execution of a motor response (Table 4.3). Except for steps 1 and 6, each division of Dejerine's scheme can be considered a higher mental process; steps 3, 4, and 5 are clearly associated with the mental representation of motor activity.

More recently, Marsden (1982) suggested that the neural process occurring between perceptual recognition and motor action could be called *motor planning* and divided into three stages: (1) perceptual judgment of the relevant external circumstance, the present motor state, and past experience; (2) formulation of a motor plan, most often consisting of sequences of routine or almost routine motor programs operating serially; and (3) execution of a smooth, ballistically balanced sequence of motor programs delivered through the motor output pathways. Basic to Marsden's approach is his recognition that most, if not all, routine motor programs are the product of the striato-pallidal-nigral system and its connections. But stage 2, the formulation, and stage 3, the execution of the motor plan, demand nonroutine motor activity. The higher mental processes (i.e., control, thinking) of stage 2 act on both the novel volitional and the more overlearned, automatic motor mechanisms to carry out stage 3.

Evidence supporting a key role for the basal ganglia in routine, overlearned motor activities and the need for cortical motor control when novel actions are performed comes from the demonstration by Mazziotta, Phelps, and Wapenski (1985) of quantitative differences in metabolism in these two regions of the brain depending on the degree of automaticity of the motor response. Using glucose metabolism techniques pioneered by Phelps and colleagues (1979), Mazziotta and his colleagues had subjects perform one of two motor acts: (1) consistently write their signature for over 30 minutes; (2) tap the thumb serially with each of the four fingers of the right hand constantly for 30 minutes. When writing their signatures, one of the most overlearned activities in the human motor repertoire, only

Table 4.3. Steps in the Execution of an Act

1 Sensory excitation
2 Mental representation
3 Representation of the act (response)
4 Activation of appropriate motor images for act
5 Discharge of cerebral motor area
6 Motor act (response)

Adapted from Dejerine, 1914/1977.

the left basal ganglia area showed increased metabolism. With the finger tapping act, simple but not overlearned, both the left basal ganglia and the left motor and premotor cortical areas showed increased metabolism. Even with cautious interpretation, this study supports previous assertions (Denny-Brown and Yanagisawa, 1976; Martin, 1967) that routine, overlearned motor acts, even those producing language symbols, are initiated and can be carried out by subcortical motor systems.

Apraxia, an inability to carry out purposeful movements on command that cannot be explained by sensory, motor, or language dysfunction, provides a potential avenue for study of thought/motor correlation, but the topic is complex, the proposed mechanisms are controversial, and the disturbance is not fully defined. Reviews of apraxia have been published by Geschwind (1965, 1967b, 1975b), Hécaen (1981), Heilman (1979), Liepmann (1905), Luria (1966), and Stuss and Benson (1986).

CLINICAL EXAMPLES

Case 4.1

A 54-year-old man suffered rupture of an aneurysm of the anterior cerebral artery. The aneurysm was corrected surgically but recovery was slow, eventually leaving the patient with a disabling gait disturbance, dementia, and incontinence. There was a generalized hyperreflexia but no focal motor, sensory, or visual field defect. The most prominent movement disturbance was an inability to alter postures voluntarily. The patient could neither stand up from a sitting posture nor sit down from a standing posture without physical guidance from others. The clinical phenomenon called *magnetic gait* was clearly present—when asked to walk he acted as though unable to lift his foot from the floor, but, if aided (pushed slightly), he made stepping movements and, with a short series of completed steps, he no longer needed aid to continue walking. Related problems were present in the upper extremities, notably a tendency to grasp objects and an inability to release this grasp. Brain imaging (see Fig. 4.4) revealed obstructive hydrocephalus (normal pressure hydrocephalus), and a ventriculoperitoneal shunt was placed. All evidence of the magnetic gait and the grasp reflex disappeared, and the patient improved sufficiently to return to his occupation. (DFB)

In some classifications of apraxia, a form that involves disturbed skill, speed and delicacy of performance of complex movements has been called limb-kinetic apraxia (Denny-Brown, 1958; Heilman, 1979). A compulsive exploration of the immediate environment, best characterized by forced grasping of the hand (or foot) with a latency or even total inability to relax the grasp, is notable. Head turning (rooting) or sucking movements are seen if an object touches the cheek or lips and the hand forcefully grasps at palpated objects, sometimes to the extent that the involved limb will actively pursue a visualized stimulus in order to grasp it (magnetic apraxia) (Denny-Brown, 1958). When the disturbance involves the leg, attempts to walk produce a stiffening of the involved leg(s) so that the foot appears stuck (glued) to the floor; the patient has difficulty advancing

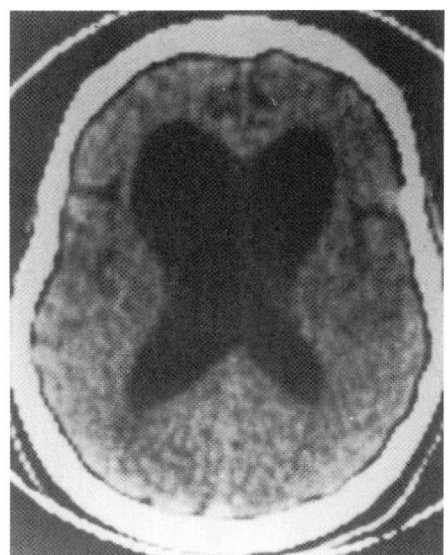
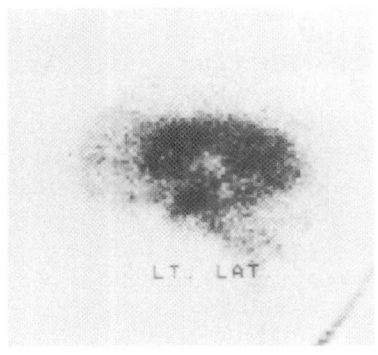

Fig. 4.4. X-ray CT scan (*left*) and isotope cisternogram (*right*) of Case 4.4. Note the massive enlargement of the frontal portions of the lateral ventricles and the trapping of the radioactive material within the ventricles. From Cummings and Benson, Chapter 7, *Dementia: A Clinical Approach,* Boston, Massachusetts, Butterworth Publishers, 1983.

the foot and making turns, but, as the magnetic posture is broken and the appropriate movements are performed repeatedly, the tendency for fixation decreases and the gait approaches normal. This characteristic gait disturbance has been called *frontal ataxia* or *frontal apraxia* (Denny-Brown, 1958; Mayer-Gross, 1935; Meyer and Barron, 1960). The problem is not paralysis (often there is no weakness at all) but a disturbance in volitional control of motility that produces a disabling motor disorder.

Case 4.2

A 59-year-old, right-handed man with a history of serious vascular disease was admitted to a hospital following the acute onset of right-sided paralysis and mutism. The paralysis improved over a few weeks so that only his right lower extremity and right shoulder were involved. Right hand strength was normal and he readily performed movements with the right hand on command, but a strong grasping tendency interfered with normal use of the hand. Even more dramatically, when he attempted to perform manual tasks with the left hand, the right hand interfered. Thus, when he attempted to write with his left hand, the right hand would forcefully take the pen away. Similarly, the right hand would steal blocks that the left hand was attempting to place in a desired design. The right hand frequently reached out and grabbed nearby items, a movement the patient was aware of but could not control except by using the left hand to force the right hand to change its position. This "alien hand" state improved over a period of several weeks. X-ray CT scan demonstrated infarction of the entire left anterior cerebral artery territory (see Fig. 4.5). (DFB)

The most dramatic example of magnetic apraxia is the relatively rare condition called the "alien hand" syndrome (Chan and Ross, 1988; Goldberg, Mayer, and Toglia, 1981; Mori and Yamadori, 1982). Patients with

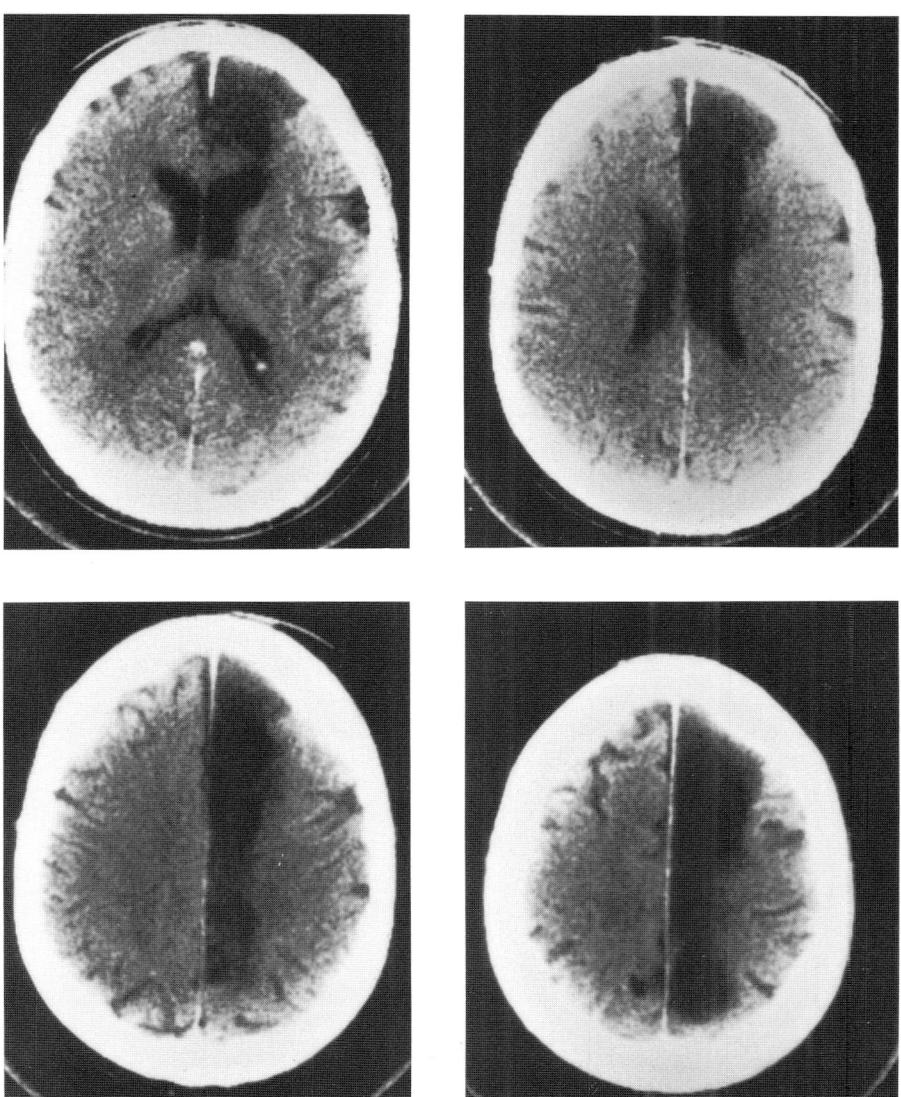

Fig. 4.5. X-ray CT of Case 4.2. Note the lucency in the territory of the left anterior cerebral artery indicating the area of cerebral destruction.

this disturbance suffer contralateral grasp reflex plus strong motor perseveration and are forced to use their obedient hand to control the other hand. The involved hand appears "alien," as if its actions were dissociated from conscious control. In the movie *Dr. Strangelove,* the title character possessed an alien hand that frequently grabbed at his throat, only to be torn away from the strangulation process by the other hand; the disorder is now sometimes called the "Strangelove effect." In this syndrome an intact, otherwise normally functioning motor response system carries out acts that cannot be controlled by the conscious, thinking brain. The independence of these complex motor acts from volitional, conscious control suggests that, while under normal conditions a strong link exists between the two systems, many complex motor functions can be performed without conscious control.

Case 4.3
A 54-year-old hypertensive man sustained a small cerebrovascular accident (CVA) that involved tissues just beneath the supramarginal gyrus on the left side (as eventually demonstrated at postmortem examination; Fig. 4.6). Despite good comprehension of spoken language, he was unable to make a fist, salute, or demonstrate use of hammer, comb, or teaspoon on command, and he even had great difficulty in imitating these movements. In contrast, he handled utensils without difficulty and was accurate in selecting the desired body movement for the command if multiple examples were presented by the examiner. There was neither paralysis nor sensory loss to explain the movement problem, and he used his limbs normally, without clumsiness, in everyday activities.

Months after the CVA occurred, the patient was asked to protrude his tongue as part of a follow-up evaluation. He immediately made body and facial movements, opened and shut his mouth, squinted his eyes, and grimaced for a full two minutes before protruding his tongue. Then he stopped, smiled, and said, "I knew

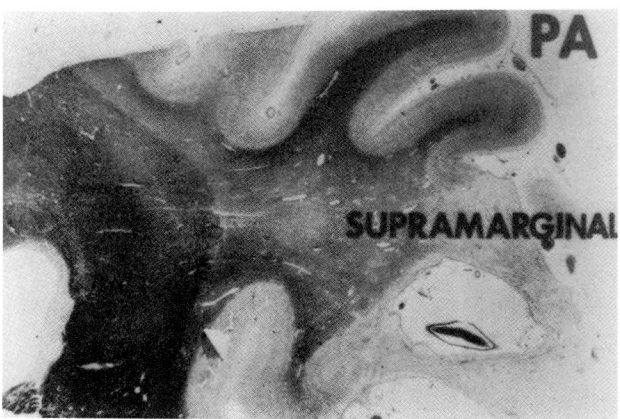

Fig. 4.6. Low-power view of brain tissue in Case 4.3 showing structural damage to both the cortex and the subcortical white matter of the supramarginal gyrus. From Benson et al., 1973.

you were going to ask me to do that; I've been practicing." Within 30 seconds he spontaneously licked his lips, showing that no motor weakness was present to explain the hesitation in complying with the command. (Benson et al., 1973)

In Case 4.3 neither primary motor disability nor primary sensory loss interfered with responses, as demonstrated by the patient's easy ability to perform all actions under nondirected circumstances. Only when a movement was verbally commanded did he fail; testing revealed that he fully comprehended the command. While he received and interpreted the verbal direction fully, this information could not be transmitted to the appropriate motor effectors. This is a syndrome of cerebral disconnection.

Case 4.4
A 42-year-old man (who is also described as Case 3.8) sustained a lesion in the deep white matter just lateral to the genu of the corpus callosum on the right side (probably vascular as suggested by disappearance of the lesion on serial radioisotope brain scans). The initial left hemiparesis rapidly improved, with complete return of elementary motor function; no basic language disturbance was ever noted. The patient easily carried out commanded motor actions with his right upper and lower extremities but failed totally in attempting the same commanded activities with the left limbs unless first allowed to make the appropriate movement with the right limb so that he could imitate it with the left limb. Thus, while able to salute, make a fist, snap his fingers, imitate writing, hammering, and so forth with his right hand, he performed only a single stereotyped waving movement when given similar commands to be performed by his left hand. In addition, he could write meaningful language in a legible script with his right hand but produced only stereotyped scribble when asked to write with his left hand. No matter what word was dictated, his left hand always produced the beginning of his name and after a few letters trailed off and stopped. He could copy with the left hand, although this was slow and the output was clumsy. (DFB)

Case 4.4 resembles Case 4.3 in the inability to carry out commanded movements, but in Case 4.4 only the left limbs were affected. There was clear evidence of adequate comprehension, as the commanded movements were readily performed by the right limbs; only the left limb failed. A disconnection between the left and right hemisphere motor association areas was postulated, a clinical variation on the callosal surgery discussed in Chapter 2.

By far the best recognized and most common variety of apraxia features an inability to carry out, on verbal command, an act that is easily carried out spontaneously. Most often this disorder has been called *motor apraxia* or *ideomotor apraxia*. Hughlings Jackson (1878/1915) described the inability of some of his patients to protrude their tongues, and this phenomenon is regularly observed in neurological clinics. Before motor apraxia can be diagnosed, motor, sensory, and language disorders sufficient to block the commanded movement must be excluded.

The disturbance has been most forcefully defined as a separation of language comprehension from motor response (Ettlinger, 1969;

Geschwind, 1965, 1967b), but alternative explanations such as disruption of necessary motor engrams, selective release of inhibitory activity, and unbalanced interhemispheric rivalry have also been suggested (de Ajuriaguerra and Tissot, 1969; Heilman, 1979; Morlaas, 1928). Motor apraxia can involve both limbs (Case 4.3) or the left limbs only (Case 4.4); Critchley (1953) defined the latter as a pathological impairment of the nonpathological left side. One of three neuroanatomical sites is damaged in cases of ideomotor apraxia: (1) white matter beneath the left supramarginal gyrus (involving the arcuate fasciculus) (Case 4.3); (2) dominant hemisphere motor association cortex (usually involving Broca's area and/or adjacent motor association cortex); or (3) anterior corpus callosum or adjacent interhemispheric pathways connecting left and right motor association areas (Case 4.4). A neural system consisting of the posterior language areas, the dominant, usually ipsilateral, motor association area, and the homologous motor association areas of the opposite hemisphere with their connecting pathways appears essential for carrying out a verbally commanded motor activity. While the basic neural system underlying this task can be diagrammed simply (see Fig. 4.7), there are many opportunities for relationships between this relatively elementary system and higher conscious or unconscious volitional command activities (thinking). Apraxia results from damage somewhere along the system that links language processing units with the primary motor cortex; the performance of at least some motor acts demands processing beyond the immediate motor reflex systems.

Ideomotor apraxia is relatively common in patients with left hemisphere language disorder (motor apraxia was demonstrated in 40 percent of aphasics admitted to the Boston Veterans Administration Hospital Aphasia Research Center in 1973 and 1974). In most cases, one of the three sites outlined above is involved. Ideomotor apraxia demonstrates interference with the neural processing needed for an appropriate motor response to spoken language, a disturbance of thought processing.

Other forms of apraxia have been described. In Liepmann's original discussions of apraxia (1900, 1905) and in many subsequent publications (Benson and Geschwind, 1985; De Renzi, Pieczuro, and Vignolo, 1968; Heilman, 1973; Wilson, 1908), a type of response impairment in which the patient cannot maintain a sequence of movements despite demonstrated ability to carry out each individual movement has been described under the name *ideational apraxia*. The disorder is frequently defined by example. Thus, a patient is presented with a pipe, tobacco pouch, and matches and told to fill the pipe, light it, and smoke it. While capable of performing each step, somewhere in the sequence a step may be omitted so that the patient puffs on an empty, unlit pipe. While the patient appears to comprehend and can perform any individual step on direct command, the process fails through omission of some portion of the sequence, a disturbance defined as a loss of the "idea" of the act.

Ideational apraxia is either extremely uncommon in focal brain disorder or its presence is hidden. Over the years several sites have been

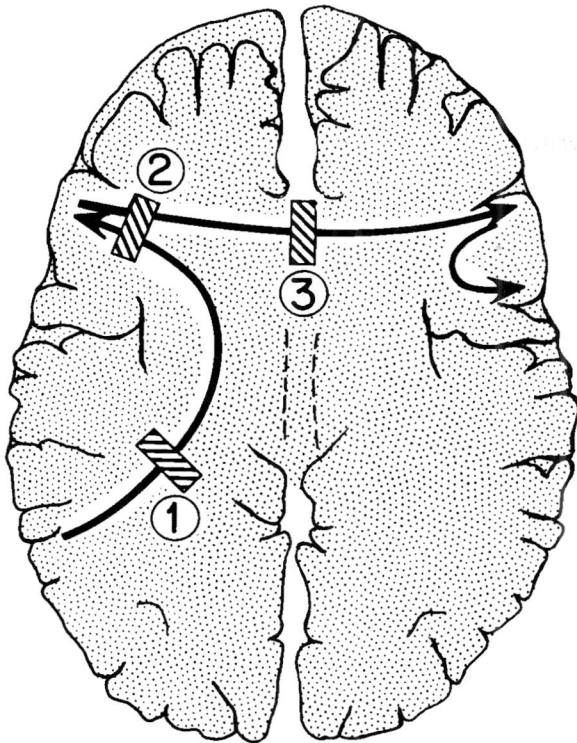

Fig. 4.7. Graphic presentation of the elementary disconnection explanation of ideomotor apraxia. 1 = arcuate fasciculus; 2 = dominant premotor cortex; 3 = corpus callosum. Arrows indicate direction of information flow to carry out a commanded movement with the left hand. From Benson and Geschwind, 1985.

posited, but as yet there is no accepted localization for ideational apraxia. On the other hand, the clinical characteristics described are not difficult to demonstrate, particularly in patients with widespread cortical degenerative disorders such as Alzheimer's disease. Almost every victim of Alzheimer's disease will suffer the disordered control of sequential actions called *ideational apraxia* at some time during the course of the disease.

One elementary explanation for ideational apraxia stresses impairment of the ability to handle sequential motor activities in proper serial order, now considered a prefrontal disturbance (Fuster, 1980; Stuss and Benson, 1986), but others have suggested parietal dysfunction as the cause of ideational apraxia (Heilman, 1973; Liepmann, 1905, 1908; Wilson, 1908). Either explanation would be consistent with the known loci of cortical pathology in Alzheimer's disease.

Several neuropsychologists have described a different operational disability under the name *ideational apraxia* (De Renzi, Pieczuro, and Vignolo, 1968). In this disturbance the patient cannot handle a real object as well as he can mime the use of that object, the opposite of motor apraxia.

This variation of apraxia can be demonstrated in the clinic, but available evidence fails to indicate focal pathology. In two cases that fit the second definition of ideational apraxia that were personally evaluated by the author, one had sustained bilateral parietal infarctions producing sensory deafferentiation sufficient to preclude tactile knowledge of the object being manipulated, and the other showed evidence of bilateral subcortical motor disturbances, primarily involving the basal ganglia, producing a motor dyscoordination that increased when the actual object was manipulated. Although consistent with the second operational description of ideational apraxia, neither of these clinical states can be considered a true apraxia, as each patient had motor and/or sensory disturbance that precluded successful object manipulation. The possibility that a disturbance of motor response not based on either sensory or motor disorder (a true apraxia) can occur on an ideational basis remains plausible nonetheless.

Clinical examples of motor disorder in which impaired ideation can be invoked are not common, and, when closely scrutinized, a nonideational basis is usually demonstrable. Nonetheless, cases such as those described here amply demonstrate the strong relationship between the complex processes of thinking and the final motor response. Some instances of apraxia (e.g. Case 4.2) appear to be based on malfunction within nonmotor neural systems that influence the motor systems. French clinicians (Lhermitte, Pillon, and Serdaru, 1986) described a condition in patients with severe frontal lobe pathology (see Case 11.6) in which a virtually intact sensorimotor system is not inhibited sufficiently to control motor responses.

NEUROANATOMICAL SUBSTRATE

In an attempt to integrate higher mental functions with the intricacies of motor function, in this discussion the motor system will be divided into five parts: lower motor neuron, brain stem motor nuclei, cerebellum, basal ganglia, and cortex. The lower motor neuron will not be discussed, though its influence on the upper parts of the final motor response pathway is of consequence to the neurology of thought.

Brain Stem Motor Nuclei

Most motor responses are directly controlled by subcerebral motor systems emanating from sets of nuclei spread along the brain stem. One group, known as the ventromedial brain stem nuclei, includes the reticulospinal, tectospinal, vestibulospinal, and interstitial–spinal nuclei. A second set, the lateral brain stem nuclear group, includes the rubrospinal nuclei (Kuypers, 1981, 1985; Peterson, 1979). The ventromedial brain stem system promotes basic movements, including maintenance of erect posture, integrated body and limb movements, synergistic movements of individual muscles and muscle groups, and the progressive course of such movements. The lateral brain stem system aids in all of the above functions but superimposes a capacity for independent use of the extremities, particularly their distal portions, in routine limb movements. Finally, the cortico-spinal pathway augments the motor control functions of the lateral brain stem pathways but permits further fractionation of movements, particularly the fine movements of the hand digits. All movements are performed under the control of these brain stem nuclei, which provide a consistent influence on the spinal cord and lower brain stem motor nuclear centers (for motor functions controlled by the cranial nerves). These activities have long been classed as reflex motor functions (Sherrington, 1906). In this view, only the cortico-spinal motor system would subserve higher integrative functions and thus be involved in the motor activities related to thinking (integrative motor acts). Three additional motor units—cerebellar, basal ganglia, and cortical—each apparently operating within limited confines, exert important influences on motor activity.

Cerebellum

The cerebellum, a massive neural structure, represents a second motor system, supraordinate to the brain stem motor nuclei but operating independently. The cerebellum receives proprioceptive input from all muscle groups, and its output tracts go to both the thalamus (and from there to the basal ganglia and cortex) and the brain stem motor nuclei. While a complex group of functions has been outlined for the cerebellum (Brooks and Thach, 1981; Gilman, 1985), the major activity appears to be integrative in nature, coordinating the innervation of individual muscles and muscle groups to provide smooth movements of controlled magnitude for tasks requiring activation of different muscle groups throughout the body (Gilman, 1985). As currently understood, the functions of the cerebellum do not appear to enter into the thinking process, although cerebellar dysfunction may decrease the speed of information processing (Botez et al., 1985), and abnormal mental functioning occurs in some cerebellar disorders (Schmahmann, 1991).

Basal Ganglia

The motor functions of the basal ganglia have been studied intensively in recent years, prompted by the surgical and drug treatments for Parkinson's disease. During much of this time the functions of the individual nuclei that make up the basal ganglia remained unknown, and conflicting opinions were often expressed (Denny-Brown, 1962; Martin, 1967). The conflicts have not disappeared, although considerable information on functions of the individual nuclear centers of the basal ganglia is now available. Figure 4.8 gives a relatively current view of the many nuclei in the basal ganglia and their network of interconnections. Despite the richness of this network, known connections with descending pathways, particularly with the brain stem nuclei, are relatively limited. Most of the influence of the basal ganglia on motor activity appears to be mediated through connections with the thalamus and premotor cortex.

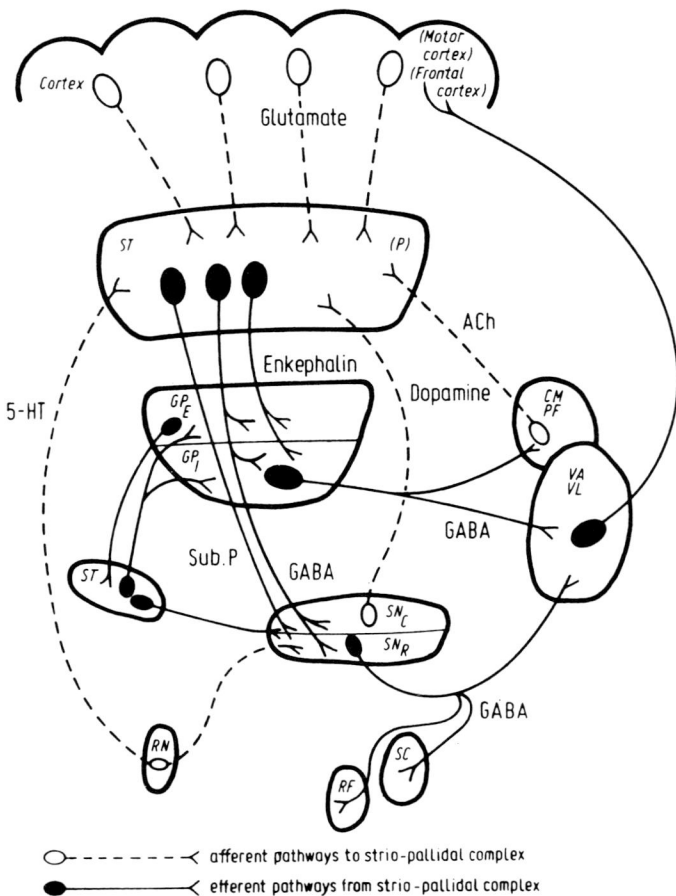

Fig. 4.8. Conception of the interconnections of a number of basal ganglia with indication of the major neurotransmitter functions involved in synaptic transmission. From Marsden, 1985.

Marsden (1985) suggested that the basal ganglia "allow automatic execution of learned motor plans." Others (Lidsky et al., 1985) believe that these subcortical motor nuclei may act to gate (control) sensory influences on the motor system. The basal ganglia apparently monitor current motor states and determine the advisability of corrective movements and then direct their output toward the thalamus and thence to the motor network in the frontal lobes capable of altering motor programs. While much evidence supports this theoretical framework, new information is constantly being gathered (Albin, Young, and Penney, 1989). Both clinical and pathological studies and associated laboratory research during the past three decades demonstrate that the basal ganglia do play a key role in motor activities and that they have rich interconnections with the cerebral cortex.

Cortex

Many different areas of cortex have been shown to influence motor responses, either directly or indirectly. In fact, strict criteria are necessary for the designation of *motor cortex*, because most areas of cortex are involved to some degree with motor response. Only those cortical areas now considered specific for motor function will be discussed here; Figure 4.9 graphically illustrates the best recognized areas. Brodmann area 4, the precentral gyrus, has long been designated *primary motor cortex* and is the location of the large pyramidal neurons thought to send axons through the brain to the anterior horn cells of the spinal cord. The distribution of neurons in Brodmann area 4 is functionally discrete so that motor nuclei affecting tongue, lips, and mouth are located low on the convexity of the cortex; thumb, hand, and arm are higher in Brodmann area 4; and hip and leg effectors are found in the superior cortex or in the medial sagittal region, an inverted homunculus similar to the sensory homunculus illustrated in Chapter 3. Following the original demonstration by Ferrier (1886) that electrical stimulation of selected areas of the exposed cortex produced movement, others (Foerster, 1936a; Penfield and Rasmussen,

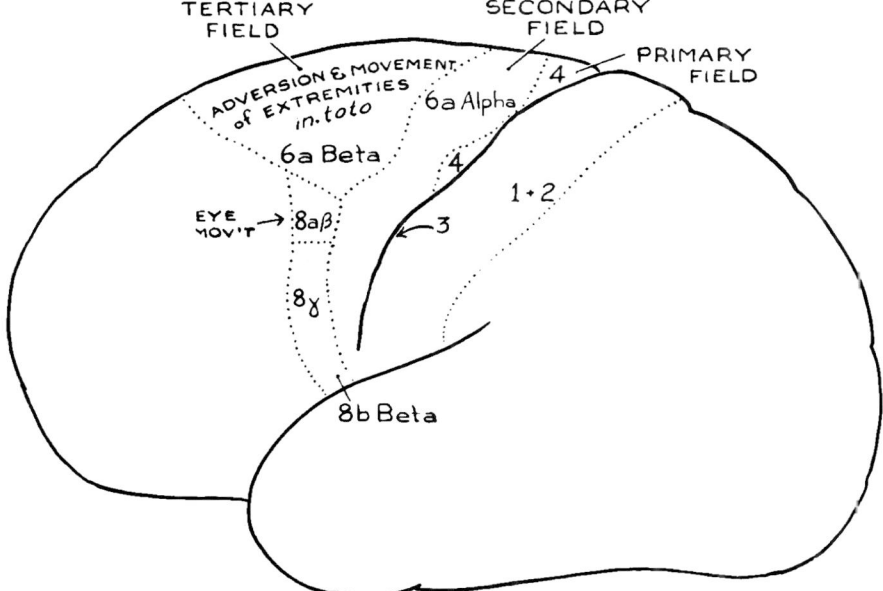

Fig. 4.9. Outline of left cerebral hemisphere indicating the major motor areas. Particularly note the association of areas 4, 6, and 8. From Penfield and Jasper, 1954.

1950) have demonstrated that discrete electrical stimulation along Brodmann area 4 produces movement of individual muscles or muscle groups. Figure 4.10 is a somewhat fanciful representation of the consensus on the cortical areas that provide direct motor control. Note the discrepancy between the large areas subserving tongue, buccofacial, and finger movements in comparison to the limited areas subserving more basic motor regions (e.g., shoulder, leg). Tongue, lips, and finger digits apparently receive the lion's share of Brodmann area 4 outflow, in keeping with their heavy load of finer, more precise motor actions.

Brodmann area 6, the premotor cortex situated just anterior to Brodmann area 4, is considerably larger and, while also having considerable functional specificity, shows a less distinct localization of function. Electrical stimulation of area 6 produces movement of groups of muscles rather than of the individual muscles activated by stimulation of nuclei in area 4 (Penfield and Rassmussen, 1950). Brodmann area 6 appears to deal with integrated movements that involve larger body units, while area 4 appears to control fine individual movements.

Brodmann area 8, sometimes called the *frontal eye fields*, resembles Brodmann area 6 cytologically and probably also affects broad body

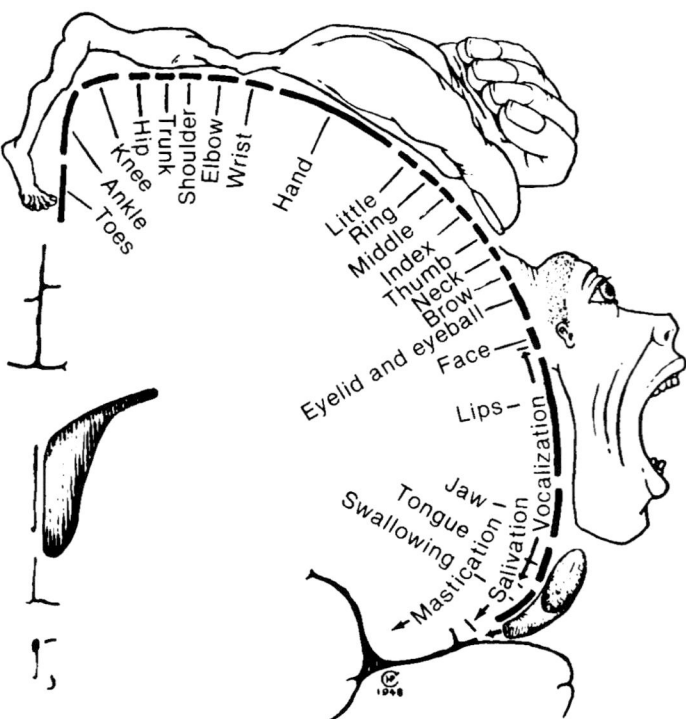

Fig. 4.10. Classic representation of the cortical homunculus for motor activity as distributed in Brodmann area 4. From Penfield and Rasmussen, 1950.

movements, particularly movements involved in rotation toward a stimulus. Stimulation of area 8 produces a turning of eyes to the opposite direction, frequently accompanied by head and shoulder rotation in the same direction. Conversely, damage to area 8 produces conjugate deviation of the eyes (and of body movements) toward the side of the lesion, a useful observation in the evaluation of focal brain damage.

The supplementary motor area (SMA), located in the medial sagittal region just beneath the premotor and precentral cortices, is now recognized as an important motor region. Stimulation and ablation work by neurosurgeons (Foerster, 1936a,b; Penfield and Welch, 1951) plus clinical/anatomical correlation studies (Brinkman, 1981; Damasio and Van Hoesen, 1980; Tanji and Kurata, 1983) have helped to characterize the role of the SMA in motor function. The specific function of the SMA, however, remains controversial. On the basis of radioactive blood flow studies, Roland and colleagues (1980) suggested that the SMA acted in the programming of a motor task; specifically, they suggested that recall of the memory of a motor sequence, the assembly of the "queue of time ordered commands" necessary for completion of the command, and the presentation of this material to the motor cortex were activities of the SMA. A somewhat different pacemaker function for the SMA has been proposed (Botez and Barbeau, 1971; Schiff et al., 1983). Clinical observations of individuals after anterior cerebral artery territory infarction had produced SMA damage (Freedman, Alexander, and Naeser, 1984) suggest that the supplementary motor area is needed to initiate motor tasks, including both body movements and speech.

The frontal cortical motor areas, particularly Brodmann area 6, receive information from many sources. The basal ganglia are strongly connected to area 6, indirectly via the thalamus and directly from cortex to the caudate nucleus. Area 6 receives input from each of the sensory association areas, providing data on environmental influences. In addition, area 6 receives major input from the prefrontal cortex and the insula, where information from the somatosensory cortices is integrated with that from the limbic and visceral systems (H.J.W. Nauta, 1986; W.J.H. Nauta, 1971). Prefrontal input represents a major correlation of thinking with the motor responses system and will be discussed in greater depth in Chapter 11.

Figure 4.11 presents a schematic six-part view of the major functional components of the motor response. The most inferior section represents basic reflex activity at the spinal cord level; the next lowest section contains the brain stem centers that directly influence the spinal reflex system. Individual muscle fibers and fiber groups are controlled by these two distal motor neuron sections. At an intermediate level the cerebellum, basal ganglia, and thalamus, interconnected both rostrally and caudally, provide a synergistic, coordinated, ballistic movement program. At the cortical level the most medial motor areas (Brodmann area 8 and the supplementary motor area) command important postural movements, and the SMA appears to participate in the activation of all cortical motor activities. The more posteriorly located cortical motor centers (Brodmann areas 4 and 6),

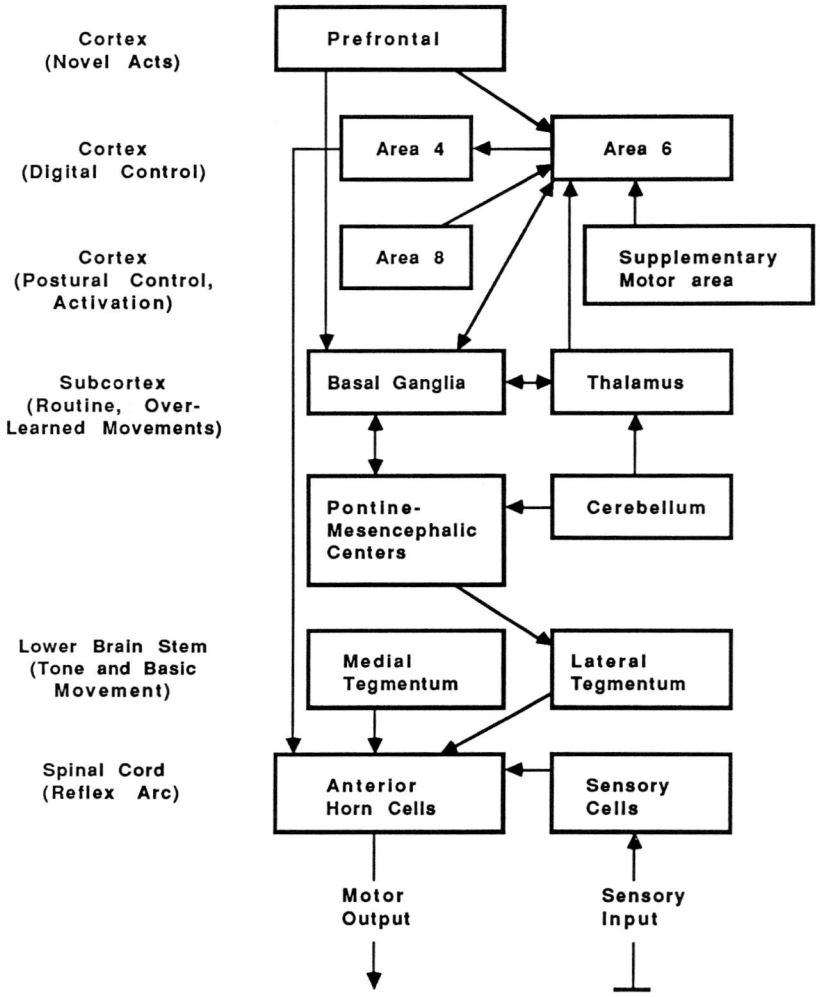

Fig. 4.11. A schematic representation of the interconnections of the major neuroanatomical entities involved in motor processing. (See text for description of activities within the component sections.)

with input from the prefrontal cortex, program novel, nonroutine motor responses.

THE NEURAL BASIS OF MOTOR ACTIVITY

Most motor response functions can be subsumed under one of three overall activities:

1. Analysis of incoming data, both exteroceptive and interoceptive

2. Formulation and monitoring of a response plan
3. Execution of the plan

The analysis step is primarily a sensory input function, and much of the final motor execution step appears to be carried out without activating thought processes. Neither, however, operates entirely without higher influence. The middle step can be considered thought processing. Although most motor activities, with the exception of those carried out by the lateral cortical motor areas, are performed without conscious awareness, noncortical motor centers should not be excluded from consideration in the thinking process. Monitoring of all motor response activities occurs constantly, and almost any activity of the ongoing process can be called into conscious awareness if needed.

Based on the anatomical data presented in the previous section, the observations of motor systems disorders presented in the clinical section, and the three steps outlined above, a neural basis for the relationship of motor function with thought can be postulated. To accompany this hypothesis, three rather gross divisions of motor response are proposed—reflex, automatic, and command motor activities (Table 4.4).

Reflex System

The most primitive motor system manages a significant majority of all motor activity in an efficient, almost fully reflex, operation. Three stages are evident—sensory excitation, motor representation (the preparation of

Table 4.4. Varieties of Motor Activity

Functional Level	Functional Activity		
	Analysis	Formulation	Response
Reflex	Sensory excitation	Motor representation	Motor response
Automatic	Sensory excitation	Formation of motor images	Motor response
	Recognition of sensorimotor state	Discharge through cerebral motor area	
Command	Sensory excitation	Representation of motor response (anticipation, program formation)	Motor response
	Representation of sensorimotor state	Monitoring of proposed motor images	
		Activation of motor act	
		Discharge through cerebral motor area	
		Monitoring of motor performance	

a response plan), and motor response. These operate in a learned, mechanical manner to produce most motor movements. Only vaguely, through conscious effort, does awareness of reflex activities arise. For instance, the reflex motor system commands multiple individual effectors that, synergistically, maintain bodily equilibrium. The individual is not aware of these effectors as they function; only by focusing attention on the maintenance of posture or specific movements can one become aware of the influence of this basic neural system. Purposeful alteration of these reflex movements demands intervention of higher control systems but often remains unconscious.

Automatic System

The second system, operating through a number of diencephalic nuclear centers plus the cerebellum, with connections to both cortical and mesencephalic areas, exerts superordinate control over the reflex system to produce well-coordinated, ballistically smooth, purposeful movements. The functions of this automatic system are considerably more complex than those of the reflex system and involve five distinguishable steps of neural processing: (1) sensory excitation, (2) recognition of the current sensorimotor state, (3) formation of a neural pattern representing the motor response, (4) transfer of this pattern to the appropriate brain stem and cerebral motor areas, and (5) activation of the motor response. This system provides *postural* control and commands well-rehearsed, *automatic* movements. Again, most activities of this system are performed without conscious thought; in contrast to the reflex system, however, activities of the automatic system are readily and frequently monitored in conscious thought. Thus, while the individual movements needed for walking on a path are not consciously noted, a careful monitoring of the ongoing process is being performed; any transgression from the anticipated movement will immediately enter conscious awareness.

Command System

The third system, operating primarily through the cortical motor areas but possessing close, reciprocal interconnections with the reflex and automatic systems, deals with the monitoring/control of purposeful motor responses and with the development of novel movements. The sequence of neural processing involved in the command system shares the first three steps of the automatic system (sensory excitation, mental representation of the sensorimotor state, and initial mental representation of a motor response), but the subsequent motor representation includes formation of a motor response program before activation of the motor act, as well as monitoring. Monitoring, leading to fine-tuning alterations, occurs both before and after the actual motor response, and the command system entails far more ongoing awareness of motor activities than the automatic system. In fact, most commanded activity is available for conscious review during and for at least a short period after the act. This makes the relationship between the command system (in both its programming and its monitoring function) and the thinking process apparent. Novel motor acts and their essential precursory steps are clearly connected with thinking.

The richness of interaction within the motor system increases with higher levels of activity. While the reflex motor system and, to a more limited degree, the automatic motor system can operate independently, the command system cannot perform its functions without complex connections, not only with the lower motor systems but also many other neural systems. For the highest level responses (novel motor programs), the integrated input of many cortical and subcortical areas is essential.

Damage to the motor system produces characteristic clinical patterns that reflect, with considerable accuracy, the level of control that has been impaired. The clinical examples provided in this chapter represent only situations in which some aspect of the mental control of motor acts was disrupted, causing negative (e.g., the failures of ideomotor apraxia) or positive (e.g., the uncontrolled actions of the alien hand) motor symptoms. In both instances an otherwise normal motor system has been isolated from either basic sensorimotor information (e.g., ideomotor apraxia) or higher mental control (e.g., alien hand syndrome). Additional examples of abnormal motor responses, based on malfunctions in other functional systems, will be presented throughout this book. In these instances, however, the disorder of the specified system will be stressed as the source of the inadequately controlled motor response. In most such instances the motor system itself will be responding correctly to an incorrect command.

5

The Neurology of Basic Mental Control Disorders: Alertness, Attention, Mental Tone

> . . . we have overlooked the circumstance that for scientific purposes "consciousness" never was anything but a heterogenous group of behavioral operations, and have fallen into the delusion of supposing that because the group possesses a name it corresponds to a unit function the neural center for which, like some uncharted island, now only awaits discovery.
>
> —R. MEYERS, 1951

AXIOMS/POSTULATES

Awareness is an essential component of thought processing; conscious awareness, in contrast, is not.

Awareness has two distinct aspects—arousal and attention; both have general and selective aspects.

While intricately interwoven, the different forms of awareness arise from functionally independent neuroanatomical systems that utilize some common neuroanatomical sites.

Basic to all high-level brain functions including thought is a property that can be called *awareness*—a complex, multifaceted activity that involves both conscious and unconscious measures to control and respond to stimulation. Two chapters of this book will be devoted to awareness; this one will deal with some pertinent aspects of basic mental control, and Chapter 11 will discuss higher level mental control mechanisms.

VARIETIES OF BASIC MENTAL CONTROL

Numerous classifications and a plethora of terms have been devised to characterize the brain activities that will be presented here under the rubric of *basic mental control*. Salient features recur, however, and three major divisions can be accepted: (1) alertness, the state of awakeness;

(2) attention, the ability to maintain coherent mental function; and (3) mental tone, the variable levels of awakeness and attention.

Alertness

Many words, often impressionistic, characterize degrees of impaired (less than full) alertness. *Drowsy, lethargic, stuporous, semicomatose, obtunded, sleepy,* and *comatose* all represent physiological states of less than full alertness or awakeness. Specific parameters for any of these terms are almost nonexistent. Guidelines for staging decreased alertness have been proposed (Plum and Posner, 1972; Teasdale and Jennett, 1974), but they rarely have the exactness essential for clinical description. At best, descriptive terms only portray the patient's appearance at a given time. Impaired awakeness must be recognized, serially measured, and recorded, since decreased awakeness significantly alters all aspects of mental life, including thought.

Accurate delineation of the degree of alertness is not easy. The best system utilizes the stimulus → response paradigm of the behaviorists. Both variables can be measured. The *degree* of stimulation necessary to produce the *degree* of response observed can be assessed with some accuracy. If a patient is asleep but awakens when his name is called and remains fully aroused, this fact can be recorded. If the patient remains somewhat drowsy and tends to drift back to sleep, requiring additional alerting stimuli such as repeated calling of the name, raising one's voice, or physical stimulus such as touching the leg or slapping the face to reestablish full contact, both the level of stimulation and the degree and duration of revived awakeness reflect the state of alertness. Greater degrees of obtundation demanding more aggressive physical stimuli (e.g., shouting, clapping the hands, pinching the Achilles' tendon) to produce lesser degrees of response such as a short mumbled reply, merely opening the eyes and looking about, or just a slight withdrawal of the limb or grimace of the face indicate greater degrees of impairment.

Alterations of the awake state (sleep) are normal and essential for health. The quantity of sleep needed varies considerably, both with age and between individuals; for most persons, sleep consumes approximately one-third of the day. Jones and Oswald (1968) recorded normal individuals with sleep durations ranging from three or less to twelve or more hours daily. Considerable decrease of optimal sleep time can be tolerated but eventually leads to behavioral disorders (e.g., hangover, decreased concentration). Investigators have outlined the stages of sleep and demonstrated that altered sleep staging is controlled by the neurotransmitters norepinephrine and serotonin, products of brain stem nuclear centers (Hobson, 1974). Thought processing is altered (but not nonexistent) during sleep, and disordered sleep patterns, usually reflecting altered neurotransmitter function, can alter thinking processes in the awake state (e.g., the hangover/sleep withdrawal state). Even subtle problems of alertness may lead to difficulties in maintaining attention.

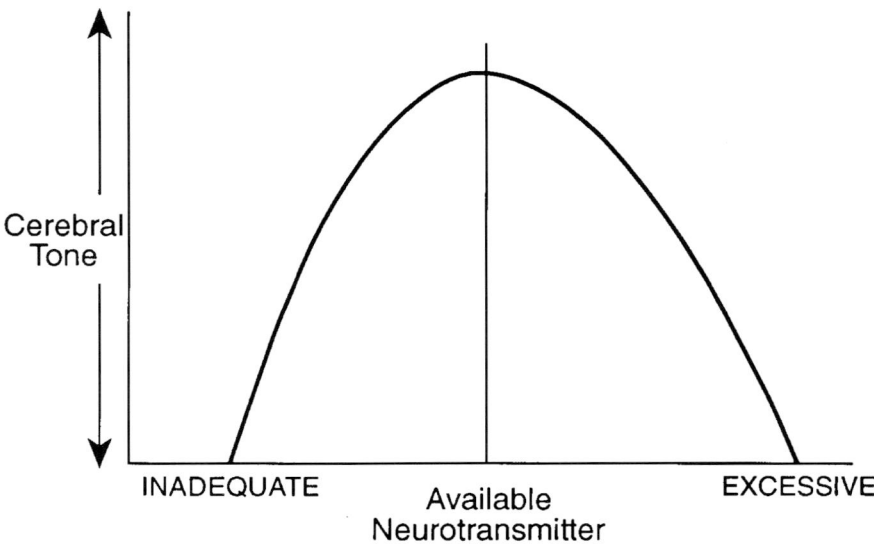

Fig. 5.1. The inverted U concept illustrating alterations in cerebral tone produced by increasing levels of neurotransmitter.

Attention

Even when fully awake, some individuals will have difficulty maintaining attention. The concept of attention is not adequately understood; however, two dichotomies can help to define the problem. One distinguishes between general attention (the ability to maintain coherent thought [Geschwind, 1982]) and selective attention (the ability to focus on a single stimulus to the exclusion of others). The other distinguishes general (overall or bilateral) disturbances from unilateral inattention (compromised ability to attend to stimuli coming from one side of the body or extrapersonal space).

Mental Tone

The concept of cortical tone, the development and maintenance of an optimal state for higher cortical operations, originated with Pavlov (1941) and remained basic to Russian psychology (Luria, 1973). Originally conceptualized with little confirming evidence, it was validated by two advances in neuroscience. The first was the demonstration by Magoun (1950), Moruzzi and Magoun (1949), Lindsley (1958), Nauta (1973), and others (French, 1958; Yingling and Skinner, 1975) of the midbrain reticular system's role in maintaining the state of awakeness. The second was the demonstration that the level of mental tone reflects neurotransmitter activity (Bachman and Albert, 1984; Chu and Bloom, 1973; Ljungberg and Ungerstedt, 1976). This influence is not merely more-is-better; the inverted U concept (Fig. 5.1) illustrates that either inadequate or excessive quantities of neurotransmitter can alter, usually decrease, mental tone. Mental tone is a real psychobiological concept that remains difficult to characterize and measure. Descriptions of clinical disorders that affect one or more aspects of basic mental control will help to characterize this elusive concept.

CLINICAL EXAMPLES

Case 5.1

A 31-year-old, modestly obese man sought medical attention because of excessive sleepiness. He was employed as a steward aboard a merchant vessel with several hours of duty at each of the three meal settings every day. After being awakened by his alarm clock, he was immediately alert, arose, and performed his duties. During the meal service he would have periods of sleepiness but remained sufficiently occupied to preclude drifting off. At the end of the meal he would return to his bunk and sleep until the alarm awakened him for the next meal service. Again, he would be alert and awake, would complete his task, and then return to bed, with a similar program for all meal services. With minor exceptions his entire day was spent either working at the meal service or asleep. During shore leave he tended to fall asleep while watching TV, during conversations with his friends, during meals, and even while sitting in his car stopped at a red light. Full neurological examination and routine EEG study results were within normal limits. A wake–sleep EEG test, however, demonstrated the presence of an immediate transition from the wake electrical pattern to the rapid eye movement (REM) sleep pattern. A diagnosis of *narcolepsy* was made, and the condition was successfully treated with stimulant medications. (DFB)

The best-defined sleep disorder is narcolepsy, a malady characterized by uncontrollable episodes of sleep occurring multiple times throughout the day (Dement, 1976). Multiple short episodes of true sleep, ranging from a few seconds to 15 minutes or more, occur; the need to sleep is overwhelming, but after a short sleep the individual awakens refreshed only to need another short sleep in several hours (Guilleminault, Dement, and Passouant, 1976). Narcolepsy is frequently associated with other paroxysmal behavioral disorders. *Cataplexy,* a short, transient paralysis of somatic musculature, is often precipitated by acute emotional outbursts such as laughter, anger, or fright; the paralysis of cataplexy can occur at any time and represents a potentially dangerous disability. Short periods of paralysis at the time of falling asleep (hypnagogic) or of awakening (hypnopompic) are, on some occasions, accompanied by vivid, dream-like experiences (hypnagogic or hypnopompic hallucinations).

Polysomnography (sleep EEG) reveals that patients with narcolepsy pass rapidly from a normal awake EEG pattern to a stage featuring REM. REM occurring within 15 minutes of sleep onset is considered pathognomonic of narcolepsy (Zarcone, 1973) and indicates a pathological imbalance in the neurochemical systems that control wakefulness, REM sleep, and non-REM sleep. While extremely bothersome, narcolepsy and its accompanying disorders (except for cataplexy) are benign and, to a degree, can be modulated by medication. If untreated, narcolepsy is disabling, since the multiple, unplanned periods of somnolence interfere with continuity of life.

Sleep deprivation, prolonged periods during which normal sleep cannot be obtained, produces unpleasant side effects, including marked alterations in thinking. Humans deprived of sleep for periods of 60 or more hours experience fatigue and irritability, altered and labile mood states, difficulty in concentration, inaccurate perceptions, and difficulty performing any but routine tasks. Incentive to work is decreased, and the maintenance of general attention becomes progressively more difficult. Psychosis, the inability to maintain contact with reality, may develop. Sleep deprivation produces a significant alteration in mental tone (disordered attention and lapses in awakeness—microsleeps), but the condition is corrected by several nights of normal sleep (Hauri, 1982).

Case 5.2

A 41-year-old man was admitted to the hospital because of his acutely altered mental state. He had suffered severe vomiting and diarrhea over a period of approximately 36 hours before admission, becoming weak and confused. By the time he arrived on the ward, blood tests had revealed a significantly low sodium level (112 mg). The hyponatremia was corrected by control of the diarrhea and by cautious infusion of hypertonic saline. A mental status evaluation performed shortly after admission, before the sodium level had been corrected, showed no evidence of paralysis, sensory loss, or visual field defect.

The patient appeared fully awake, was intently interested in his surroundings, and chattered continuously. Language function was intact, but he constantly diverted from the selected topic; he could not maintain a coherent line of thought. He failed memory tests because he could not maintain information for more than a few seconds. His digit span was limited to 2 or 3 forward, and this was only achieved intermittently. The examiner frequently presented his own name, which the patient retained only momentarily and never could reproduce after several minutes. He failed other tests demanding attention such as the serial subtraction of sevens from 100, reverse digit span, and reverse spelling. A diagnosis of *acute confusional state* based on electrolyte imbalance was made.

The patient recovered rapidly and was next seen by the examiner three days later, in a section of the hospital distant from the site of the original examination.

Table 5.1. Acute Confusion: Clinical Characteristics

Rapid development
Fluctuating status
Altered arousal
Inattention
Incoherent speech, thought, action
Impaired memory and intellectual function
Perceptual distortions
Emotional lability

When he saw the examiner he stared and then stated: "I know who you are—you are Dr. Benson." The acute confusional state had grossly compromised his learning ability (and other thought processes), but a limited degree of memory function had been retained. (DFB)

In Case 5.2 the primary disturbance was an inability to maintain a coherent line of thought, a disorder of general attention. The patient was fully alert (awake) and retained most high-level mental functions (language, learning ability), but all functions were compromised by inability to maintain attention. Terms such as *acute confusional state, delirium, toxic encephalopathy,* and *metabolic encephalopathy* have been used to label this problem.

Clinically, the *acute confusional* state involves a broad spectrum of mental functions. Table 5.1 lists the major characteristics seen in the disorder. As the name indicates, the onset is sudden and dramatic. It may develop in a matter of moments (e.g., after head injury) or over several days (e.g., with drug intoxication, febrile illness), but the key characteristic, the inability to maintain coherence of mental functions, always appears over a relatively short time span. Some degree of altered awakeness, ranging from mild drowsiness and lethargy to total coma, is usual, but in exceptional situations (such as with Case 5.2) the patient remains fully awake despite the serious attention difficulty. Almost all acutely confused individuals suffer altered sleep/wake cycles, particularly a tendency to be restless at night and to sleep heavily during the day. A broad range of mental abnormalities result from impaired attention and concentration. Thus memory, judgment, cognition, visual–spatial function, and even interpersonal relationships will be suboptimal.

In contrast, basic sensory and motor functions remain intact. Language may also be intact (at least there is no overt evidence of aphasia), but the pragmatic quality (meaningfulness) of the verbal output betrays the patient's problem in maintaining coherency. Objects may be misidentified (Cummings, 1985a; Weinstein and Kahn, 1952), and confabulations may occur (Bleuler, 1975). Rambling, indecisive, tangential conversational speech, interrupted by spells of decreased awakeness, is common. Dysgraphia, a disturbance in the ability to produce written language, is almost always present (Chedru and Geschwind, 1972). Both thought processing and thought content are affected.

Hundreds of etiologies can lead to an acute confusional state in the human. Table 5.2 presents some common causes. At the turn of the century Bonhoeffer (1912) clearly demonstrated that the mental concomitants of the acute confusional state are not specific to the disease process. Rather, the same clinical state can arise from many different medical causes (Bleuler, 1975). Thus disorders as divergent as cerebral mass lesions, hepatic failure, drug intoxications, or systemic infection with high fever can produce the acute confusional state.

Management of the acute confusional state depends on proper diagnosis and treatment of the underlying disorder and is often successful

Table 5.2. Major Causes of Acute Confusion

Drugs
  Prescription/nonprescription
  Abuse/withdrawal
Surgery
  Anesthesia and recovery
  Blood loss
  Systemic/metabolic alterations
Systemic disorders
  Infections
  Toxic/metabolic disorders
  Sleep disorders
Neurological disorders
  Brain trauma
  Structural damage (e.g., stroke)
  Epilepsy

(Lipowski, 1990; Strub, 1982). The prognosis is generally favorable in young, healthy individuals but is more guarded for the very young and may be quite grave for the elderly. Lipowski (1980) estimated that from 25 to 40 percent of individuals over age 65 years admitted to the hospital with or treated in the hospital for acute confusional state will die of the underlying disease process.

Case 5.3

A 31-year-old woman was seen for neurobehavioral diagnosis and treatment. History revealed that she had had a disturbed youth. By age 25 years she had run away with a motorcycle gang, had abused drugs and alcohol, and had once seriously attempted suicide by slashing her wrist. One year before this admission, she had been admitted to another hospital in a deep coma, apparently caused by excessive alcohol plus a variety of street drugs. She awakened in six days, and her degree of responsiveness improved somewhat until discharge two weeks after admission. By that time she could help others move her in bed, would occasionally talk, and would swallow food, but remained incontinent of both urine and feces. With the care of her parents she slowly improved, walked independently, became somewhat helpful about the house, fed herself, and gained control of her bowels, although bladder incontinence persisted. She tended to wander away, necessitating custodial measures. The family believed that these restraints angered the patient so that she regressed, rarely talking or moving, refusing to help in the house, not eating unless fed, and again becoming doubly incontinent.

Background history included a father who was a "skid row" alcoholic, a paternal uncle with manic–depressive illness, and a maternal aunt and maternal grandmother who had needed psychiatric care for depression.

On evaluation the patient sat immobile in a chair, rarely moved, and did not speak. Neither paralysis nor sensory loss could be demonstrated. Although closed at most times, her eyes occasionally opened and moved conjugately. She occasionally mumbled some words, but neither her movements nor the speaking were based on external stimulation. A CT scan was read as normal, an EEG showed mild, diffuse bilateral slowing, and an MRI showed small, bilateral increased signal intensities in the basal ganglia, compatible with old infarction. A diagnosis of *akinetic mutism* was made by the neurology service, while a diagnosis of organic depression with catatonic features was made by the psychiatry service. Treatment with a variety of drugs was unsuccessful except for two episodes when, following intravenous benzodiazepine administration, the patient awakened, moved about, and spoke spontaneously but in a few hours reverted to the original akinetic and mute state. Further treatment with the same and other drugs was ineffective. (Benson, 1992)

Cairns and colleagues (1941) described a condition they called *akinetic mutism* in patients with colloid cysts located in the anterior part of the third ventricle. The condition is now defined as "a state of unresponsiveness to the environment with extreme reluctance to perform even elementary motor activities" despite absence of significant motor paralysis (Segarra and Angelo, 1970). Nielsen and Jacobs (1951) described a similar state following bilateral damage to the cingulate cortex. Over the years additional cases of akinetic mutism have been reported (French, 1952; Klee, 1961; Segarra, 1970; Thompson, 1951), and two phenomenologically distinct forms have been suggested (Segarra, 1970). In one form, the patient appears somnolent (eyes closed, divergent squint when the lids are retracted), whereas in the second the eyes are open and move in a conjugate manner. The first has been termed *somnolent akinetic mutism* and the second *vigilant akinetic mutism*, with the term *coma vigil* suggested for the latter.

The patient with somnolent akinetic mutism is silent and immobile despite apparent wake–sleep cycles. The patient with vigilant akinetic mutism appears alert but presents almost no evidence of physical or mental activity. Both may show occasional limited movement and/or vocalization in response to strong external stimuli, but more often the actions occur spontaneously and are not repeated on request. Vigilant akinetic mutism based on medial frontal brain damage includes a characteristic motor disturbance—paralysis of one or both legs but normal strength in the arms and hands. Akinetic mutism based on a mesencephalic disturbance is associated with complete or partial paresis of cranial nerve III, IV, or VI. In neither variety of akinetic mutism is motor paralysis sufficient to produce the degree of immobility or mutism noted. In fact, immobility and mutism based on upper motor neuron paralysis is a distinct disorder with its own name, the *locked-in syndrome* (Plum and Posner, 1972).

Akinetic mutism can result from either focal structural or nonstructural pathology. When a focal cause is identified for somnolent akinetic mutism, the mesencephalic reticular area is the site. When focal damage is identified in vigilant akinetic mutism, the medial frontal lobe, either the inferior frontal region (subcallosal) or the cingulate region (supracallosal), is the site. More often, focal damage occupies an interim area (e.g., hypothalamus or third ventricle) (Ross and Stewart, 1981), producing a mixed akinetic/mute picture. Even more common, however, is a nonstructural cause such as drug intoxication.

A variety of disorders have been reported as the cause of akinetic mutism—mass lesions, intracerebral hemorrhage, cerebral infarctions, intracranial infections, and even the retraction of the medial frontal lobes during surgical section of the corpus callosum (Bogen, 1987). As with most neurobehavioral disorders, it is the location of the lesion, not the etiology, that is most important.

While akinetic mutism is considered a neurological disorder with specific pathology, psychiatrists define a broader but related state under the term *catatonia*. In its broadest use, catatonia refers to any type of movement disorder associated with psychiatric disturbance (Gelenberg, 1976; Taylor, 1990); in a more restricted use, catatonia designates the limited motor activity, limited vocalization, waxy flexibility, and motoric negativism in cases of schizophrenia (DSM-III-R) (American Psychiatric Association, 1987), but modern diagnostic studies suggest that depression is more common than schizophrenia as the cause of catatonia (Abrams, Taylor, and Stolurow, 1979; Taylor, 1990). While catatonia has been ascribed to purely psychogenic causes, many of these patients suffer concomitant organic problems such as metabolic disorder, chemical intoxication, or partial vegetative states. How a psychogenic disorder can cause catatonia remains unknown.

The two types of akinetic mutism, somnolent and vigilant, bear a more than vague resemblance to the two basic variations of mental control—awakeness and attention. Somnolent akinetic mutism relates to the disturbed awakeness associated with mesencephalic reticular pathology, and vigilant akinetic mutism resembles the awake but inattentive state. Akinetic mutism provides a reasonable clinical model for the major disorders of basic mental control. Table 5.3 highlights the two varieties of akinetic mutism.

Case 5.4

A 51-year-old man was hospitalized following the acute onset of right hemiplegia, right hemisensory loss, right visual field disturbance, and severe nonfluent aphasia. A strong conjugate deviation of the eyes to the left allowed the patient to follow moving objects only to the left of midline. He did not respond to visual stimuli presented on the right side, and loud auditory stimuli, no matter where presented, produced head and eye movement to the left. Both isotope brain scan and EEG demonstrated a single lesion in the posterior superior frontal region on the left side.

Within several days, the degree of paresis decreased and the sensory abnormality became less pronounced. The patient could move his eyes somewhat to the right of midline, but the right visual fields remained hemianopic. After another few days both motor and sensory functions improved greatly, and he could move

Table 5.3. Akinetic Mutism

Type	Characteristics	Locus of Damage
Somnolent	Unresponsive, inactive, eyes closed, dysconjugate eye movements	Mesencephalic reticular area
Vigilant	Unresponsive, inactive, eyes open, conjugate eye movements	Bilateral midline, frontal (from septal area to cingulate cortex)

his eyes fully to the right but could not maintain them there. He now responded to stimuli presented in the right visual field but neglected them when stimuli were presented simultaneously to both visual fields. Similarly, he would fail to respond to right-sided somesthetic or auditory stimuli presented in competition with left-sided stimuli. Approximately ten days after-onset he regained full eye movements (except for residual mild right gaze paresis) and full somesthetic, auditory, and visual sensory appreciation. (DFB)

Figure 5.2 shows a radioisotope brain scan of a patient with signs and symptoms similar to those of Case 5.4 (Heilman and Valenstein, 1972) except that the inattention affected the left side. In Case 5.4, a cerebral infarction involving the left posterior superior frontal cortex (approximately Brodmann area 8) produced an apparent hemiplegia and hemisensory loss (including hemianopia), which disappeared within two weeks. While the findings were real, they were not based on damage to primary motor or sensory functional systems. Instead, Case 5.4 represents a dramatically severe example of unilateral inattention/inintention that was transient.

Attention disorders are common but often hidden by a confusional

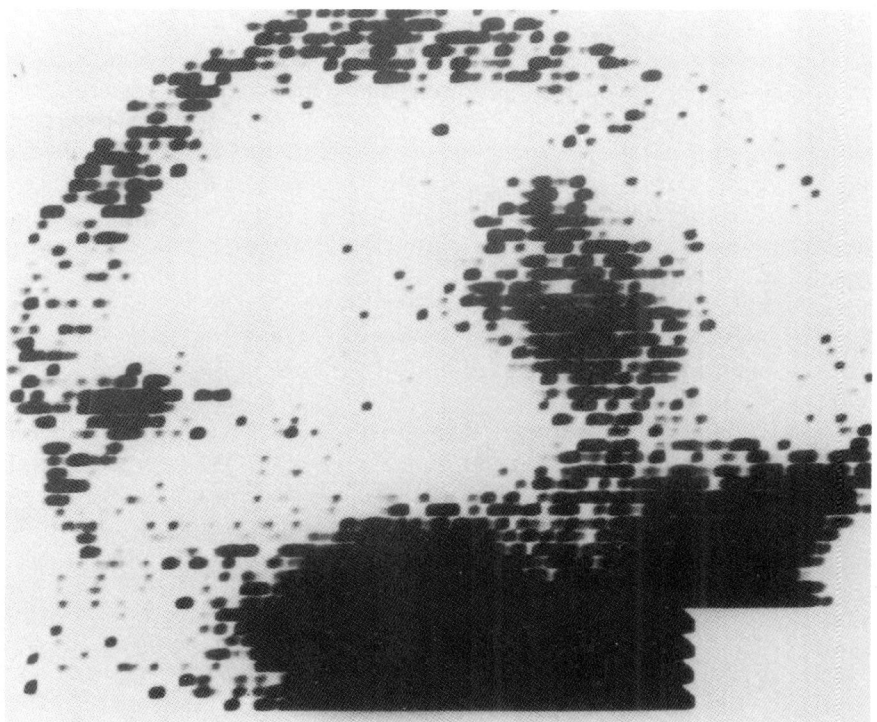

Fig. 5.2. Radionuclide brain scan of a patient with severe unilateral inattention/inintention following right posterior frontal infarction demonstrated by the isotope scan. From Heilman and Valenstein, 1983.

state or disruption of primary sensorimotor function. Although recognized for the past century (Anton, 1896; Loeb, 1886; Oppenheim, 1889; Poppelreuter, 1917), only in the past few decades have these disorders been analyzed sufficiently to escape status as behavioral curiosities and allow insight into the underlying neural mechanisms.

As with most behavioral abnormalities, various labels have been applied to disturbances of attention. Two terms, *inattention* and *neglect*, are synonymous. Closely related, but theoretically separate, is *inintention*, a disturbance of the ability to initiate movement, also known by terms such as *hypokinesia, akinesia,* and *abulia*.

The most readily observed example of attention disorder is unilateral neglect as seen with double simultaneous stimulation. When tactile, auditory, or visual stimuli are presented simultaneously in opposite sensory fields, a patient with unilateral inattention reports only one, neglecting the other. Increasing the relative degree of stimulation on the neglected side (e.g., wiggling the fingers in one visual field, waving the arms in the other) often overcomes the problem. Unilateral inattention indicates opposite hemisphere abnormality but attempts to localize the disorder to a single anatomical site (e.g., parietal lobe) have failed. Unilateral neglect can occur after damage to a number of brain areas (Heilman et al., 1983, 1985a,b; Mesulam, 1981).

The etiology of unilateral inattention is variable, (e.g., stroke, trauma, tumor). Based on clinical observations, many investigators (Brain, 1941; Critchley, 1953; McFie, Piercy, and Zangwill, 1950) postulated parietal dysfunction, and later CT correlation studies (Heilman, 1983) confirmed that neglect was often associated with temporal–parietal lesions. Identical neglect syndromes, however, may follow damage to the brain stem (particularly the mesencephalon), the thalamus, the cingulate gyrus, the superior dorsal–frontal cortex, and the posterior parietal cortex. Most investigators now believe that a complex neuroanatomical network connecting all of these areas subserves attention to sensory stimuli arriving from the opposite environmental field (Heilman et al., 1985a,b; Mesulam, 1981, 1985a, 1990).

Closely related to unilateral inattention is the concept of *unilateral inintention,* a tendency to utilize motor responses on one side of the body in preference to the other without motor paralysis to explain the preference. Thus, as in Case 5.4, the limbs on the side opposite the lesion remain immobile even though not paralyzed. The affected limbs do move during bilateral activities or when specifically ordered. Similarly, the eyes often move freely in one direction but are limited and impersistent in the opposite direction (gaze paresis), even though full lateral extraocular excursions may be possible. The point separating sensory neglect (inattention) from unilateral akinesia (inintention) is obscure, and in most clinical situations some combination of the two is present.

Another related but clinically distinct unilateral attentional disturbance is called *hemispatial neglect* (Bisiach et al., 1979). The affected individual not only fails to respond as well to stimuli in a given visual field (visual neglect), but also cannot visualize from memory as well in that visual field. Bisiach and Luzzatti (1978) described two patients with right hemisphere damage who when asked to describe, from memory, the buildings surrounding the main square in Milan from two different spatial perspectives—facing the cathedral, and facing away—could recollect most of the details but tended to omit most landmarks to the left in the revisualized image in both recollections (see Fig. 5.3). Thus, in addition to the unilateral sensory inattention and motor inintention, a disturbance of unilateral revisualization was demonstrated; similar unilateral sensory memory disorders probably affect the other major sensory systems. Thus, beneath each hemisphere's attentional competency lies a complex matrix involving sensory input, manipulation of memories, and motor responses.

Many observations suggest right hemisphere predominance for clinical

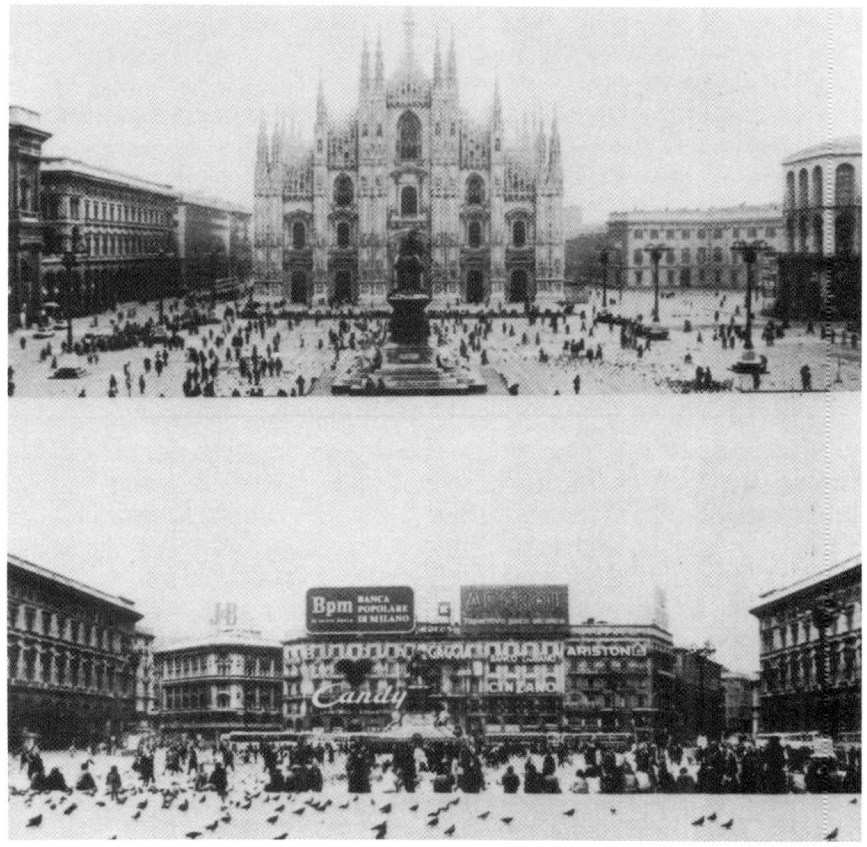

Fig. 5.3. View of the square in front of the cathedral in Milan from opposite sides of the square. In reproducing details from memory, the two patients reported by Bisiach and Luzzatti (1978) excluded most of the details located to the left on either of the views. From Bisiach and Berti, 1989.

neglect (Critchley, 1953; Heilman, 1979; Hier et al., 1977; Weinstein and Kahn, 1955). While simple sensory neglect (e.g., unilateral extinction of bilateral simultaneous stimulation) can result from damage to either hemisphere, more complex forms of inattention are more frequently reported with right hemisphere pathology. The apparent right hemisphere prevalence may be an artifact, however, particularly if the task demands identifying the location of the stimulus in extrapersonal space (the right hemisphere appears dominant for visual–spatial discrimination) or if aphasia obscures the left hemisphere responses.

Case 5.5

A 61-year-old man suffered acute left hemiplegia. An initial confusional state with decreased mental awareness cleared rapidly, leaving him alert and fully responsive. Both motor and sensory losses were dense on the left side, but only a poorly defined and inconsistent visual field defect was demonstrated. While there was no language disturbance, decreased ability to learn new information was obvious. The patient remained disoriented, unable to remember the name of the hospital, his doctor, or even that he was a patient in a hospital. He consistently denied the marked paralysis of his left side, insisting that he was physically normal, that he could get up and walk about if he desired, and that he was moving his left limbs on command even though they remained immobile. If told of the paralysis or if it was shown that he could not move the left limbs on command, he accepted the information; but within a few minutes, if asked directly, he again denied paralysis. *Anosognosia* (the denial of hemiplegia) was diagnosed, and a cerebral infarction involving deep white matter structures (the right internal capsule) was suspected. The source of the amnesia was not evident. Both the amnesia and the denial syndrome persisted, eventually necessitating transfer to a nursing home for ongoing care. (DFB)

Active denial of obvious defect (anosognosia) represents the most severe degree of inattention (see Table 5.4) and invariably indicates the presence of additional mental disorder such as confusional state or amnesia. Case 5.5 had a combination of nondominant motor and sensory pathway lesions plus amnesia; language function was normal, but the memory disorder abolished the patient's ability to remember that he had the hemiplegia/hemisensory disorder.

Case 5.6

A 59-year-old man was admitted to the hospital following injuries to his limbs and trunk sustained in a mugging. There was no evidence of basic neurological defect, but, because of a period of unconsciousness, a carotid angiogram was per-

Table 5.4. Hierarchical Stages of Attention Deficit
Neglect
Unconcern
Unawareness
Anosognosia

From Benson and Geschwind, 1975.

formed. No evidence of intracerebral bleeding was found, but a right middle cerebral artery aneurysm was noted. Surgical treatment of the aneurysm was performed about two weeks after the original injury. The patient had been awake and alert and had made his own decision to undergo the operation. The surgical procedure was complicated and in the postoperative state the patient not only had a residual left hemiplegia, but he denied its existence (anosognosia).

Neurobehavioral consultation was requested about two weeks later. When asked at that time why he was in the hospital, the patient replied that brain changes had paralyzed his left side. The anosognosia had disappeared. A digit span of 6 forward was demonstrated, and the patient conversed coherently. Additional testing was performed, and after ten to fifteen minutes his conversation became loose, he appeared fatigued, and his attention wandered. Digit span was now limited to 4. When asked why he was in the hospital, he now replied that he was there for treatment of a viral influenza. He adamantly denied any weakness on his left side and, when shown his paralyzed left side, denied ownership of the limbs. The anosognosia had reappeared. (DFB)

Case 5.6, like Case 5.5, involves denial of hemiplegia (anosognosia), but in Case 5.6 the behavior was intermittent, a product of the combination of acute confusion brought on by fatigue with unilateral inattention/inintention.

Case 5.7
A 71-year-old man was hospitalized following the acute onset of confusion. Clinical examination revealed no abnormality involving either motor or somesthetic sensory systems, but a severe problem in visual function was present. While his pupils reacted to light, the patient appeared blind, was unable to identify objects, and could not even distinguish light from dark. His condition was diagnosed as *cortical blindness*. He adamantly denied any visual problems, often complaining that the light was poor in the room, that he did not have his best pair of glasses with him, or that it was nighttime. Along with the blindness there was a full amnesia syndrome (see Case 9-5). A diagnosis of *Anton's syndrome* (the denial of blindness) (Anton, 1896) was made, and an isotope brain scan confirmed the suspected bilateral infarction in the territory of the posterior cerebral arteries. The patient's condition remained static through several years of follow-up; the amnesia persisted, and he continues to deny, downplay, or rationalize his blindness.

It was assumed that posterior visual cortex damage produced the cortical blindness and medial temporal area damage was the source of the amnesia. The patient was literally unable to remember that he was blind. (DFB)

In Case 5.7, Anton's syndrome followed damage to the primary visual cortex and to the medial temporal regions of both hemispheres. The denial of blindness, like the denial of hemiplegia in Case 5.5, resulted from a combination of sensory loss and memory disorder.

Disturbances of unilateral (and bilateral) attention mechanisms are almost always complicated. In most cases basic motor and/or sensory functions are damaged, and disorders of language, memory, and other higher order functions add to the complexity. Not infrequently, the attention disturbances are masked by signs and symptoms produced by damage to neighboring brain areas; only when basic sensorimotor disturbances are combined with some disturbance of mental clarity do striking clinical syndromes such as anosognosia occur. Table 5.4 presents a simple hierarchical representation of attention deficits ranging from simple neglect to anosognosia. The key finding underlying all anosognosic phenomena is neglect, the disturbance of attention/intention. When neglect is unilateral and occurs in a clear state of consciousness, it is easy to demonstrate. With alteration in the degree of awareness, however, complex variations of attentional disorder appear. One common variant is the appearance of unconcern. The patient acknowledges the physical deficit but is unable to register or maintain an appropriate degree of concern for the disability. Such patients act as though there was no disability and show only grudging interest when it is brought to their attention, a response easily misinterpreted as a psychological defense mechanism. Another variant is apparent unawareness of the deficit. These patients ignore the involved limb. The affected limbs may remain in an uncomfortable position and can even be damaged with little reaction by the patient. When told of their deficit, these patients acknowledge the problem but immediately resume behaviors that demonstrate decreased awareness of the deficit.

The final variant in Table 5.4, anosognosia (Babinski, 1914, 1918), is the active denial of the defect. A patient with a hemiplegia will deny any weakness (Case 5.5) and may even deny ownership of the involved limb. Thus, when asked whom his paralyzed arm belonged to, one patient replied that it must have been left by his sister who had visited earlier in the day (Weinstein and Kahn, 1955). Anosognosia is so dramatic that its relationship with unawareness, unconcern, and the neglect state is often overlooked. Similarly, Anton's syndrome, a dramatic example of anosognosia, is rarely discussed as such. Instead, the visual disturbance is stressed. Explanations based on both psychodynamics (Battersby et al., 1956; Weinstein and Kahn, 1955) and brain localization studies (Heilman et al., 1983; Kennard, 1939; Welch and Stuteville, 1958) have been offered for anosognosia; but the crucial factor, the disturbance of awareness (called *clouding of consciousness* in the older literature), receives limited attention. Patients with full denial (anosognosia) have either amnesia (Cases 5.5 and 5.7) or some degree of confusion (Case 5.6).

Denial of left hemiplegia is far more frequently noted than denial of right hemiplegia, a fact that suggested correlation of anosognosia with right parietal disorder (Babinski, 1914; Critchley, 1953). Geschwind (1982), Mesulam (1985a), and others have proposed that the left hemisphere has competency to explore and maintain awareness of only the right side of space while the right hemisphere can respond to both left and right aspects of external space and maintains awareness of stimuli coming to both left and right hemispheres. Most data supporting this unilateral dominance theory is anecdotal, stemming from observation of patients with anosognosia and related phenomena. In one of the few semicontrolled studies of anosognosia and related phenomena (Cutting, 1978), the right hemisphere preponderance was only partially supported. By testing stroke patients within one week of onset, Cutting demonstrated either outright denial (anosognosia) or some related disturbance (anosognosic phenomena) that indicated decreased awareness in 87 percent of patients with right hemispheric lesions compared with only 24 percent of those with left hemispheric strokes. However, when the individuals with acute left hemispheric defect in whom aphasia precluded meaningful response (57 percent) were added to those who were able to deny their problem, the number of patients with left hemisphere damage who did not report their problem rose to 81 percent. Stated another way, in the first week following an acute brain injury (stroke) only 13 percent of right hemisphere and 19 percent of left hemisphere subjects reported full awareness of their deficit.

Case 5.8

Two weeks after undergoing coronary bypass surgery, a 52-year-old, left-handed man was found unresponsive at home. He was hospitalized in coma and only gradually recovered consciousness. A CT scan of his head performed ten days following onset showed bilateral medial thalamic lacunar infarctions (Fig. 5.4). His recovery was slow and incomplete, complicated by difficulty in learning new information, altered sleep/wake cycles, and frequent periods when he was difficult to mobilize.

When examined, the patient appeared drowsy unless stimulated but was readily alerted with verbal stimulation. He followed commands reasonably well, but all of his reactions were slow and halting. He had frequent flashes of anger, but these were always short lived. Although disoriented for time and place, he could repeat seven digits, perform simple arithmetic sums, and interpret similarities and differences. He was not, however, able to copy a three-dimensional cube or draw the face of a clock. He failed to remember any of four unrelated words in three minutes and confabulated freely. While he was capable of carrying out most daily living activities (e.g., dressing, toilet care), these were not performed unless specifically commanded. Without directed stimulation he remained immobile and did not converse. His status improved over the next few months, but he remained largely immobile. (*Courtesy of Emre Kokmen, M.D., Mayo Clinic, Rochester, Minnesota*)

In Case 5.8, bilateral thalamic damage produced a severe degree of inintention. Although the patient could perform most tasks without evidence of motor or sensory disturbance, movements were rarely made unless specifically commanded by another person.

Over the years a small number of cases of progressive dementia associated with degeneration of the thalamus have been reported (Martin et al., 1983; McDaniel, 1990; Stern, 1939). While the clinical picture varies, the most consistently reported problem is slowing of physical and mental functions, psychomotor retardation so severe that it can prove fatal (Lugaresi et al., 1986). A similar syndrome can occur with bilateral thalamic hemorrhage. Patients with this syndrome fail to respond to most external (and probably internal) stimuli. Nonresponse is not total, but an apathetic, laconic abulia is notable (Case 5.8). Whether pathology

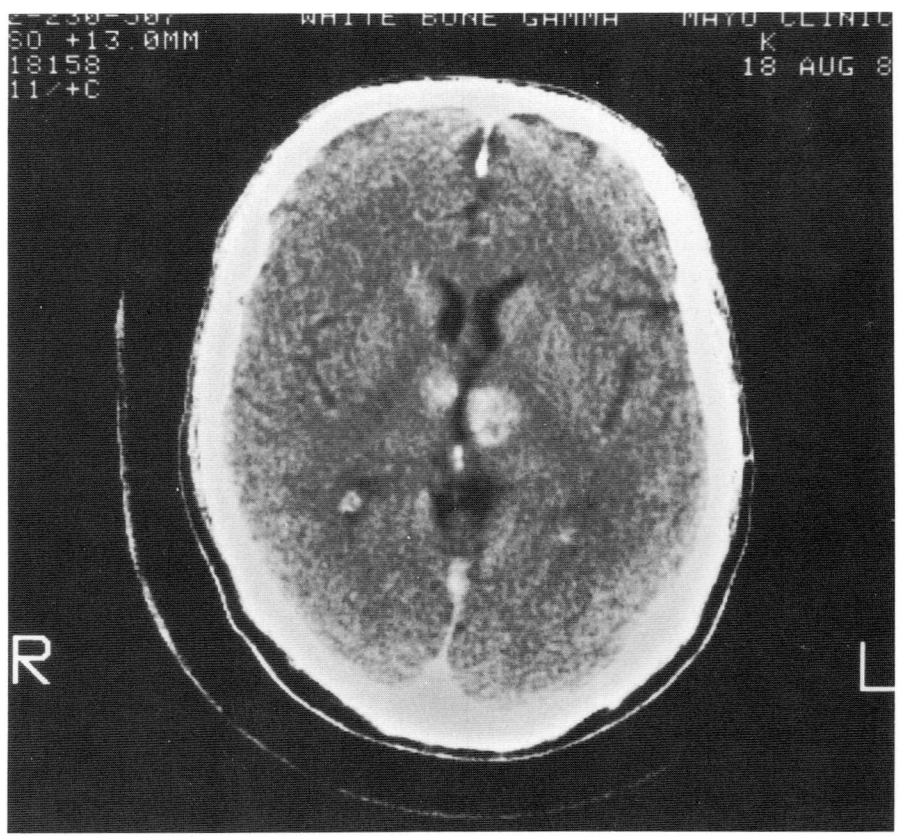

Fig. 5.4. X-ray CT scan of Case 5.8 illustrating hemorrhagic infarctions involving bilateral medial thalamic structures. Courtesy of Dr. E. Kokmen.

Table 5.5. Neuroanatomical Network for Attention/Intention
Mesencephalic reticular formation
Thalamic reticular nuclei
Thalamic relay nuclei
Selected midline limbic nuclei
Parietal–occipital association cortex
Frontal association cortex
Connecting pathways

involves only the thalamus remains an unsettled question, but it clearly centers on thalamic structures and produces a picture of severe subcortical dementia (Cummings and Benson, 1983).

NEUROANATOMICAL SUBSTRATE

Clinical studies correlating brain and behavior, augmented by animal experiments, indicate that a rich, primarily basal network of nuclear centers and their connections maintains basic mental control. Table 5.5 lists the anatomical areas known, or strongly suspected, to be associated with some aspects of basic mental control; most are reciprocally linked. While these areas are extensive, much of the brain, particularly cortical structures, can be damaged without altering arousal or most aspects of attention.

The neuroanatomy of sleep is a good starting point to explore the neuroanatomical network subserving basic mental control. F. Bremer (1935) suggested that the diencephalon–upper brain stem junction was crucial to sleep–wakefulness, contradicting the accepted view of diffuse cortical/subcortical control. In 1962 M. Jouvet demonstrated an REM sleep-inducing system in the upper pons. This led to a theory that two neural systems control REM and non-REM cycles (Hobson, 1974; Hobson, Lydic, and Baghdoyan, 1986). Figure 5.5 outlines these systems. The first system (REM-off cells) includes the dorsal raphe nuclei (serotoninergic), the locus coeruleus (nonadrenergic), and several additional brain stem nuclei that discharge during wakefulness, decline in activity during non-REM sleep, and almost cease discharge during REM sleep (Chu and Bloom, 1973). The second is a cholinergic (REM-on) system located in mesencephalon, medulla, and pontine tegmental fields. These cells discharge at the lowest rate during wakefulness, increase during non-REM sleep, and have high firing rates during REM sleep. Interaction between the two opposing systems appears to control alterations in the sleep/wakefulness cycle (Jouvet, 1972), but other neurotransmitters may also play a part. Cells of the frontal forebrain, posterior hypothalamus, and particularly the superchiasmatic nucleus of the hypothalamus (Hanada and Kawamura, 1981; Jacobs, 1985) influence wake–sleep cycle activation.

One aspect of phasic arousal, the degree of responsiveness to external stimuli, is related to activity of the mesencephalic reticular formation and selected sites of its upward projection (thalamus, hypothalamus, frontal septal region). The reticular formation is a network of short, multisynaptic neurons that respond to external and internal stimuli. Moruzzi and Magoun (1949) demonstrated that bilateral damage to the mesencephalic reticular region (in animals) produced a state resembling sleep without normal waking response to sensory stimuli, even though the primary sensory and motor pathways appeared intact (see Fig. 5.6). This led to intense investigation of the reticular activating system (Anokhin, 1961; Bowsher, 1961; French, 1958; Magoun, 1963), focused largely on bilateral reticular system damage. In 1974, Watson and colleagues demon-

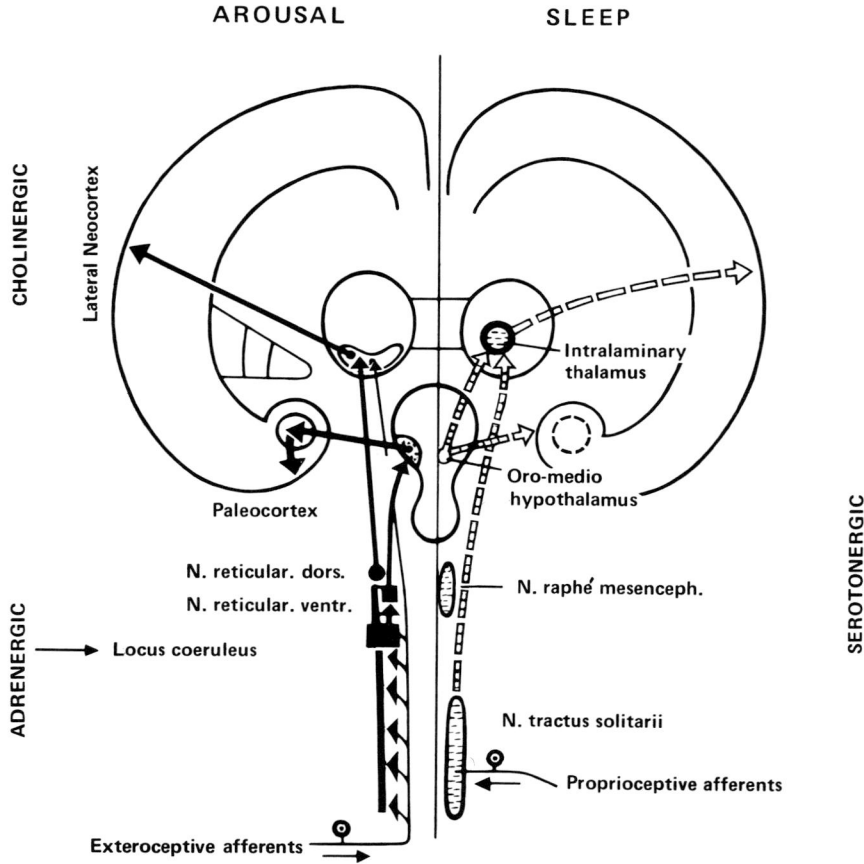

Fig. 5.5. Artistic rendition of the three systems (cholinergic, serotonergic, and adrenergic) involved in sleep–wakefulness. From Chase, 1972.

strated that unilateral damage to the mesencephalic reticular formation could produce a strong, permanent unilateral neglect syndrome in the monkey. Following such a lesion the animals appeared unaware (lacked appreciation) of the opposite side of their body in space, and a disturbance of attention (unilateral inattention) was inferred. A phasic (attention), not tonic (alertness) disorder was present. Two systems—a tonic factor associated with sleep, alertness, wakeness, and arousal; and a phasic system governing attention to sensory input—interact to provide the arousal aspect of basic mental control.

Both attention and response can be altered by disturbance of the sensory input system (Battersby et al. 1956; Denny-Brown and Banker, 1954) or the motor output channels (Heilman and Van den Abell, 1979), but damage to specific parietal or frontal association areas with no direct sensory or motor functions can also produce striking attentional problems.

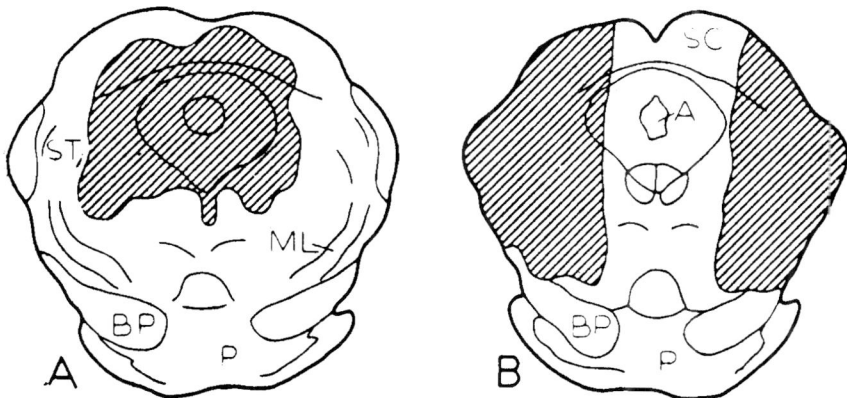

Fig. 5.6. Graphic outline of site of lesions in the brain stem capable of affecting response to environmental stimuli. A demonstrates reticular lesions that produced chronic sleep but no paralysis. B represents lateral mesencephalic lesions which produced sensory and motor loss but no alteration of sleep cycle. From Moruzzi and Magoun, 1949.

Figure 5.7 graphically illustrates the tonic arousal and the sensory attention pathways suggested. Figure 5.8 presents an outline of the motor activation programs for intention (Watson, Valenstein, and Heilman, 1981). Although obviously complex, both diagrams represent simplifications of the complicated network involved in the phasic aspect of mental control.

The neuroanatomical aspects of attention illustrated in Figures 5.7 and 5.8 can be subdivided into three major functional systems: (1) midline structures significant for the tonic aspect of attention, (2) nuclear networks that subserve basic sensorimotor functions, and (3) two cortical areas that act as staging areas for the response to external stimulation. Each system plays a vital role in attention.

Three major anatomical groups constitute the midline (tonic) system: selected thalamic nuclei (Dempsey and Morrison, 1943); the mesencephalic reticular formation; and certain midline frontal structures including the septal and subcallosal cortex, the anterior cingulate gyrus, and possibly the supplementary motor area. Bilateral damage to these structures (Cases 5.8, 11.2, and 11.4) produces severe disability in both attention and intention (decreased cerebral tone).

Superimposed on the tonic system is a neural network that handles routine (reflex) sensory input and motor output, as described in Chapters 3 and 4. Damage that affects the operation of either the primary motor or sensory cortices themselves or their external connections disrupts a finely tuned, hemispheric response system. Damage to the basic sensorimotor system decreases responses on the side opposite the damage (amorphosynthesis) (Denny-Brown, 1963). An important factor in many cases of unilateral neglect is unilateral damage to the primary sensory or motor neural system.

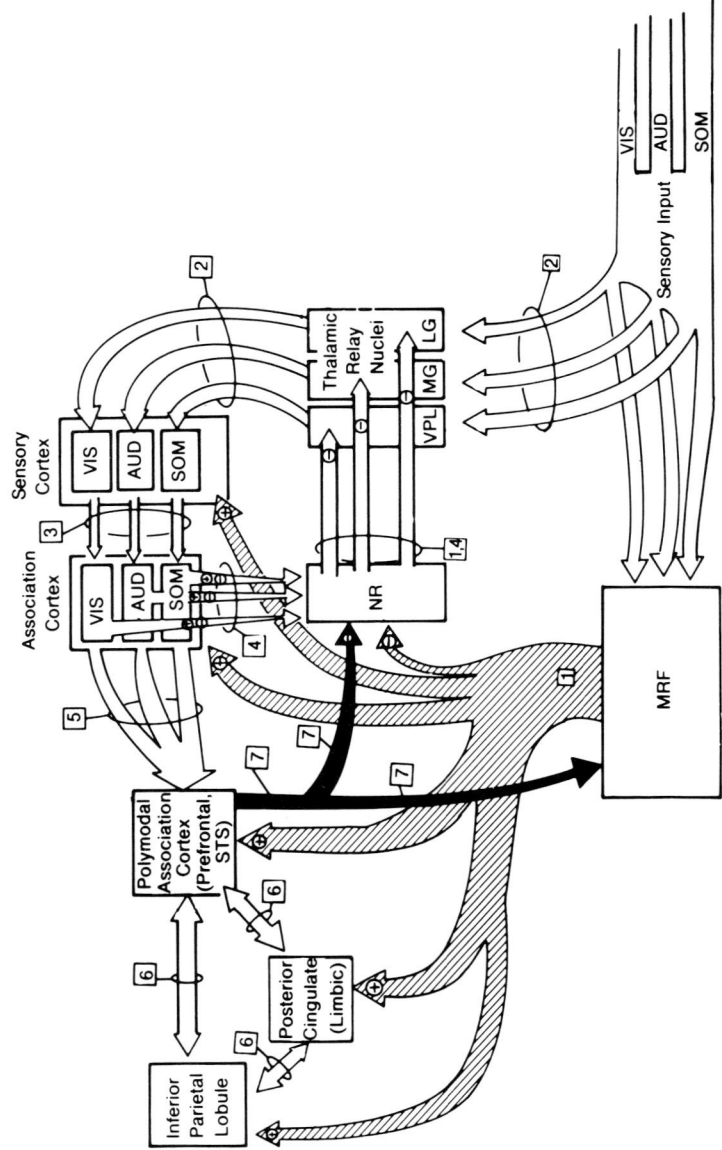

Fig. 5.7. Graphic illustration of the sensory attention pathways and tonic arousal system. MRF = mesencephalic reticular formation; NR = nucleus reticularis. Arrows indicate direction of information flow; numbers indicate which disconnection can alter attention. From Watson et al., 1981.

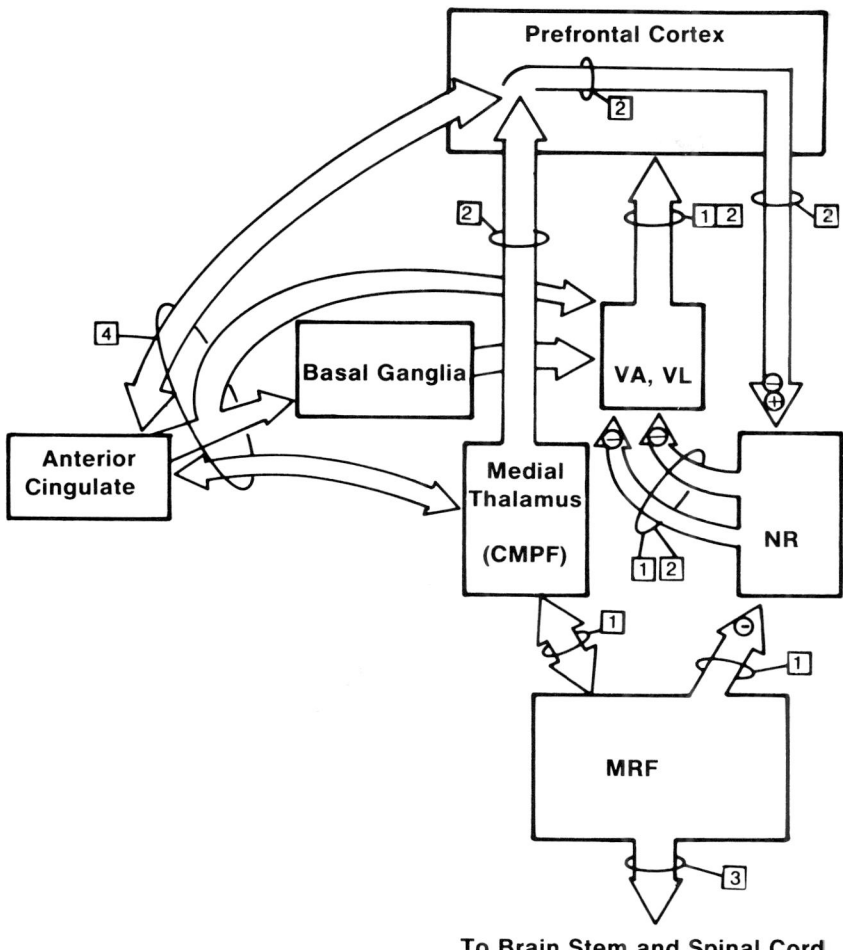

Fig. 5.8. Graphic illustration of motor activation programs for intentional movements. MRF = mesencephalic reticular formation; NR = nucleus reticularis. Arrows indicate direction of information flow; numbers indicate areas in which disconnection can alter motor response. From Watson, Valenstein, and Heilman, 1981.

Clinical correlation studies have shown that a third attention activity—unilateral attention—has a different anatomical base. Two cortical areas appear to act as staging areas for unilateral attention. One, located in the parietal–occipital cortex (Brodmann area 19), deals with sensations received from the contralateral side in space, particularly stimuli that direct visual attention (head and eye movements) in space (Crosby, Humphrey and Lauer, 1962). Damage limited to the parietal region produces a transient inability to attend to stimuli, particularly visual stimuli, from the opposite field. A second cortical area, the frontal eye field (Brodmann area 8), receives input from all association cortices that process external sensations (Pandya, Dye, and Butters, 1971). Damage to the frontal eye field of one hemisphere produces a transient unilateral neglect that can involve all sensory systems (Case 5.4). Both animal ablation studies (Bianchi, 1895; Kennard, 1939) and clinical cases (Damasio, Damasio, and Chui, 1980; Heilman and Valenstein, 1972) (Case 5.4) illustrate the importance of Brodmann area 8 for unilateral attention. Lesser degrees of damage to Brodmann area 8, the parietal–occipital junction area, or their major connections can produce subtle defects of attention that are often overlooked.

THE NEURAL BASIS OF BASIC MENTAL CONTROL

Basic mental control is not a neat, unitary function but rather the varied product of a complex neural network. Figure 5.9 presents one hypothesis for the neural basis of attention (Mesulam, 1985a) in which many different but functionally interrelated brain areas are involved.

It can be seen that the two levels of basic mental control—arousal and attention—can be further subdivided into tonic and phasic activities. The

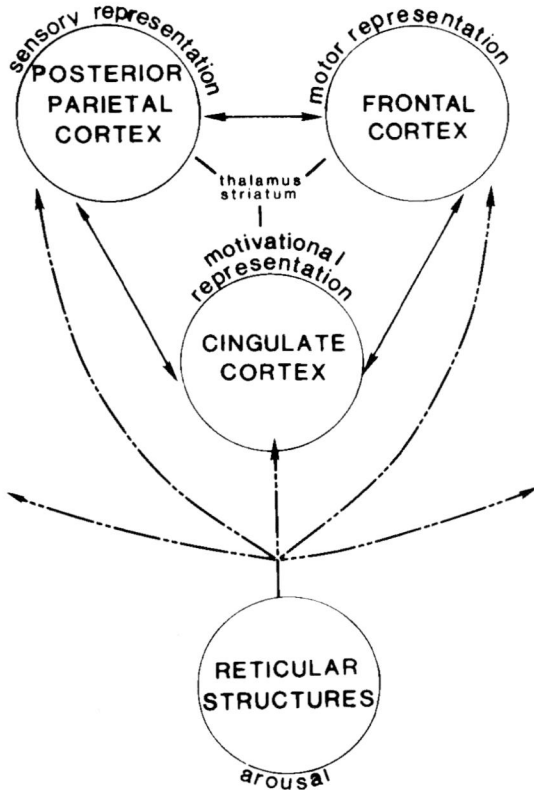

Fig. 5.9. Graphic conceptualization of the interrelated neural structures involved in attention. From Mesulam, 1981.

tonic aspect of arousal includes three stages—awakeness, non-REM sleep, and REM sleep. The resulting cerebral tone reflects interrelated biochemical and physiological alterations arising largely from the brain stem. Conscious awareness and therefore thinking are strongly influenced by these fluctuations.

The phasic aspect of arousal responds to basic sensation (somesthetic, auditory, visual) and the reticular system. The reticular system alerts the higher nervous system and also modulates the sensory input available for processing into thought.

The tonic aspects of attention are subserved by midline structures (thalamic, hypothalamic, and midline frontal) that focus or modulate sensory input and motor response (intention). *Drive* (motivation) is the term most often used to define the tonic aspect of cerebral attention, but this activity also encompasses higher level control functions that will be discussed in Chapter 11. Basic to drive, however, is the fundamental ability to maintain attention. The combination of basic attention with higher level control functions provides the tone for conscious attention, a significant aspect of thought processing.

The phasic aspect of attention, like the phasic aspect of arousal, reflects interaction between two functions. One is the constantly active reception/association function of the basic sensorimotor systems that provide between-hemisphere comparisons of stimuli and responses, the perceptual rivalry described by Denny-Brown (1963). A stimulus presented to the sensory system of one hemisphere is recognized as identical to the same stimulation presented to the other hemisphere. Imbalance in function of appropriate cerebral systems leads to unilateral neglect (Riddoch, 1917). The second aspect concerns unilateral direction of attention, a function of the parietal–occipital junction and frontal eye field cortices. Both areas direct awareness to the locale of incoming sensory stimuli, and both areas command motor responses, but on a supraordinate, not a fundamental, level.

Finally, the neural basis for the direction and control of attention deserves consideration. Some ability to exclude from higher level attention most of the stimuli constantly bombarding the sensory organs is essential. Few of the stimuli that enter the neural circuits reach conscious awareness. Gating mechanisms for pain were discussed in Chapter 3, but higher level gating mechanisms have also been posited, e.g., thalamic gating (Scheibel, 1980), hypothalamic gating (Damasio, 1979), basal ganglia gating (Oberg and Divac, 1979), and frontal gating (Fuster, 1980). The best defined is the nucleus reticularis of the thalamus (Scheibel and Scheibel, 1967), which is thought to act as a feedback control mechanism capable of inhibiting or facilitating the sensory impulses that reach synapses in the thalamus (Scheibel, 1980). Feedback to the nucleus reticularis from the prefrontal areas can either facilitate or block conduction of sensory stimuli, thus selecting the stimulus attended to in conscious awareness. At this step, a combination of basic and higher level mental control mechanisms is operative.

Thus, while basic mental control may be discussed as a single module of brain activity, the process acts through multiple integrated neural systems that subserve individual functions. Separately and in combinations, these basic control systems powerfully influence the processing of mental associations.

6

The Neurology of Emotional Disorders

> . . . of how much more Passion than Reason has Jupiter compos'd us?—Besides, he has confin'd Reason to a narrow corner of the brain, and left all the rest of the body to our Passions.
> —DESIDERIUS ERASMUS
> *IN PRAISE OF FOLLY*, 1514/1942

AXIOMS/POSTULATES

Emotion cannot be regarded as a unitary function.

Emotional response reflects the interaction of many different influences including mood, verbal and nonverbal affect, drive and cognitive control.

Emotional influences reflect neuroanatomically discrete but functionally integrated neural systems.

The integrated product of the emotional functions influences thought processing.
The opposite is also true.

Emotion has been recognized for millennia as a vital component of mental life that colors thinking. One enduring contribution, traced from Empedocles through Hippocrates and Galen and on to the seventeenth century (Needham, 1978), was the typology of four humors—sanguine, choleric, melancholic, and phlegmatic—thought to circulate within the body cavities and to characterize human temperaments. Later, emotional problems were linked to deeply embedded memories (Benedikt, 1894; Freud, 1938; Jung, 1954). Psychophysiological speculations such as the James-Lange theory (James, 1890) and Cannon's stress/homeostasis theory (1927) emphasized visceral and autonomic influences on emotional response. Many "personality disorders," clusters of emotional behaviors, have been described: depressive personality, hysterical personality, obsessive–compulsive personality, inadequate personality, paranoid personality, and so forth (American Psychiatric Association, 1957, 1968, 1980a; Cloninger, 1987; Spitzer and Wilson, 1975; World Health Organization, 1977). Few individuals, however, have the specific cluster of traits described for any personality type, undermining the validity of such classifications.

Psychological research has utilized several opposing dichotomies: pain–pleasure, happy–sad, neuroticism–psychoticism, extroversion–introversion, and, more recently, right hemisphere–left hemisphere. No single dichotomy has proved sufficient for characterizing human emotion, and a circular model may be more useful (Leary and Coffey, 1955; Plutchik, 1980) (Fig. 6.1). One approach to assessing emotional status is based on profiles derived from responses to questions (e.g., the Minnesota Multiphasic Personality Inventory [Hathaway and McKinley, 1951]). Such forced responses, however, are readily misinterpreted.

Emotional disorder following unilateral brain damage has often been reported. Broca (1865), Jackson (1864), and later figures correlated emotional changes with left hemisphere damage. Others (Babinski, 1914; Bleuler, 1951; Kraepelin, 1921) suggested that either hemisphere could be involved. Goldstein (1940) described a catastrophic reaction in brain-damaged patients, an inability to cope accompanied by frustration, negativism, withdrawal, refusal to communicate or even self-care, and severe

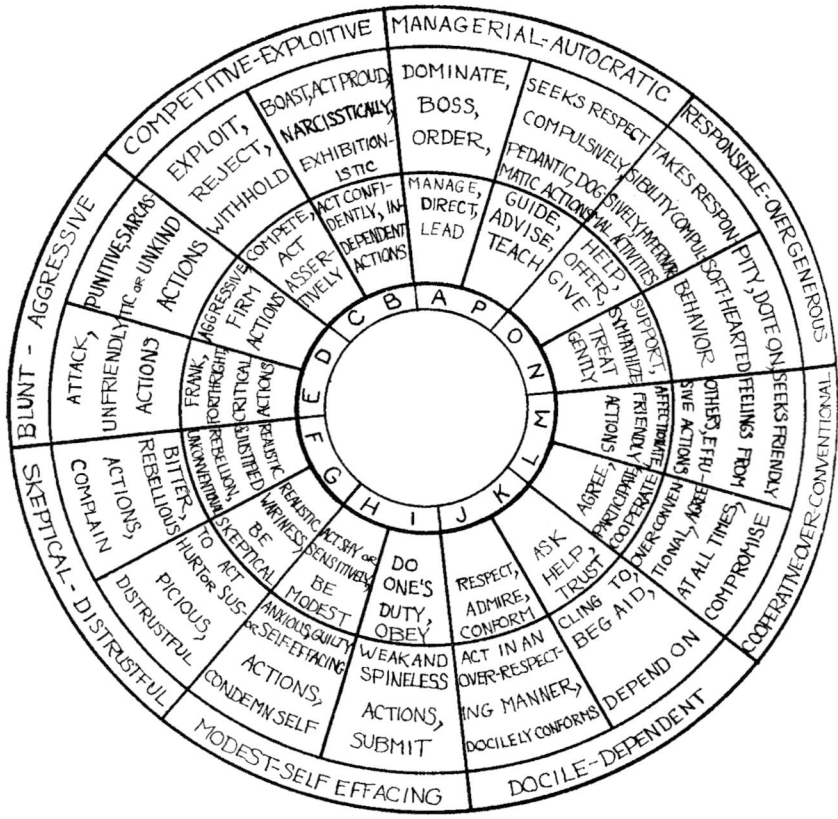

Fig. 6.1. A circular representation of diametrically opposed emotional reactions. From Leary and Coffey, 1955.

depression with crying, anger, and hostility. The opposite, an organic indifference reaction, has also been described (Babinski, 1914; Denny-Brown, Meyer, and Horenstein, 1952; Hécaen, 1962), and the two different emotional responses—indifference and catastrophic reaction—have been related to unilateral hemispheric dysfunction. Catastrophic reaction is found more often in patients with left hemisphere damage, while indifference tends to follow right hemisphere damage (Gainotti, 1972). In another approach, Papez (1937) proposed that the limbic system was the cerebral base of emotion (Pincus and Tucker, 1985). MacLean (1949, 1954, 1958) demonstrated the importance of the limbic system for emotional response, but the neural basis of emotion is considerably more complicated.

VARIETIES OF EMOTION

One basic aspect of emotion is *mood,* which has been defined as a subjective feeling tone (Hinsie and Campbell, 1970; *Oxford English Dictionary,* 1979), a frame of mind, or the emotional state of a person (*Oxford English Dictionary,* 1979; *Stedman's Medical Dictionary Illustrated,* 1979). Everyone experiences various moods (e.g., anger, joy, depression), and one's mood may oscillate or swing easily. In this chapter, *mood* will refer to a relatively pervasive but often impersistent internal disposition, an internal feeling tone, and it will be considered distinct from the external manifestations of emotion.

A second basic term, *affect,* represents the observable physical manifestations of emotion (*New Webster's Dictionary,* 1975; *Oxford English Dictionary,* 1979; *Stedman's Medical Dictionary Illustrated,* 1979). Descriptions of affect emphasize the outward appearance (e.g., lively, jolly, sullen, apathetic). The observed affect may not coincide with the underlying mood, however. Discordance of mood and affect is common (an affective facade) and may be dramatic in some neurological conditions such as the euphoria that may accompany advanced multiple sclerosis despite an underlying mood of severe depression (Surridge, 1969). Even more blatant are the wild emotional overflows of pseudobulbar palsy (Lieberman and Benson, 1977). *Affect* refers only to the external expression of feelings; it may reflect the underlying mood but is often colored by additional factors.

A number of ill-defined terms characterize the energy of the emotions. *Drive* has been defined simply as a force that activates human impulses (*Dorland's Illustrated Medical Dictionary,* 1974), as an urgent, basic, or instinctual need (American Psychiatric Association, 1980b; *Webster's New Collegiate Dictionary,* 1979) or as the strength of the motivating force needed to produce an organized effort (*New Webster's Dictionary,* 1975). In psychoanalytic theory, drive is a mental constituent, probably genetically determined, that produces a state of tension sufficient to impel the individual to act in a manner to alleviate the tension (Freedman, Kaplan, and Sadock, 1975; Hinsie and Campbell, 1970). It is generally agreed that drive can be distinguished from *instinct,* a more basic force, in that drive can be influenced by learned incentives (American Psychiatric Association, 1980b). A related term, *motivation,* can also be defined as a force that regulates, impels, or induces behavior or that provides incentives to act (*Dorland's Illustrated Medical Dictionary,* 1974; Freedman, Kaplan, and Sadock, 1975; *New Webster's Dictionary,* 1975; *Webster's New Collegiate Dictionary,* 1979).

As a source of energy for propelling an organism to seek a goal or to satisfy a need, motivation is a broader concept than drive (Hinsie and Campbell, 1970). It often includes cognitive recognition of the goal to be attained (forethought, planning, and anticipated gratification).

Emotion itself is difficult to define; at best, the term is used broadly. Emotion has been called "the affective state of consciousness in which joy, sorrow, fear, hate and the like is experienced" (*New Webster's Dictionary,* 1975). Some suggest that the term should refer primarily or exclusively to consciously perceived feelings and their external manifestations (Hinsie and Campbell, 1970); others disagree. Benson (1984) defined emotion as the behavioral attribute that reflects the inner feeling tone modified by verbal and nonverbal affective influences, by the power of drive and by cognitive control measures.

Finally, a composite of behavioral characteristics, *personality,* has been defined simply as a sum of qualities that make an individual a unique self and an intelligent being (*Oxford English Dictionary,* 1979; *Stedman's Medical Dictionary Illustrated,* 1979; *New Webster's Dictionary,* 1975). Personality reflects a broad variety of behaviors, including attention, memory, self-reflection, mood, affect, and emotion. Hinsie and Campbell (1970) suggest that personality represents a compromise between inner drive and learned control. It is widely held that personality develops through experience and learning, but an individual's personality tends to remain consistent, little affected by efforts to change it.

CLINICAL EXAMPLES

While traditionally classed as psychiatric disturbances, many emotional disorders have an obvious neurological basis. To illustrate the range of brain-related emotional disorders, four categories of disorder—of mood, affect, drive, and cognitive control—will be used here. Few clinical problems are pure examples of any single category, but many do have characteristics that fall *primarily* within one or the other.

Disorders of Mood

Case 6.1

At age 31 years, a right-handed woman in the sixth month of pregnancy suffered a generalized seizure followed by lethargy, somnolence, and confusion that progressed to coma. Cerebrospinal fluid (CSF) studies revealed increasing lymphocytosis, normal glucose levels, and elevated CSF protein level (192 mg/100 ml). Fungal and bacteriological studies of CSF and serum were negative. An EEG showed generalized slowing with left-sided slow wave activity and spiking, and a radionuclide scan demonstrated a left frontotemporal abnormality. A presumptive diagnosis of herpes simplex encephalitis was made.

One month after delivery of a stillborn child the patient became alert and ambulatory, but her behavior remained markedly inappropriate. She did not recognize family members or friends. She lost her ability to speak English, and was severely aphasic in her native Spanish. Her verbal output was incoherent, repetitive, and irrelevant, consisting mainly of neologistic jargon. Her sexual behavior changed. She showed no interest in intercourse with her husband but would comply with his sexual advances; in contrast, she made inappropriate sexual advances to female attendants, both physically and verbally. She was constantly chewing and swallowing, and all objects within reach were placed in her mouth. She ate both food and non-food items, including toilet paper and feces. She gained 50 pounds in a short time, and her caloric intake was controlled only by chaining the refrigerator shut and providing toilet paper (bought by the case) and chewing gum (by the carton) for her to chew. Learning could not be demonstrated. She appeared unable to recognize objects or people and showed compulsive manual and oral examination of visualized objects. Emotional placidity was evident: her behavior was characterized by a pet-like compliance and passivity. A behavioral diagnosis of Klüver-Bucy syndrome was made. (Lilly et al., 1983)

Klüver and Bucy (1937, 1939) described striking behavioral abnormalities in monkeys following bilateral anterior temporal lobe resection: "psychic blindness," strong oral tendencies, an irresistible urge to touch items in the environment, hypersexuality, and a loss of normal anger and fear responses. The latter, an uncharacteristic placidity in the monkeys, represented a dramatic alteration of emotional response. Normally aggressive rhesus monkeys became calm, allowed the handler to touch and fondle them, and lost much of their irritable defensive attitude. These observations were subsequently replicated by a number of investigators (Akert, Gruesen, and Woolsey, 1961; Gross, 1973), and it was determined that the placidity could follow either inferotemporal or amygdala excisions (Horel, Keating, and Misantine, 1975; Schreiner and Kling, 1953).

The Klüver-Bucy syndrome was originally considered only a laboratory phenomenon, but human case reports resembling the syndrome have appeared sporadically (Marlowe, Mancall, and Thomas, 1975; Terzian and Dalle Ore, 1955). The human syndrome has been considered either incomplete or obscured by additional brain disturbances. In each reported subject, however, altered emotional behavior described as apathetic or placid was noted. R. Lilly et al. (1983) reported twelve personally examined cases of Klüver-Bucy syndrome and noted that the syndrome in the human was complex, with prominent aphasia, dementia, and amnesia. All twelve patients showed a blunted affect with apathy and pet-like compliance. While a number of different etiologies were recorded (brain trauma, herpes encephalitis, Alzheimer's and Pick's degenerative dementias), all had pathology that involved anterior temporal lobe structures bilaterally, implying a relationship between placidity and bilateral anterior temporal damage.

Case 6.2

A young man was first seen at a VA hospital at age 26 years and was followed for several more years. He came from an educated, professional family but had never been successful, graduating from high school only after considerable family intervention. He was also unsuccessful as an infantryman in Vietnam, eventually being discharged for the convenience of the service. During his military career a number of short episodes of nonresponse (absence) were recorded, but no seizures were recognized. Shortly after discharge, medical evaluation indicated a covert seizure disorder, and EEG revealed epileptic discharges, most prominent in the left temporal region. The patient's behavior, always a problem, became increasingly difficult, prompting his family to supplement his military disability payments sufficiently to allow him to maintain himself in a city over a thousand miles from their home.

Clinical examination revealed no overt neurological defects, but a number of striking behavioral abnormalities were noted. All conversations were extensive, featuring detailed, overinclusive responses (circumstantiality) frequently supplemented by quantities of written material (hypergraphia). When the patient became interested in a topic he tenaciously demanded its discussion (viscosity). He had no interest or experience in sex and denied any sexual desires (hyposexuality). Much of his conversation concerned topics of an obscure, controversial nature such as minor legalities or philosophical issues (intensification of intellectual life). His behavior and conversations were disturbing; he was contentious, irritable, and almost invariably expressed intense personal concerns (intensification of emotional life). A diagnosis of epilepsy with interictal personality disorder (Geschwind syndrome) was made. The seizures were readily controlled with appropriate anticonvulsant medications, but the behavioral abnormality remained intractable and disabling. (DFB)

H. Gastaut and colleagues (1956) noted that the interictal personality of some epileptics (now called *Geschwind syndrome* [Benson, 1987]) seemed the opposite of that described in Klüver-Bucy animals. Table 6.1 compares pertinent findings of the two syndromes and indicates that the emotional reactions are indeed in sharp contrast. While the Klüver-Bucy patient is placid and compliant, the interictal personality is characterized by intensified emotional responses. Bear (1979a,b) suggested that the epileptic emotional state could be considered a hyperconnection syndrome, a result of excessive neural activity; in contrast, he regarded the Klüver-Bucy syndrome as a hypoconnection syndrome resulting from destruction of the anterior temporal region.

While Table 6.1 implies that the opposite personality traits represent

Table 6.1. Temporal Lobe Personality Disorders

Klüver-Bucy Syndrome	Geschwind Syndrome
Hypermetamorphosis (constantly changing attention)	Circumstantiality (over-inclusive attention)
Hypersexuality	Hyposexuality
Emotional placidity	Emotional intensity
Anterior temporal destruction	Anterior temporal hyperactivity

opposite pathologies affecting temporal structures (quite probably true), not all instances of interictal personality disorder are based on anterior temporal seizure foci (Trimble, 1983). Well-defined examples of the Geschwind syndrome have been noted when the seizure focus affects limbic structures distant from the temporal lobe (e.g., insula, cingulate gyrus). The interictal personality syndrome remains controversial (Hermann and Stevens, 1980; Stevens, 1966) but enjoys increasing acceptance as one of the more consistent "organic" personality disorders (Bear, 1979b; Benson, 1991; Blumer and Benson, 1975).

Case 6.3

A 55-year-old man was brought to a hospital emergency room because of outbursts of raucous laughter that had commenced earlier that day. The episodes were intermittent, typically lasting between 10 and 30 seconds, and occurred as often as every 20 to 30 minutes. Between episodes the patient was noncommunicative, making only rare verbal responses. Emergency room evaluation, including medical screening and neurological examination were unremarkable but, except for a few faint responses to personal questions, and an occasional nod of the head, there was no communication from him.

The patient had suffered a minor head and low-back injury approximately four years earlier and several months later had experienced a "manic episode." An EEG at that time demonstrated occasional sharp waves in both temporal areas, but a CT scan was negative. He was started on anticonvulsants and responded well. The anticonvulsants were discontinued, and three successive EEGs were considered normal. He remained well until the onset of the laughter.

He was discharged from the emergency room but a few hours later was brought back because of continued abnormal behavior, including additional episodes of raucous laughter. An EEG showed almost continuous seizure discharge emanating from both anterior temporal regions. Treatment with intravenous anticonvulsants at first produced an agitated confusional state, but the patient slowly calmed. He next demonstrated paranoia, but this also resolved within a day. After return to normal emotional status he was completely unable to remember anything that had occurred during the three days in question. (Glassman, Dryer, and McCartney, 1985)

Pathological laughter and, to a lesser degree, pathological crying, can result from focal brain disorder (Cantu and Drew, 1966; Ironside, 1956; Martin, 1950; Swash, 1972) and can be differentiated from other episodic emotional outbursts such as pseudobulbar affect, *risus sardonicus, Witzelsucht,* and depression (Poeck, 1969). Pathological laughter is paroxysmal and episodic, unrelated to environmental stimulus, and uncontrolled by the patient. In some instances the patient has no memory of the outbursts, a characteristic suggesting seizure discharge. At postmortem, cases with pathological laughter, almost without exception, have focal pathology involving the junction of the midbrain and the diencephalon (Ironside, 1956; Martin, 1950). Davison and Kelman (1939) collected fifty-three cases of pathological laughter from the literature and noted that the hypothalamus or tissues with direct connections to hypothalamic structures were involved in all. K. Poeck and G. Pilleri (1964), however, reported 10 cases of pathological laughter, all with subcortical lesions but none involving the hypothalamus itself. Six were left sided, four were right sided; none involved cortex. A variety of etiologies have been noted, including tumors, abscesses, or trauma; it is the location of the disturbance along subcortical midline or limbic structures that appears crucial to the development of pathological laughter.

Other emotional experiences may be reported with epilepsy. The most common is an overwhelming feeling of fear, but embarrassment, anger, and depression also occur as preictal feelings (Williams, 1956). The emotional alteration is sudden in onset, unrelated to environmental context, follows a stereotyped pattern for the individual, and is often followed by a partial or generalized seizure. Such emotional auras are not uncommon (Daly, 1958; Stevens, 1975; Williams, 1956), but a consistent seizure focus has not been correlated with a specific emotional aura. Based on a sizable seizure surgery experience, Penfield and Kristiansen (1951) localized many epileptic auras, but for those that were purely emotional they could make only a general localization within the cortex. A limbic localization is now inferred (Gastaut and Broughton, 1972; Weiser, 1979) for seizures that commence with emotional symptomatology.

Disorders of Affect

Case 6.4

A 63-year-old man was transferred to a VA hospital from a mental institution for a neurobehavioral evaluation. The patient had no history of psychiatric problems. He had been admitted one month earlier with a relatively short history of apathy, withdrawal, and negativism. A diagnosis of depression had been entertained, but he failed to respond to antidepressant medications and was transferred to rule out an organic mental problem.

The patient was a well-developed, healthy male without acute medical problems. The basic neurological examination, including motor strength, sensation, and reflexes, was entirely normal, but his behavior was unusual. His entire day was spent sitting in a somewhat slumped posture with almost no movement to his face (masked facies) and little or no gesture. Mental status evaluation demonstrated that he was oriented to both time and place, could maintain a coherent conversation, had a digit span of 6 forward, could retain three words over a period of five minutes, and used language in a normal manner. He could copy two- and three-dimensional drawings, although the latter were performed poorly. There were no delusions, hallucinations, or evidence of disturbed insight.

The most striking abnormality concerned verbalization. His voice was so soft that it demanded close attention. While the syntactic and semantic content appeared normal, there was no melody. All verbal production was a soft monotone. When asked to sing familiar melodies such as "Jingle Bells" or "Happy Birthday," he recited the lyrics accurately but without melody. Even more striking, when asked about his recent mental hospitalization, he responded (in flat monotone and without gesture) that he was extremely angry at his children who had put him into that _____-_____ hospital and when he got out he was going to get after the little _____s for throwing him into the mental hospital. The verbal content was strongly emotional but was delivered in a monotonous, unemotional manner without facial expression or gestures.

A CT scan demonstrated a small but distinct defect, probably a recent infarction, in the right posterior inferior frontal lobe, the area analogous to Broca's area of the left hemisphere. (DFB)

Ross and Mesulam (1979) described two individuals who were unable to express emotion through either gesture or vocal tone following damage to the posterior inferior frontal cortex (Broca's area) of the right hemisphere. They suggested that the right frontal opercular area is essential (dominant) for emotion, a theory later refined and enlarged under the term *aprosodia* (Ross, 1981; Ross, Harney, and de LaCoste-Utamsing, 1981). These authors described individual patients who either failed to understand the emotional quality of the examiner's vocal output or were unable to repeat and/or vocalize emotional prosody. Right hemisphere perisylvian localizations were suggested—an anterior (emotional expression)/posterior (emotional comprehension) division—mirroring the localization of language expression and comprehension in the left hemisphere (Ross, 1981). Despite their inability to display emotion, these patients could harbor strong feelings. It was only the ability to express emotion through speech or gesture that was associated with focal damage in the right posterior–inferior frontal region.

Bear (1983), citing earlier cerebral pathway studies (Mishkin, 1972; Ungerleider and Mishkin, 1982), suggested that language-based cognitive activities of the left hemisphere demand so many sensorimotor pathways that few remain for emotional responses, and therefore emotion was a product of the neural structures of the right hemisphere. Whether this simple neuroanatomical basis for emotion can be accepted, clinical evidence indicates that the right hemisphere frontal cortex and immediate subcortical structures are important for prosodic and gestural elements of emotional display. This can be considered nonverbal affect.

Case 6.5

A 68-year-old, retired salesman was admitted to a VA hospital for language therapy. Approximately four weeks earlier he had suffered acute onset of right hemiplegia and aphasia.

On admission, physical examination revealed evidence of atrial fibrillation and peripheral atherosclerosis, but the patient was otherwise healthy. Neurological examination showed a dense right hemiplegia and a mild hypalgesia and hypesthesia that involved the entire right side. No visual field defect was evident, but the patient was unable to maintain his gaze to the right (gaze paresis). Language examination showed a nonfluent aphasia. The patient could read individual words but not sentence-length material, and he was unable to write.

He was placed in an intensive rehabilitation program and improved for about one month, particularly in physical activities, so that he was walking with minimal aid. During this period he appeared optimistic and cheerful. Over the next few weeks, however, he seemed to become depressed. He became withdrawn, lost motivation for therapy, and talked of personal uselessness and the hopelessness of his situation. For several weeks he remained withdrawn and negative and expressed suicidal thoughts on several occasions. He was treated with antidepressant medication and was regularly counseled; the rehabilitation therapists encouraged him in his activities, pointing out and praising him for the gains that he was making. The depression slowly dissipated until he was again cheerful, moderately optimistic, fully cooperative, and well motivated (see also Case 12.4). (DFB)

Within the variety of emotional responses that can complicate aphasia following left hemisphere damage, a dichotomy can be seen (Benson, 1973, 1992). One common syndrome features frustration/depression/catastrophic reaction and primarily occurs with anterior aphasias (e.g., Broca's aphasia). The other features unconcern/unawareness/paranoia and is almost exclusively associated with temporal lobe damage (e.g., Wernicke's aphasia). A simple explanation for the dichotomy may be offered. Patients with anterior aphasia are usually aware of their disorder, frustrated by their limited ability to communicate, and painfully aware of their limitations. They recognize the problem as their own, and this inward-looking state leads to depression. Patients with posterior aphasia, on the other hand, are incompletely aware of their difficulty; they tend to be unconcerned and often interpret their communication problems as the fault of others, an outward projection leading to paranoia. While this explanation seems reasonable, emotional reactions following left hemisphere damage may also have a more direct anatomical/functional correlation (see Case 12.5 and subsequent discussion).

Depression is more common in stroke victims than in individuals with similar (or even greater) disability due to orthopedic problems (Folstein, Maiberger, and McHugh, 1977). In stroke patients, Robert Robinson and colleagues (Robinson and Benson, 1981; Robinson and Price, 1982; Robinson and Szetela, 1981) have demonstrated that depression is much more common if the stroke, as demonstrated by CT scan, involves left anterior more than left posterior tissues. In fact, the more anterior the extent of the cerebrovascular lesion in the left hemisphere, the more likely a significant depression. Right hemisphere strokes do not show this anatomical predilection, although a tendency for right posterior cerebrovascular accidents to be associated with depression has been suggested. Robinson and colleagues (Robinson and Chait, 1985) conjecture that the tendency for depression to follow left frontal but not right frontal damage may indicate asymmetry of noradrenergic neurotransmitters, a theory yet to be confirmed. For whatever reason, depression is associated with damage to the left anterior hemisphere.

Positron emission tomography has demonstrated alterations in glucose metabolism in patients suffering acute depression (Baxter et al., 1985; Schwartz et al., 1987). While cerebral hypometabolism is widespread in depression, a greater degree is present in the left hemisphere than in the right and is more pronounced in frontal than in more posterior areas of the left hemisphere. Concomitant alterations occur in left caudate metabolism (Baxter et al., 1989). Following successful treatment of the depression, cerebral glucose metabolism returns to normal and the hemispheric asymmetry disappears. A right–left asymmetry of cerebral dysfunction in patients with depression is also suggested by evidence from other studies including focal neurological signs (Freeman, et al., 1985), EEG alterations (Flor-Henry and Koles, 1980; Rochford, Wineapple, and Goldstein, 1981) and neuropsychological test results (Wexler, 1980). While inconsistent and less powerful, these studies also imply that left hemisphere dysfunction is greater than right in serious depression and that the prefrontal areas are most involved. Abnormal left frontal cortex function appears to be associated with depressive emotional behavior.

G. Gainotti (1972) evaluated a sizable number of hemiplegics for evidence of either indifference (anosognosia) or depression (catastrophic reaction) and reported a significant hemispheric variation. More patients with damage in the right hemisphere reported some type of anosognosic phenomenon, while more patients with left hemisphere damage reported some degree of depression. Damage in the left hemisphere produced a strong emotional response (depression), while damage to the right hemisphere reduced emotional response (indifference, anosognosia), implying right hemisphere dominance for emotion (Bear, 1983; Geschwind, 1977). Additional support for right hemisphere dominance of emotion comes from studies showing that patients with right hemisphere damage have difficulty recognizing emotion that is expressed either visually or vocally (DeKosky, Heilman, and Bowers, 1980; Heilman, Scholes, and Watson, 1975; Van Lancker and Canter, 1982). Other studies (Ross, et al., 1981) (Case 6.4), however, suggest that the observed emotional loss is more apparent than real. Patients with right hemisphere disturbance may have difficulty comprehending and expressing emotion through visual, melodic, gestural, or other nonlinguistic verbal means despite the presence of strong feelings. Thus nonverbal affect, not emotion, appears to be the function altered by unilateral right hemisphere structural damage.

Emotional expression also depends on the selection of words, for both semantic and syntactic use. Language impairment can lead to verbal responses that suggest abnormal affect and that are easily misinterpreted as altered emotional status. Attempts to correlate brain damage with emotion tend to utilize questionnaires; by this method both depression (Gainotti, 1972) and schizophreniform disorder (Flor-Henry, 1969) appear more common with left hemisphere pathology, but it is quite possible that these results reflect impaired ability to comprehend and/or express the verbal connotations of feeling rather than true alterations of mood. As noted in Case 6.4, the linguistic expression of emotion (verbal affect) can be separated from prosodic and gestural (nonverbal affect) expression.

Bear and Fedio (1977) collected a number of behavioral abnormalities that are often reported in the interictal state of epileptics and, based on their study of individuals with either right- or left-sided epileptic foci, suggested that the emotional disorders differed depending on the side of the focus. Previous studies (Flor-Henry, 1969; Serafetinides and Falconer, (1962) also had revealed right/left differences in patients with epileptic foci, possibly based on an altered language status in patients with left temporal lobe foci (Bear and Fedio, 1977; Blumer and Benson, 1982). Sherwin and colleagues (1982) postulated that ongoing subclinical seizure discharges involving left temporal lobe structures could interfere with normal language circuitry and cause intermittent problems in both comprehension and production of language. Such a seizure-based language impairment was conjectured as the source of the loose associations of the schizophrenia-like behavior reported in some long-term epileptics (Hill, 1962; Slater, Beard, and Glithero, 1963; Trimble, 1982). Bear and Fedio (1977) found that patients with a right temporal lobe focus tended to downplay (deny) their problems, while McIntyre, Pritchard, and Lambrusco (1976) suggested that right temporal lobe epileptics reacted more physically to emotionally charged situations. These observations have not been fully accepted, however (Mungas, 1982; Rodin and Schmaltz, 1984).

While complicated and difficult to interpret, observations from diverse sources indicate that considerable differences in the expression of emotional behavior exist and to some extent are attributable to the hemisphere involved.

Case 6.6

A 62-year-old man was admitted to a VA hospital for evaluation and possible therapy after probable stroke. He had a long history of arteriosclerosis with complications, including hypertension, myocardial infarction, and atrial fibrillation. At least three episodes of suspected cerebrovascular accident were reported, and it was conjectured that additional cerebral damage had occurred during periods of cardiac dysrhythmia.

On examination, the patient's strength was adequate in all four extremities, although he appeared somewhat weaker on the left, particularly in the upper extremity. Deep tendon reflexes were generally hyperactive, and there was an unsustained clonus at the left ankle. The jaw jerk was strongly positive. Both toe signs were extensor, and Hoffman's sign was present bilaterally. Testing of sensation did not reveal pertinent lateral asymmetry.

The patient told of occasional swallowing difficulty and choking episodes. He had no significant language impairment, but his verbal output was slow, he performed below anticipated levels in confrontation naming, and on request he produced only five animal names in 60 seconds.

The most dramatic observation concerned the patient's affective state. With attempts at conversation he almost invariably grimaced, started sobbing, and formed true tears. The crying spells would last for 60 to 90 seconds and tended to recur as the conversation continued, but if the topic could be shifted in a particularly pleasant direction (e.g., questions concerning his wife and children), the crying would not only stop but be replaced by a smile or light laughter. Return of the discussion to less pleasant topics such as his current status or his need for hospitalization would again elicit exaggerated crying. When asked about his mood during these crying spells, the patient insisted that he was not as unhappy as it appeared; his strongest feelings were of embarrassment at his inability to control the emotional outbursts. This condition, *pseudobulbar affect*, appeared to be based on bilateral cerebral vascular lesions. (DFB)

The dramatic display of emotional expression called *pseudobulbar affect* is characterized by a gross exaggeration of normal emotional display. The patient may produce uproarious, uncontrolled laughter lasting for many seconds or minutes or the opposite, an equally lengthy, uncontrolled bout of crying with real tears. In either instance, the mood expressed (happiness, sadness) is usually appropriate; it is the intensity of the response that is pathological. A strong, uncontrolled emotional outburst occurs when a mere smile or frown would be appropriate.

Many explanations have been offered for pseudobulbar affect, including psychiatric (e.g., psychotic breakdown) and psychodynamic (e.g., a means of psychic defense) theories. Others consider the excessive emotional display of pseudobulbar affect similar to pathological laughter (Case 6.3). It has been suggested that pseudobulbar affect follows bilateral damage to frontal/brain stem pathways, decreasing inhibition (control) of the degree of emotional response (Lieberman and Benson, 1977). In most instances pseudobulbar affect accompanies pseudobulbar palsy, a state in which bilateral upper motor neuron disturbance involves the bulbar musculature (Tilney and Morrison, 1912). Bilateral upper motor neuron disorder can cause bulbar musculature weakness (paucity of facial movements, hoarseness, hypophonia, and swallowing difficulties), as well as bilateral motor problems of the limbs (weakness, spasticity, hyperreflexia), but the degree varies; the disinhibited affect may be far more prominent than the motor disturbances. Pseudobulbar affect demonstrates that emotional display (affect) may inaccurately reflect the underlying feeling tone.

Many theories of emotion neglect the basic observation that the affective quality of an emotional alteration following brain damage varies with the neuroanatomical site and the hemisphere involved.

Disorders of Drive and Cognitive Control

Case 6.7

At age 58 years, a man was admitted for evaluation of the long-term effects of a leucotomy performed almost 30 years earlier. He had originally been hospitalized while in military service, had been discharged to a VA hospital, and had remained under care for a psychotic disorder diagnosed as schizophrenia. He had not responded to the available treatments, and, after several years of incapacitating psychosis manifested by delusions, command hallucinations, negativism, blocking, and so on, the decision was made to perform a leucotomy. After surgery the patient underwent social rehabilitation and was eventually discharged to a board-and-care home. His subsequent psychiatric status remained stable with sufficient improvement so that he could care for himself and hold a job.

When the patient was hospitalized for the follow-up evaluation, a CT scan revealed large bifrontal leucotomy lesions (see Fig. 6-2), and an extensive neuropsychological examination revealed that his IQ and most other basic mental functions were normal for his age and educational level. He was clean, neatly dressed, spoke freely of his life and experiences, and denied significant psychotic symptoms. There was, however, a degree of unreality to his conversation, and the history revealed that he had never been able to develop close relationships or maintain friendships. While socially appropriate, his conversation tended to be idiosyncratic and lacked appreciation of the feelings of others. He tended to be

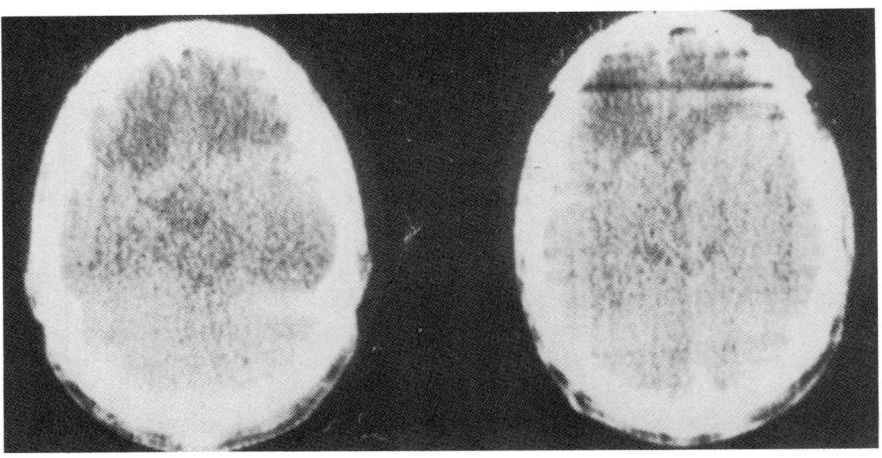

Fig. 6.2. X-ray CT scans demonstrating the large prefrontal lucencies produced by leucotomy surgery performed many years earlier. From Naeser et al. 1981.

sarcastic and cynical, describing his own feelings and actions and those of others with brutal frankness; extended discourse with him created unpleasant tension in the listener. (DFB)

Tens of thousands of prefrontal destructive lesion procedures were performed in the 1940s and 1950s (Freeman, Watts, and Hunt, 1942; Valenstein, 1980), but remarkably few details of residual emotional behavior are available. Most of the procedures were crude, so lacking in anatomical precision that the area of frontal lobe damage could only be surmised. With few exceptions, only patients with disabling emotional disorders were subjected to the procedure. Little information germane to the correlation of frontal damage and behavioral functioning could be gathered (Stuss and Benson, 1986; Valenstein, 1973). When studied, the results were vague (Malmo, 1948; Mettler, 1949; Petrie, 1952). In one sizable study, Greenblatt and Solomon (1966) noted four potential psychiatric outcomes following prefrontal lobotomy: (1) decreased drive, (2) decreased ability to plan ahead, (3) decreased concern with social restrictions, and (4) shallowing of affect.

While it was widely accepted that prefrontal surgery did influence behavior, including emotional expression (Freeman, Watts, and Hunt, 1942; Petrie, 1952; Reitman, 1946; Smith, Kiloh, and Boots, 1977), the cause of the alteration has remained conjectural. The most effective lesions disconnected prefrontal cortex from thalamus; lesions in other areas were less beneficial and tended to produce undesirable side effects such as apathy. Few studies have focused on the effect of prefrontal disconnection on emotion. In testing selected postleucotomy patients such as Case 6.7, Stuss and Benson (1983, 1986) found that the subjects could successfully match and identify emotional facial expressions but often failed to match the appropriate facial expression to an emotionally laden scene (e.g., one subject matched a happy face with a funeral scene). Their responses tended to be precipitate, poorly thought out, and almost automatic. While frontally damaged patients appeared to perceive emotion correctly, their translation into a response was often inappropriate.

Neuroimaging studies have demonstrated that a phenomenologically distinct communication disorder (*verbal dysdecorum*) may follow right prefrontal damage (Alexander, Benson, and Stuss, 1989). While damage to the right prefrontal dorsal convexity and/or the right medial sagittal frontal structures produces no fundamental language disorder, it may cause dysfunction characterized by improper, socially undesirable responses. The patient often speaks in a caustic or cynical manner with the barbs aimed at himself as often as at others. Conversations include topics usually avoided and a bluntness of response that is disconcerting. The output is jarring to the listener and irritates and eventually alienates acquaintances, friends, and relatives. The patient fails to monitor the impact of his or her conversation, a disturbance in the control of cognitive function that affects many behaviors, including emotional response. Case 6.7 suffered from this problem.

Following frontal lobe damage many patients suffer alterations in behavior, and terms such as *frontal-lobishness, frontal behavior,* and *frontal personality* have been used (see Cases 11.2 and 11.3). Some observers (Blumer and Benson, 1975; Kleist, 1934a) have noted differences in frontal personality disorders and have thought that the neuroanatomical locus of damage was crucial. One frontal personality syndrome, characterized by apathy, indifference, and abulia despite retention of intellectual competency, has been termed *pseudo-depressed* or *pseudo-retarded* (Blumer and Benson, 1975; Cummings, 1985) and is associated with sagittal, medial polar, and/or medial dorsal convexity damage (Aymes and Nielson, 1955). Most prominent is a decrease in drive that alters all behavior, including emotional response. A distinctly different frontal personality disorder, called *pseudo-psychopathic* by Blumer and Benson (1975), includes a disregard of social restrictions, a facetious, gallows-type humor, and lack of interest in anything but immediate personal pleasure, a hedonistic state. Although the patient is fully cognizant of proper behavior, the immediately desired action is not controlled by this knowledge. This inability to monitor and inhibit behaviors, including social responses, was associated with pathology involving orbital and dorsolateral frontal regions. Thus, two frontal functions—drive and cognitive control—were seen as essential for emotional response.

Case 6.8

A 28-year-old veteran was hospitalized for evaluation and management of episodes of violence. He had sustained significant head injury necessitating surgical exploration after an accident. Seizures had occurred but were fully controlled by anticonvulsants. The patient told of many episodes in which he would lose his temper. The episodes did not appear ictal, as there was a distinct build-up without overt seizure activity. The patient could remember the occurrences and was concerned about them; he felt real remorse. Otherwise, he was a healthy young man without physical or neurological disorder.

On one occasion he was critically questioned concerning his need for disability support, and after this unpleasant session a psychologist attempted to administer the Rorschach test. Following presentation of Card 3, the patient turned somewhat pale, a glare appeared in his eyes, he said, "I've had enough of this, I'm leaving," and got up and left the room. When next seen he was throwing his clothes into his suitcase and, after being observed for several minutes, turned to the examiner and said, "Get the hell out of my way." The nurses and house staff were instructed not to interfere as he might be dangerous. The patient did not, however, leave the hospital, secluding himself for several hours and then resuming normal ward activity. The following morning he waited patiently for the examiner to arrive and immediately apologized for his behavior. He gave a detailed account of his activities during the hour or so in which his behavior was out of control and potentially violent, and he expressed grave concern that he might harm someone during one of these episodes. A diagnosis of episodic dyscontrol was entertained. (DFB)

Some mental disorders include serious problems with emotional control. One such problem is called *episodic dyscontrol* (or *limbic rage syndrome*). Episodic paroxysms of dangerously violent physical or verbal outbursts are the key features. Episodic dyscontrol is characterized by short episodes of rage. While many investigators have suggested a neurological abnormality (Elliott, 1978a,b, 1992; Maletzky, 1973; Mark, Sweet, and Ervin, 1975; Pincus, 1980; Rickler, 1982), no specific pathology is known. Some cases of episodic violence are related to epilepsy, some to mass lesion (particularly when the temporal lobe is involved), and many follow brain trauma. In other cases, however, no evidence of brain disorder can be found.

NEUROANATOMICAL SUBSTRATE

Emotion is a complex mental function that reflects the coordinated activities of many parts of the brain. From the review of clinical cases, a neuroanatomical network for the control of emotional response can be suggested, correlating emotional abnormalities with neural structures.

Mood, the pervasive but only partly conscious emotional state, appears to be altered by disorders involving the base of the brain, specifically malfunction affecting mesencephalic, diencephalic, and/or basal limbic functions. Neurochemical changes are important in alterations of mood in everyday life and underlie some psychiatric disorders. Damage to certain limbic structures can produce a variety of alterations ranging from the placid, compliant state of the Klüver-Bucy syndrome to the fear and anxiety seen in some cases of limbic epilepsy. Mood seems related to the activity of basal/limbic neural structures. Most of these subcortical and brain stem structures are cell clusters with short, polysynaptic connections; many appear to influence emotion through the release of chemical neurotransmitters.

Affect, the outward expression of mood, usually reflects the underlying emotional state; damage or malfunction of basal/limbic structures alters affect by altering mood. Cases 6.4, 6.5, and 6.6, however, demonstrate that affect can also be altered by focal damage to the cerebral hemispheres. Such neurological observations indicate a correlation between the hemisphere damaged and the observed alteration of affect. One set of affective responses (amelodia, decreased affective demonstration) predominates following damage to right cortical structures; a different type of affective behavior (verbal denial, expressions of depression, and so forth) is associated with unilateral left hemisphere damage; a third emotional response syndrome (lability of emotional expression) typically follows bilateral cortical damage.

Table 6.2 presents four varieties of affect. Mood-consistent affect, of course, represents the outward expression of the mood prevalent at the moment. The other three represent alterations of emotional expression based on cortical activity, either normal or pathological. While the clinical examples of verbal, nonverbal, and pseudobulbar affective responses (Cases 6.4, 6.5, and 6.6) reflected structural brain damage, it is probable that variations of affective response resembling these three conditions also occur on the basis of neurotransmitter dysfunction.

An important but frequently overlooked aspect of emotion concerns drive, the energizing force of behavior. Clinical cases in which decreased drive/motivation follows focal brain damage usually involve damage to medial brain regions, particularly frontal tissues, including the supplementary motor area and/or the cingulate gyrus. Additional clinical observations link more inferior structures, also in the midline, such as the frontal septal area, the medial mesencephalon, and the medial thalamus, with decreased drive. All of the latter structures have strong medial frontal connections, and the entire group can be considered a medial "frontal system" (Alexander, DeLong, and Strick, 1986). This neural network influences many brain activities, including emotional response.

Finally, there is another frontal system that plays an important role in human emotional response. Clinical observations (Case 6.7) demonstrate that disconnection of the prefrontal cortex from other cerebral structures can produce a state in which the individual fails to monitor personal behavior. These patients can state, verbally, a correct response to a situation, but their actions are incorrect. The inability to utilize well-learned social restrictions represents an impairment of cognitive control. Among many behaviors influenced are the behavioral responses of emotion. Nauta (1973) said of this problem: "The failure of the affective and moti-

Table 6.2. Varieties of Affect

Mood-consistent affect
Verbally influenced affect
Nonverbally influenced affect
Pseudobulbar (disinhibited) affect

vational responses of the frontal lobe patient to match environmental situations that he nonetheless can describe accurately could thus be tentatively interpreted as a consequence of the loss of a modulatory influence normally exerted by the neocortex upon the limbic mechanisms by the frontal cortex." Cognitive control is recognized as a frontal lobe function that plays a role in the shaping of emotional behavior.

THE NEURAL BASIS OF EMOTION

Emotion is a complex behavior reflecting many interrelated neural structures and activities. For a neurological analysis, the multiple facets of emotion must be separated into meaningful, operational subunits such as mood, affect, drive, and cognitive control.

Figure 6.3 illustrates the neural continuum that controls emotional response. Whether momentary or continuing, the emotional response represents the underlying mood as altered by both verbal and nonverbal influences on expression (affect), the degree of drive excited by the occasion, and the control exerted by cognitive monitoring.

Three spheres of influence that act on the emotional response mechanisms deserve emphasis. The first represents external influences, both those from the environment and those from the visceral milieu. These are constantly changing.

A second major sphere of influence is the neural system of emotion itself, the system outlined in Figure 6.3. While most aspects of this system are subject to change in daily life, the degree and direction of alteration is relatively restricted and the response to an emotion-provoking stimulus tends to be consistent for any given individual. Damage or dysfunction of this system tends to produce emotional disorder.

The third major sphere concerns learned behavior, particularly as it influences prefrontal cognitive control functions. Knowledge of the conse-

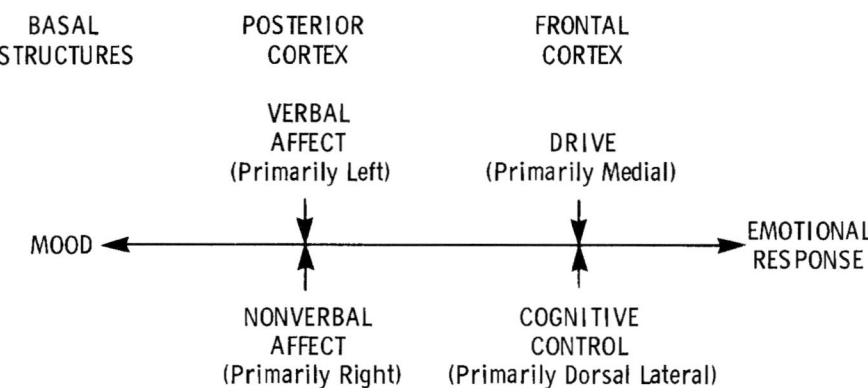

Fig. 6.3. Graphic outline of the interrelated brain activities that influence an emotional response. From Benson, 1984.

quences of actions, of social proprieties, sensitivity to the potential effect of an emotional response on others, and many similar aspects of cognitive control are modified through learning. Culturally and socially learned modifiers provide one of the more stable influences on emotional behavior. There is a sizable literature, both popular and professional, on measures designed to alter emotional behavior through learning. The limited success of any of these measures indicates how difficult it is to change one's behavior. While some emotional responses surface rapidly and appear to lack control, an individual's basic emotional response patterns are remarkably stable and resistant to change.

The behavioral entity called *personality* is usually described in terms of emotional response patterns. For any given individual, the personality represents a remarkably stable state. Attempts to alter personality by training (e.g., education, behavioral modification, psychotherapy) are largely futile. The one circumstance in which personality is often altered is brain damage, particularly damage to areas that influence emotional response. The altered personality that may follow brain damage usually remains stable, albeit different. As the midtwentieth century experience with psychosurgery demonstrated (Greenblatt and Solomon, 1966), this can be advantageous. Individuals who suffered excessive drive (obsessive–compulsive) or affective response (intractable depression), who were lost in fantasy, or who were crippled by social concern could benefit from frontal-lobe-destructive procedures (Valenstein, 1980). In too many instances, however, the "new" personality that followed brain insult was a less desirable combination of behaviors.

Most individual emotional responses are carried out unconsciously, in a manner analogous to a motor reflex, but they can be modified by conscious mental activity. An example will help to clarify this complex relationship. If a ball suddenly breaks one's window, the first response is a combination of fright and anger. This feeling is usually expressed in both verbal and nonverbal affect through angry words and gestures. The immediate response is often strong. In most circumstances, however, the initial, reflex response is rapidly modified by appropriate inhibitions, influenced by multiple internal and external factors. Whether the incident was purposeful or accidental, whether based on carelessness or bad luck, whether truly unexpected or a recognized risk, and similar factors are quickly assayed. Whether the perpetrator is known or unknown, a responsible friend or a stranger, is noted. The response of the ball-thrower will be noted; if true concern and remorse are evident, the angry outburst may be fully controlled. If disdain or flight are noted, however, the angry response may increase. Most of the emotional response operates at a rapid and unconscious level, best recognized in retrospect. The entire response will be influenced by one's background and training; whether one's behavior pattern in similar situations has been passive, turn-the-other-cheek or angry and retaliative will be reflected in the immediate reaction. The final product is a behavioral response to an emotional stimulus in which the checks and balances of both neural and social modifiers are active.

This scenario illustrates normal response modification; brain damage can alter this pattern, most notably in the direction of decreased control. An initial response surfaces but may be less modified, and remorse for any excess in the response may or may not be expressed. Alternately, brain damage may inhibit the power of the response by decreasing motivation (impaired drive), decreasing affect-laden gesture and/or vocal prosody (impaired nonverbal affect), or decreasing verbal response (impaired verbal affect). Pervasive placidity, dulling of feeling tone, or poorly controlled violence (basal–limbic dysfunction) may result. The wide range of acquired alterations of emotional response represents the malfunction of relatively discrete and selective brain mechanisms. Emotion is a multifaceted behavior based on a relatively fixed, distinctly organized, and integrated functional system.

7

The Neurology of Visual Imagery

> In looking at an object we reach out for it. With an invisible finger we move through the space around us, go out to distant places where things are found, touch them, catch them, scan their surfaces, trace their borders, explore their texture. It is an imminently active occupation.
> —RUDOLPH ARNHEIM, 1969

> Often we have to get away from speech in order to think clearly.
> —R. S. WOODWORTH AND H. SCHLOSBERG, 1954

AXIOMS/POSTULATES

Visual sensation progresses through the steps of reception, discrimination and unimodal association to form a visual percept available for thought processing.

A visual image is a visual percept augmented by appropriate cross-modal references.

Visual imagery does not require immediate visual stimulation.

One key aspect of visual sensory processing—visual–spatial discrimination—is, to a considerable degree, hemisphere specific.

The importance of visual sensory input for human thinking has always been recognized, though accorded different weight in different periods (Aristotle, 1931; Arnheim, 1969; Condillac, 1754). In fact, visual imagery loomed so large as a factor in human thought that attempts were made to downgrade its status (Ach, 1905; Humphrey, 1963; Mayer and Orth, 1901) in a counterresponse to the sensory experimentation that dominated early physiology and psychology (von Helmholtz, 1856–66; Wundt, 1873–74).

In recent years, the role of visual imagery in thinking has been underacknowledged and that of language has ascended. Because of its dominance for language, the left hemisphere has been considered the "major" hemisphere, the right hemisphere being downgraded to a "minor" status and even considered a reserve brain.

Most neurological approaches to the visual system follow two lines.

The first, neuroophthalmology, deals with pathological derangement of the visual sensorimotor system. Studies of brain lesions that produce abnormal eye movements provide insight into the neural mechanisms needed to scan space. It also involves observations of the altered size and configuration of the fields of vision following brain damage. A vast literature (Bender, 1962; Holmes, 1918; Mishkin, 1972; Troost, 1981; Walsh and Hoyt, 1969) correlates patterns of visual abnormality with specific central nervous system loci. Most neuroophthalmologists, however, refrain from following visual stimuli beyond the hard-wired, sensorimotor stages. To understand what happens to visual stimuli after they reach the cortex, the steps essential for the extraction of information from these stimuli requires a second approach, that of neuropsychology and behavioral neurology.

Most behavioral neurologists and neuropsychologists have focused on abnormalities associated with language, memory, and cognitive disorders (e.g., aphasia, amnesia, dementia), but disturbances of higher visual processing have been reported in the neurological literature for over a century and these clinical problems have been tentatively correlated with specific loci (Benson, 1988a; Brown, 1988; Damasio, 1985; Farah, 1990; Hécaen and Albert, 1978; Luria, 1959, 1966). The sophisticated correlation of anatomy and behavior that characterized the study of language disorders, however, remains tentative for visual–spatial investigations. Studies of the cortical processing of visual information remain in a formative stage.

VARIETIES OF VISUAL–SPATIAL FUNCTION

To discuss higher visual function, the pattern of sensory processing introduced in Chapter 3 will be followed. The progressive hierarchy of reception discrimination, and unimodal association will be reviewed and crucial aspects of heteromodal association presented. The final result, visually derived knowledge, will be termed *visual gnosis*.

Reception refers to the conduction of the visual stimulus, from the retina through the optic nerves, the optic chiasm, and optic tracts to the lateral geniculate nucleus of the thalamus and on, via the geniculocalcarine pathways, to the primary visual cortex (Brodmann area 17). This is no simple connection; changes in stimulus organization occur at each synapse and by the time visual information reaches the optic cortex it has been reorganized and has undergone important gating. But for this chapter these steps will be considered a single process—visual reception. Clinical disturbance along the primary visual pathways produces abnormalities of primary visual sensation. Blindness, total or partial (hemianopia, quadrantopia, scotomata), although not based on sensory processing disorders at the cortical level, frequently results from brain damage that also produces higher visual dysfunction; receptive disorders and higher visual processing disorders frequently coexist.

Discrimination, as discussed in Chapter 3, represents a comparison of sensory stimuli. *Visual* discrimination can be defined as the process of distinguishing variations in the visual stimuli received via the primary visual receptive channels. Efron (1968) defined this step as an "awareness of discriminated existents," noting not only the ability to distinguish but also an initial level of awareness of the discrimination. Rather pure disorders of visual discrimination have been recognized (see Case 7.1).

Unimodal association, the third step in sensory processing, compares (matches) discriminated percepts with prior percepts, a process of categorization (concept formation). The comparison of the concept thus formed with previously experienced visual information demands memory and represents an essential, unimodal memory function. The product is a visual percept.

Heteromodal association, the next step in visual sensory processing, is the step in which material from sensory processing, the categorized unimodal percept, is related to other sensory inputs. Information from multiple modalities that has been gathered and stored earlier is associated with the visual percept for identification/categorization purposes. Two cortical functions—cross-modal sensory processing and memory retrieval—are essential for heteromodal association.

Agnosia has accumulated a variety of meanings. The term was once used to identify almost any disorder of higher sensory processing (Nielsen, 1936/1948); this was followed by a period in which it was bluntly stated that agnosia did not exist (Bay, 1953; Critchley, 1964). In early discussions (Lissauer, 1889; Poetzl, 1928), variations of visual agnosia were postulated; Critchley (1953) defined one, apperceptive visual agnosia, as disordered perception, and another, associative visual agnosia, as disordered recognition. While controversial, the dichotomy remains alive in the literature (Farah, 1990; Grüsser and Landis, 1991).

Several other problems hinder investigation of disordered visual gnosis and deserve comment. First, most studies of visual gnosis require language-based reports. Disordered language function must be ruled out or properly separated from the visual disorder, not always an easy task. Second, a visual gnostic disorder may follow damage to several different brain areas. No single anatomical site can be related to a given visual function (e.g., color naming); instead, there is a network of interconnected cortical and subcortical structures. Third, the inherent visual competency and educational/vocational background of subjects varies considerably. A visual–spatial discrimination disturbance will be far more disabling to an artist or engineer than to a person who rarely utilizes such skills; conversely, the skilled individual may score above average on standardized tests despite significant damage. Fourth, brain damage that causes disordered visual gnosis often produces additional nonvisual symptoms that overshadow the visual problems so dramatically that they are downplayed or overlooked.

Despite these formidable problems, numerous investigators are now probing the processes of visual gnosis with encouraging results. Most concentrate on structural studies (Keating and Horel, 1972; Schneider, 1969; Ungerleider and Mishkin, 1982) and psychophysical interpretations

(Brown, 1988; Lessell, 1975; Marr and Nishihara, 1978; Mishkin, 1972). In recent years, physiological and metabolic studies have greatly enhanced the ability to analyze visual processing (Corbetta et al., 1990; Hubel and Wiesel, 1979; Phelps, Kuhl, and Mazziotta, 1981). Yet clinical observations remain a rich resource for research in higher visual processing (Farah, 1990).

CLINICAL EXAMPLES

The cases presented below have been selected to highlight pertinent features of visual gnosis. In each case there is a reasonably specific defect, but, as in most clinical situations, difficulties involving other systems are mixed with the higher visual processing disorders.

Case 7.1

A 25-year-old soldier, through a series of accidents, sustained significant carbon monoxide poisoning and developed severe cerebral edema. He remained comatose for a prolonged period and then made a slow and incomplete recovery. He was eventually transferred from a military hospital to a VA hospital with two diagnoses—blindness and chronic brain syndrome.

At the VA hospital he was alert and cooperative, gave appropriate responses to purely verbal questions, and appeared to have adequate memory and language functions. He was unable to read or write (alexia with agraphia), could not copy letters or drawing, and could not identify objects on visual confrontation, though he immediately named them if they were placed in his hand. He never recognized people by their appearance but immediately recognized them when they spoke. The findings suggested blindness, but he insisted that he could "see," and testing showed normal visual acuity (20/20 O.D., 20/25 O.S.) by indirect ophthalmoscopy. Testing of elementary visual attributes demonstrated excellent color vision, excellent ability to discriminate minimal differences of light intensity, and consistent ability to tell the direction of a movement and dimension of a presented object. The patient, however, was totally unable to identify form. Thus, when shown a pencil, comb, and toothbrush, he could not differentiate them. When presented with three figures—two circles and a cross—his ability to select the one that was different was random. Brain imaging techniques available at that time failed to demonstrate any focal area of brain damage. A diagnosis of *apperceptive visual agnosia* based on hypoxic damage to primary and secondary visual cortices was made. The patient's visual gnosis disorder remained static through a decade of follow-up examinations. (Benson and Greenberg, 1969)

The term *apperceptive visual agnosia* was applied to Case 7.1 because there appeared to be sufficient distortion of the properly received visual sensations to make identification impossible (Critchley, 1953). The patient was not blind, as he readily responded to basic visual information—color, light intensity, movement, and dimension. All four steps in sensory processing—reception, discrimination, unimodal association, and heteromodal association—appeared to function normally for these four visual elements. But the network of visual processing needed to perceive form was disrupted. The patient could not develop a visual percept for form (apperception). While not common, similar cases of apperceptive visual agnosia have been reported (Adler, 1944; Benson and Greenberg, 1969; Mendez, 1988).

Case 7.2

A 50-year-old man developed acute right-sided weakness, right somesthetic disturbance, and right homonymous hemianopia. Improvement was fairly rapid so that two months after onset the motor and somesthetic findings had completely disappeared, but the right homonymous hemianopia remained unchanged. Spoken language was normal, and the patient could spell words aloud and write to dictation. In contrast, he could not read any words (alexia), although he could copy them correctly. He could read only a few letters of the alphabet but read multidigit numbers correctly. A disturbance in color identification persisted. He was usually incorrect when asked to name colors but accurately matched and sorted colors by hue, even those with subtle differences in brightness and saturation. He correctly matched colored chips to outline drawings of objects (e.g., yellow for banana). He had no difficulty with the standard tests for color blindness and gave appropriate color names for objects such as lemon and fire engine. A diagnosis of alexia without agraphia plus color agnosia was entertained. Autopsy, several years later, demonstrated that an occlusion of the left posterior cerebral artery had produced infarction of medial occipital tissues plus infarction of the splenium of the corpus callosum. (Geschwind and Fusillo, 1966)

Case 7.2 illustrates two disorders of visual gnosis—alexia and color agnosia. The dramatic dissociation of reading and writing capabilities in this case indicates a disorder of visual, not language, processing. In the same manner, the patient's inability either to name a color or to point to the color when the name was provided despite intact color discrimination and use of color names demonstrated that the problem involved the pathways needed for association and was not a primary language disorder.

Case 7.3

A 47-year-old male physician was resuscitated from a cyanotic hypotensive episode brought on by a suicide attempt with alcohol and sedatives. Within three weeks he was fully alert, awake, ambulatory, and without elementary neurological disturbance except for a dense right homonymous hemianopia. He could write paragraph-length descriptions of his activities that were legible and accurate; in sharp contrast, he was completely unable to read even material he had just written (alexia without agraphia). Conversational speech showed a full lexicon, but he failed all attempts at confrontation naming unless he could touch the object: then he immediately spoke the correct name. He failed to recognize familiar people (e.g., his wife and children) until they spoke (prosopagnosia). He could neither name colors nor point to the appropriate color when the name was presented but easily recited the correct color names for tomatoes, fire engines, bananas, and so forth and correctly sorted colored chips into piles based on the color (color agnosia). Multiple tests of visual function demonstrated excellent three-dimensional vision, accurate performance of a multiple line maze, and fully normal performance on hidden figure puzzles. He could copy complex drawings, even though he could not name the object of the drawing (see Fig. 7.1), could produce drawings of objects on command, and easily moved about the environment with-

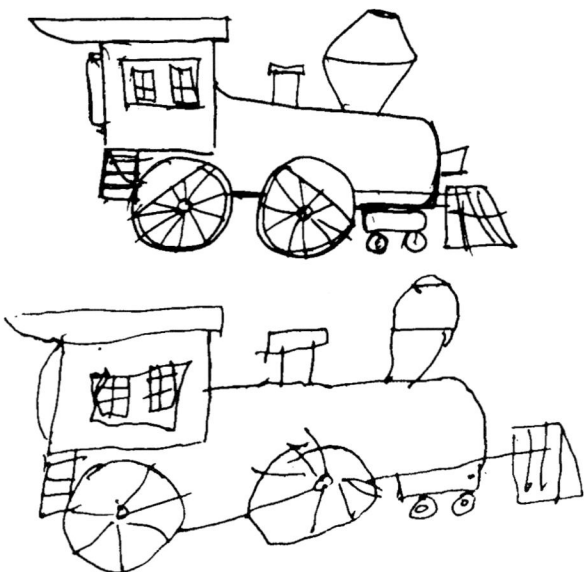

Fig. 7.1. Attempt (*lower*) by Case 7.3 to copy line drawing (*upper.*) Although the copy is successful, the patient was unable to name the object that he had copied. From Rubens and Benson, *Archives of Neurology,* 24:305–316, copyright 1971 American Medical Association.

out difficulty. An isotope brain scan demonstrated increased uptake in the left medial occipital region (territory of the left posterior cerebral artery). With time the patient learned to read individual letters and would then spell aloud to recognize the word; eventually he was able to read at a high-school level. His ability to name common objects on confrontation also improved, but the prosopagnosia remained dense. A diagnosis of associative visual agnosia was made.

Approximately three years later the patient died of laryngeal carcinoma. At postmortem study his brain had no metastases, but both posterior cerebral arteries were occluded. The anticipated left medial occipital infarction (the cause of the right hemianopia) was present, and there was evidence of an additional small, but distinct infarction in the right medial occipital region. While the left hemisphere infarction involved both the geniculocalcarine pathways and the outflow tracts emanating from the visual association cortex (the inferior longitudinal fasciculus), the smaller lesion on the right involved only the inferior longitudinal fasciculus. Figure 7.2 illustrates the sites of occipital pathology. (Rubens and Benson, 1971; Benson, Segarra, and Albert, 1974)

Case 7.3, like Case 7.1, was diagnosed as having visual agnosia, but this manifestation is obviously different. The patient accurately copied letters of the alphabet and drawings, even complex three-dimensional drawings. Both reception and discrimination of all visual parameters were intact; accurate visual percepts were formed, but this patient's ability to activate the higher level processing needed to associate faces, objects, letters, drawings, or colors with memory stores and identify the visual per-

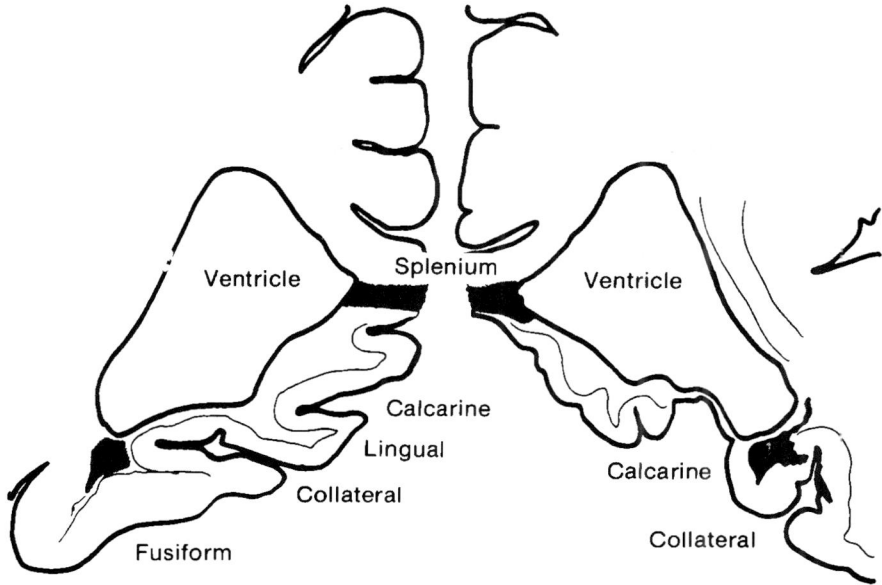

Fig. 7.2. Artist's illustration depicting the major sites of pathology found in the brain of Case 7.3. Note the bilateral occipital pathology and damage to the splenium of the corpus callosum. From Benson et al, *Archives of Neurology,* 30:307–310, copyright 1974 American Medical Association.

cept was lost. Case 7.3 illustrates breakdown at a higher level in the progression of visual–sensory processing, a disorder that did not allow recognition of a correctly processed percept. The patient's ability to use this higher order information when nonvisual stimuli were presented indicates a disconnection, a separation of the intact unimodal visual processing channels from the equally intact heteromodal processing network.

These three cases illustrate different disorders of visual gnosis. None could read, but Cases 7.2 and 7.3 showed a disturbance of visual processing in which letters of the alphabet and colors, although not identified, could be copied and matched accurately. Case 7.2, unlike Case 7.3, could identify objects, read numbers, and, in general, had a milder disturbance. Both Case 7.2 and Case 7.3 had infarctions that involved the left medial occipital region plus infarction of the splenium of the corpus callosum. Case 7.3 was different in that another infarction involved his right occipital lobe. Reading, the language-oriented visual function, was disturbed in both patients, but only Case 7.3 with bilateral infarctions showed visual agnosia and prosopagnosia as well.

It has long been contended (Dejerine, 1892; Geschwind, 1962; Hinshelwood, 1900) that alexia without agraphia indicates separation of an intact right visual sensory processing unit from an equally intact left hemisphere language area. Color naming is often disturbed in this disorder, as it was in Cases 7.2 and 7.3. Both patients, however, could match colors accurately and provide the appropriate color name for a named object, yet could not give a name when a color was presented or point to a given color when the name was presented. This two-way defect indicates separation of the visual percept from cross-modal association. There is a disturbance of neither visual reception/discrimination (as demonstrated by the ability to match colors) nor language/cognition (as demonstrated by the ability to use color names correctly). Case 7.1 stands in contrast, as he had no difficulty with either color recognition or naming. Although both Cases 7.1 and 7.3 can be said to have visual agnosia, the visual processing features are different. Case 7.1 had difficulty forming some types of visual percepts; Case 7.3 was unable to carry out higher level associations based on intact visual percepts. The former is accurately categorized as *apperceptive* agnosia, the latter as *associative* agnosia, terms suggested by Lissauer (1889) and further defined by Critchley (1953), Farah (1990) and Grüsser and Landis (1991).

Case 7.4
A 70-year-old, right-handed man noted the acute onset of headache followed by disorientation in space and difficulty reading and recognizing colors. His main complaint was an inability to differentiate and recognize faces. He could not recognize his wife or his daughter by sight, although he immediately recognized them by their voices. His own image in the mirror was unfamiliar. Facial expressions could not be comprehended, and he could not identify either familiar or famous people from their photographs. A full neurological examination was normal except for the visual fields, where a dense left homonymous hemianopia plus a partial superior altitudinopia of the right visual field was demonstrated. The patient could almost always match colors but made many errors in attempting to name colors or point to a color when the name was given. Death followed a series of strokes, but at postmortem old bilateral, cystic lesions, each involving the inferior occipital–temporal region (fusiform gyrus), were found, and the problem in recognizing faces was attributed to these defects. (DFB)

Case 7.4 illustrates the inability to recognize familiar faces (prosopagnosia), a dramatic visual gnosis disorder that has spawned a sizable literature (Bodamer, 1947; Bornstein, 1963; Damasio, Damasio, and Van Hoesen, 1982; De Renzi, 1986; Grüsser and Landis, 1991; Sergent and Poncet, 1990; Tzavaras, Hécaen, and LeBras, 1970). Prosopagnosia is a true agnosia, as the patient cannot identify previously recognized faces on visual presentation but readily names and identifies individuals from their voices or distinguishing nonfacial characteristics (e.g., clothing, hair color). While most reported cases of prosopagnosia follow right posterior hemisphere damage (Meadows, 1974), leading to claims that right hemisphere pathology alone is sufficient to produce the disorder (Landis et al., 1986b; Whitely and Warrington, 1977), every patient with a persistent prosopagnosia that has come to postmortem analysis has had bilateral occipital pathology (Damasio, 1985; Hécaen and Tzavaras, 1969; Meadows, 1974). Case 7.3 also suffered prosopagnosia following bilateral occipital pathology but was unusual in that the largest lesion was in the left hemisphere while only a small (apparently crucially located) lesion was found in the right occipital region. To diagnose prosopagnosia, sufficient reception/discrimination must be demonstrated to exclude blindness. Aphasia must also be excluded by having the patient identify a person from nonvisual stimuli. Two relatively well-defined cases (Benson, Segarra, and Albert, 1974; Lhermitte et al., 1972) both had bilateral damage to the inferior longitudinal fasciculus, the white matter tract that connects unimodal visual association cortex with the inferior temporal cortex. Bilateral inferior temporal cortex damage has been said to produce visual agnosia, including prosopagnosia (Levine, 1978; Levine and Calvanio, 1980), but to date the available case material is too limited to substantiate this hypothesis.

A closely related problem that should be distinguished from prosopagnosia is difficulty with facial recognition or matching (Grüsser and Landis, 1991). Various techniques to challenge the ability to match faces feature different angles of observation (e.g., full face, three-quarter face, profile; De Renzi and Spinnler, 1966), differences in ambient shading (Benton and Van Allen, 1969), or variation of a single feature such as eyes or mouth (Hécaen and Tzavaras, 1969). The results of these tests have been consistent—individuals with right posterior hemisphere damage have more difficulty matching faces than patients with left posterior hemisphere damage (Rondot, Tzavaras, and Garcia, 1967; Sergent and Corballis, 1990; Warrington and James, 1967). Discrimination of facial features need not be associated with prosopagnosia, however; several patients with severe prosopagnosia have performed within normal limits on facial discrimination tests (Rubens and Benson, 1971; Tzavaras, Hécaen, and LeBras, 1970).

Prosopagnosia indicates a disorder in utilizing memory of previously recognized faces (particularly notable is the inability to recognize the face or photograph of a specific family member). Facial recognition tests probe the ability to discriminate features of previously unknown faces; this is a different operation from that of recognizing a face that is well known.

Case 7.5

A 54-year-old man was admitted to the hospital following a grand mal seizure. For the previous six months he had shown forgetfulness and decreased interest in activities; for about two months he had been unable to dress himself and tended to get lost in familiar places. He had difficulty finding the apartment house where he had lived for many years and once became lost in a corridor of this building, needing aid to find his own apartment. He depended on small discriminating features such as the color of a garage door, a specific mailbox, or a distinctive doorway to orient himself. Neurological examination was normal except for a dense left inferior quadrantopia and a tendency to neglect left superior visual field stimuli. Constructional difficulties were severe, and the patient could not dress himself. He did, however, readily recognize familiar faces and quickly learned and consistently recognized the faces of hospital staff.

In the hospital, he rapidly learned to get from the bathroom to his own room by counting the number of doors between the two rooms; to go to the hospital store, he memorized the floor number and the specific right and left turns from the elevator. If he missed a turn he became totally lost and had to ask directions. After he had been in the hospital for over two months he was taken, blindfolded, to an unfamiliar section of the hospital adjacent to his own ward. It took 30 minutes of trial and error for him to find his own bed, a task that could have been accomplished in 30 seconds. CT scan (Fig. 7.3) revealed a right medial occipital abnormality consistent with an area of infarction. (Landis et al., 1986a)

Case 7.5 illustrates a phenomenologically distinct problem of visual processing—becoming lost in familiar places. Although relatively rare, the disorder has been given many names (Critchley, 1953; Hécaen et al., 1956; Landis et al., 1986a) and many interpretations (Paterson and Zangwill, 1945; Whiteley and Warrington, 1977). While unable to find his way about in familiar confines without verbal cues such as counting, Case 7.5 could accurately point to suggested places on a map and had no difficulty orienting himself on either a map or a floor plan. The restricted visual gnosis disorder he suffered has been called *environmental agnosia*.

Case 7.6

A 34-year-old man was admitted for surgical treatment of intractable epilepsy. History revealed that he had sustained a shrapnel wound in the right parietal area at age 28 years, leaving a persistent left homonymous hemianopia. Two surgical procedures attempting to control seizures had removed sizable portions of the right posterior parietal and superior occipital cortex. Figure 7.4 shows the surgeon's conception of the extent of excised brain.

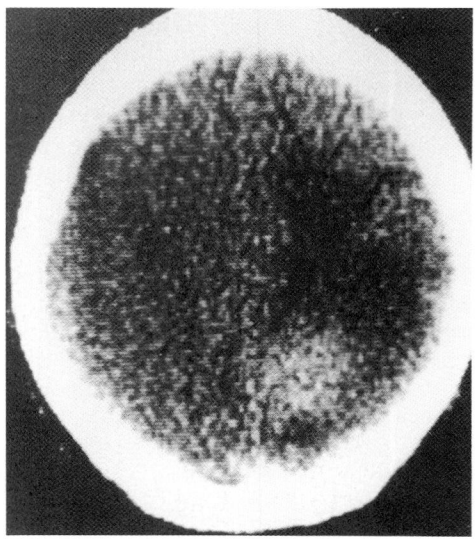

Fig. 7.3. X-ray CT scan of Case 7.5 revealing the presence of a right medial occipital area of infarction. From Landis et al., *Archives of Neurology*, 43:132–136, copyright 1986 American Medical Association.

When the patient was reexamined two and a half years after the second operation, the left homonymous hemianopia remained, but there was no disturbance of language, no problem in color naming or recognition, or in naming objects and images. He recognized faces, was lucid, well oriented, and cooperative, but described problems dressing himself, often needing help from his wife. Part of the dressing problem was a tendency to ignore the left side of his body, but this was complicated by a disorientation in space. When attempting to dress his son, for example, he put an overcoat on backwards, realizing his mistake only when his son laughed at him. He could perform some simple constructional tasks but failed all attempts to draw to command or to copy three-dimensional figures. Despite the unilateral neglect, he seemed aware of his own left body and the left side of space. He had no impairment in environmental memory (he got about his home and the hospital without difficulty) but was unable to orient himself on a map and could not trace even a simple route (topographagnosia). In fact, when his home city of Montreal and the Laurentian Mountains were put on a map, he was unable to suggest where the St. Lawrence River would be located. (Hécaen et al., 1956)

Case 7.6, in contrast to Case 7.5, suffered disability in orienting himself to an abstract spatial representation such as a map or a floor plan, a disturbance called *topographagnosia* (Critchley, 1953; Landis et al., 1986a). Clinical distinction of environmental agnosia (Case 7.5) and topographagnosia (Case 7.6) is only infrequently made, and, unfortunately, the two terms are often interchanged. The presence of one without the other, as illustrated by Cases 7.5 and 7.6 and others in the literature (Macrae and Trolle, 1956; Semmes et al., 1963), suggests that the two disorders of orientation in external space follow damage to different neural systems. All cases of environmental agnosia reported by Landis et al. (1986a) had pathologies that involved the right medial occipital area. In contrast, reported cases of pure topographagnosia (Hécaen et al., 1956; McFie, Piercy, and Zangwill, 1950; Paterson and Zangwill, 1944) have

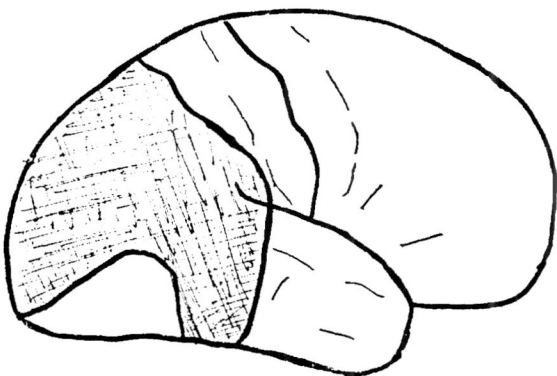

Fig. 7.4. The surgeon's conception of the extent of excised cortex in Case 7.6. From Hécaen et al., 1956.

had pathology that involves the dorsal convexity of the right parietal lobe. Thus, it appears that the two spatial orientation processes—orientation in actual space (environment) and orientation to spatial representation (map)—operate through different neural circuits.

Case 7.7

A 40-year-old man was evaluated because of episodic recurrence of visual images long after removal of the original stimulus. Six years earlier a biopsy had demonstrated gliotic changes in the right parietooccipital region. After the surgical procedure the patient noted persistence and recurrence of visual images in the blind left visual field. When he attended to a visually presented object and looked away, an image persisted. The "afterimage" would gradually fade over 30 to 90 seconds, but if he moved his eyes it could be rejuvenated. The image was more likely to persist if the object was brightly colored or seen against a bright background. It would move in the direction of gaze when he moved his eyes, and if one eye was shut the image remained visible to both eyes. While present in both visual fields, the persistent image was particularly strong on the left side. On two occasions the patient experienced a similar persistence of tactile sensation, the rough texture of a table and the shape of a piece of a sculpture.

Examination demonstrated a dense left homonymous hemianopia, but there was no indication of left neglect and the patient successfully copied three-dimensional representations. Clinical testing revealed significant problems in retaining (learning) nonverbal information but he did well on tests of verbal learning. A CT scan (Fig. 7.5) revealed a large cystic lesion that involved much of the right occipital lobe and extended into the right temporal lobe. (Cummings et al., 1982)

In Case 7.7, a blind visual field "sees" an image, a disturbance called *palinopsia* (Bender, Feldman, and Sobin, 1968; Michel and Troost, 1980). Almost invariably, the palinopic image is a continuation of an image correctly visualized in the intact visual field. At times, however, the image may persist and even become multiple (*visual allesthesia* [Jacobs, 1980; Kawamura et al, 1987]). In palinopsia and related disturbances some stages of visual processing, particularly percept formation and hetero-

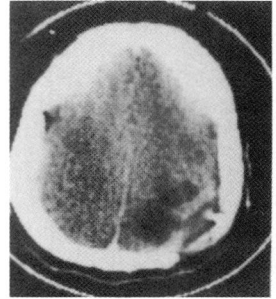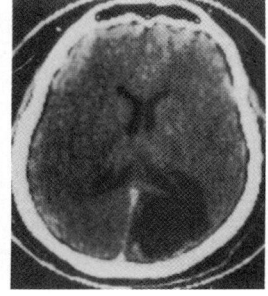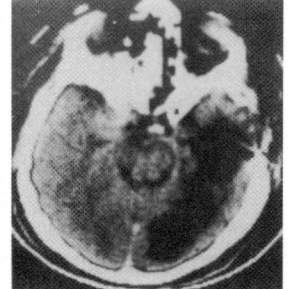

Fig. 7.5. X-ray CT scan demonstrating the large lucency in the occipital lobe of Case 7.7. From Cummings et al., 1982.

modal association, are functioning. The lesion that has produced a blind visual field obviates reception of external stimuli in one hemisphere's visual cortex, but visual processing mechanisms farther along the neural chain of that hemisphere may accept signals from the opposite hemisphere and enter this information into higher level processing channels. A palinopic image is an external stimulus appropriately received and processed by the visual network of the opposite hemisphere. Whether the appearance of the image in the blind field is considered a product of *covert seizure discharge* (Jacobs, Feldman, and Dimond, 1973; Swash, 1979) or a *release phenomenon* (Cummings et al., 1982), a palinopic image represents activation of the higher visual-processing network of a hemisphere that has lost reception of visual input.

Case 7.8

At age 64 years, a former bank executive was referred for evaluation of a slowly progressive disorder of vision and language. Eight years earlier he first noted difficulty in reading. At that time he could still write (alexia without agraphia) and remained on the job by having his secretary read to him. Over time, however, he lost the ability to write, had difficulty finding his way in familiar places (environmental agnosia), and his performance in all visually mediated tasks deteriorated. Eventually his ability to express himself became limited, but his family insisted that he understood conversations.

Examination revealed an alert, attentive, and healthy man who was cooperative and had excellent insight into his problems. His verbal output was fluent, but there were conspicuous word-finding problems. Visual confrontation naming was severely deficient, but naming became normal if he was allowed to touch the object (visual agnosia). He could not read letters, numbers, or words and could write only a few words to dictation.

The neurological examination was normal except for a right lower quadrant visual disturbance and a notable eye movement disorder. The visual field problem could be demonstrated only by double simultaneous stimulation and was inconsistent. The patient walked as though partially blind. While he could navigate through doors and through a room without collision, he had difficulty orienting himself to pieces of furniture. His gaze tended to remain fixed on an object (sticky fixation), although, when he was asked to follow a moving object, both lateral and vertical gaze were full. When asked to touch a stationary object held in front of him, he consistently missed by inches (ocular dysmetria), and, if he was asked to note a number of objects in an array, he usually found only one or two (simultanagnosia).

Both CT and MRI revealed bilateral symmetrical atrophy, most prominent in the posterior parietal and occipital regions (see Fig. 7.6). The EEG showed a 6–7 Hz slowing.

Over the next two years the patient slowly deteriorated, became more demented, and died about 10 years after the onset of visual problems. At postmortem his brain showed focal atrophy involving occipital and parietal tissues. Microscopic examination revealed deterioration of lamina II of the cortex with spongiform degeneration of the cortical and immediate subcortical tissues and considerable proliferation of reactive gliosis. A diagnosis of subcortical gliosis was made. (Benson, Davis, Snyder, 1988)

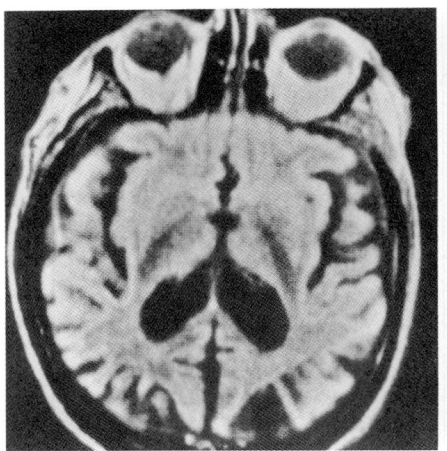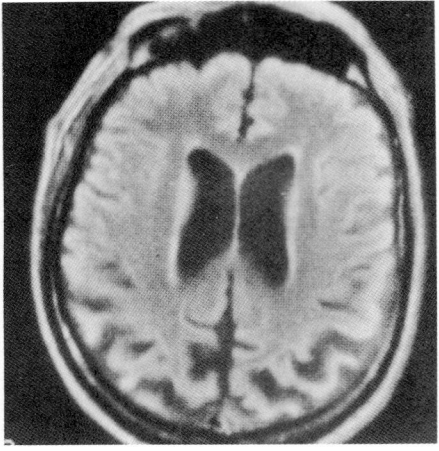

Fig. 7.6. Magnetic resonance scan of Case 7.8 demonstrating marked increase in the size of the posterior ventricles and greater atrophy in posterior than anterior cortex. From Benson, Davis, and Snyder, *Archives of Neurology*, 45:789–793, copyright 1988 American Medical Association.

In Case 7.8 a degenerative process primarily affecting the visual system caused a slow, progressive dissolution of visually oriented activities that led to disordered communication and abnormal movements. Only the handling of visual information was affected in the early stages. Visual reception remained intact far into the disease progression (evidenced by full visual fields to confrontation testing), whereas almost all purely visual associations degenerated early and severely. The disorder in Case 7.8 and similar cases has been labeled *posterior cortical atrophy* (Benson, Davis, and Snyder, 1988) with the suggestion that a lobar cortical degenerative process differentially affects the posterior sensory association cortex. Starting with alexia, Case 7.8 eventually developed a full panoply of higher visual gnostic disorders: object and color agnosia, environmental disorientation, topographagnosia and prosopagnosia, and eventually the full Balint syndrome (Balint, 1909; Damasio, 1985; Hausser, Robert, and Girard, 1980; Hécaen and de Ajuriaguerra, 1954)—optic dysmetria (a tendency to misdirect the hand when reaching for an object in space), sticky fixation (an inability to move the eyes between two objects in space), and simultanagnosia (a tendency to concentrate on a single or a few visualized objects to the exclusion of surrounding objects)—were demonstrated. Far along in the disease course, many years after the visual processing disorder had disabled him, Case 7.8 retained insight into his predicament, had normal language except for word-finding problems, showed considerable memory competency, and demonstrated only minimal alterations of personality. Only at a very late stage of the disease were more widespread mental changes noted, and even then the primary visual, auditory, somesthetic, and motor systems remained functional.

Case 7.9

A 46-year-old man was seen for neurobehavioral evaluation. At age 19 years he had sustained a head injury in World War II. After the injury he developed an intractable seizure disorder, which was eventually treated by section of the corpus callosum (Bogen and Vogel, 1962). The seizures were controlled, and the patient suffered no gross neurological or behavioral abnormalities consequent to the procedure. When evaluated for more subtle disturbances, he showed the manifestations commonly reported with callosal section (see Case 4.4), including ideomotor apraxia that involved only the left limbs, agraphia with the left hand, tactile naming disturbance of the left hand, and extinction of the left ear stimulus when double simultaneous auditory stimuli were presented.

A unique abnormality of constructional ability was found. The patient could copy script and both two- and three-dimensional drawings with either hand but performed these tasks best with his left, nondominant hand. His ability to copy with the left hand contrasted sharply with a total inability to write or draw with that hand to verbal instruction. A striking dissociation was noted when he was asked to construct a visualized block design pattern. If both hands were free, he placed blocks into position with his left hand and the right hand then removed them. If one hand was kept from the task, the other attempted to copy the design. The left hand alone copied a four-block design with the appropriate number of blocks but usually erred in design pattern. In contrast, the right hand alone often used the wrong number of blocks and placed them in a scattered, random-appearing way that, nonetheless, often approximated the desired design pattern. (DFB)

Case 7.9 has many important features. First, the classic split-brain findings demonstrating the inability of the right hemisphere to benefit from language-based instructions are present. In addition, there is a complex and variable difficulty with construction. Both hands (both hemispheres) failed, but their failures were fundamentally different. The left hand (right brain) correctly performed the outline but failed to reproduce the inner detail, whereas the right hand (left brain) did the opposite. Some have suggested that the right hemisphere is dominant for constructional tasks (Benton, 1967; Bogen and Gazzaniga, 1965); others consider the right hemisphere more competent (dominant) at visual–spatial discrimination while the left hemisphere excels at the motor response (execution) of visually guided tasks (Benson and Barton, 1970; Warrington and James, 1967). Both hemispheres apparently play significant roles in constructional tasks, a premise that receives support from the widely made observation that constructional tasks are sensitive screening tests for brain damage (Hécaen and Assal, 1970; Luria and Tsvetkova, 1964; Dee, 1970; McFie and Zangwill, 1960). Nahor and Benson (1970) demonstrated that damage to any of the three superior cortical areas (frontal, parietal, occipital) in either hemisphere led to disturbed ability to copy relatively simple three-dimensional drawings. Temporal lobe structural damage, on the other hand, did not interfere with constructional tasks.

These selected cases illustrate a variety of clinical abnormalities that can be traced to pathological involvement of the higher level visual system; the symptoms depend on the part of the visual processing network that is involved. While these cases show that elements of the visual pro-

Table 7.1. Disorders of Visual Gnosis

Visual Function	Disorders Involving Unimodal Visual Acts	Disorders Involving Heteromodal Visual Acts
Color	Achromatopsia	Color agnosia
Language		Alexia, Anomia
Memory		Nonverbal learning disorder
Spatial	Amorphosynthesis Constructional disturbance Dressing disturbance	Hemi-inattention Constructional disturbance Dressing disturbance
Geographical	Environmental agnosia,	Topographagnosia
Object	Apperceptive visual agnosia Visual hallucinosis	Associative visual agnosia Visual hallucinosis Visual allesthesia Palinopsia
Face	Facial matching	Prosopagnosia

Motor		Balint's syndrome
		  Ocular dysmetria
		  Sticky fixation
		  Simultanagnosia

Overall		Posterior cortical atrophy

Adapted from Benson, 1988a.

cessing system are indeed separable, they are also highly interrelated. In the clinic, most higher visual system problems are mixtures of processing abnormalities, frequently complicated by problems involving other functional systems. Relatively distinct examples of the kind described in this chapter are the exception.

Table 7.1 outlines a number of higher visual-processing disorders. Disturbances of basic visual functions such as extraocular movement disturbances or visual field disorders have been excluded, as has blindness. Higher visual disturbances have been divided into two groups—unimodal (perceptual) disorders and heteromodal (recognition) disorders. Although admittedly artificial, Table 7.1 helps to categorize these confusingly intermixed conditions.

NEUROANATOMICAL SUBSTRATE

Eye movements, which are crucial for many visual functions, depend on a complex group of nuclei and pathways in the brain stem with reciprocal connections to sensory and motor areas of both hemispheres. These nuclei and their connections have been thoroughly studied (Cogan, 1966; Troost, 1981; Walsh and Hoyt, 1969). While the brain stem systems managing eye movement are crucial to optimal visual function and clearly responsive to high-level mental control, disorders of these systems are of limited significance to the neural basis of thinking and will not be reviewed here.

A second hard-wired eye movement system influences sensorimotor responses. The cortical eye areas—anterior (Brodmann area 8) and posterior (Brodmann areas 18 and 19) are relatively well demarcated (see Fig. 7.7). Visual input to the posterior area activates the conjugate, directional eye movements needed to track a moving object (i.e., when an object moves across the visual fields, this cortical area commands the eye and body movements needed to follow the object's trajectory). The frontal area participates in "volitional" eye movements; i.e., when a verbal command is given to look in a specified direction, this area directs the brain stem operations needed for the movement (Holmes, 1921; Teuber, Battersby, and Bender, 1949). Difficulty in a single directional eye movement, such as a unilaterally disturbed visual following movement, can be present on clinical examination and indicates the functional distinctness of the cortical eye movement areas.

The third hard-wired ophthalmic system includes the nuclei and tracts that transmit visual stimuli to the cortex via the pathway sketched in Fig-

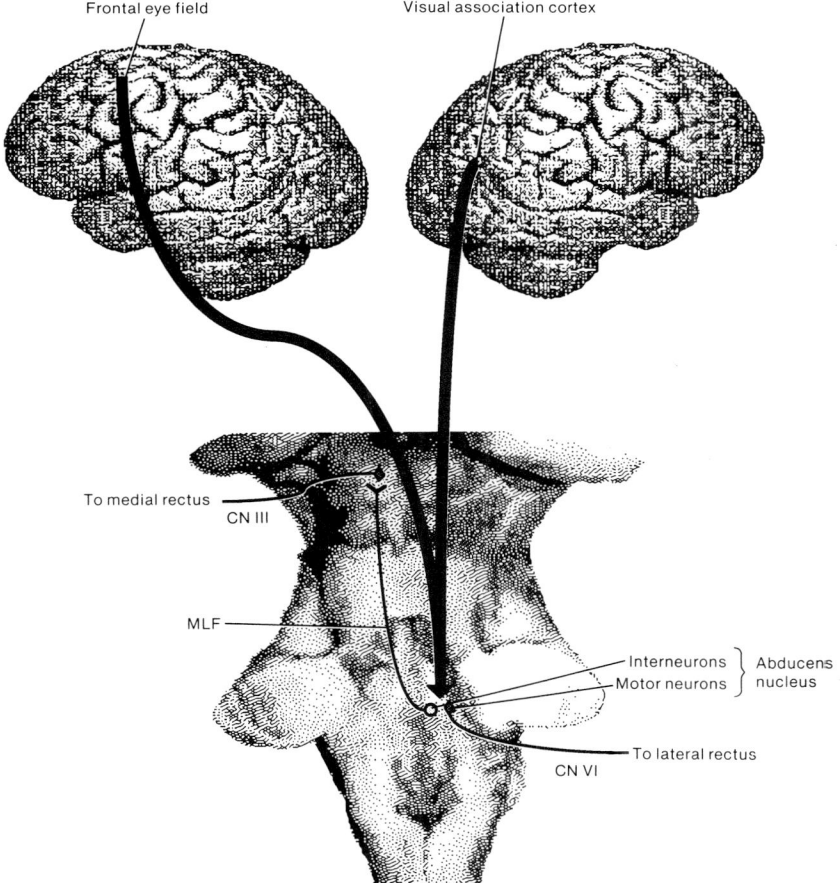

Fig. 7.7. Artist's illustration of the two cortical eye fields and their connection to the oculomotor system of the brain stem. From Nolte, 1988.

ure 3.5. Abnormal visual fields (e.g., hemianopia) indicate damage to this pathway (Halstead, 1943; Kaul et al., 1974; King, 1967; Weiskrantz et al., 1974). Visual field defect was carefully considered in early visual behavior studies (Benton, 1967; Arrigoni and De Renzi, 1964; Gloning, Gloning, and Hoff, 1968), but the correlation with higher visual function has not been consistent. While of unquestionable importance in providing partially processed visual information to the cortex, the conduction pathways participate only indirectly in higher visual processing; they affect thinking only by providing the material for visual imagery.

Much less is known about the anatomical basis of higher visual processing than about the basic visual functions. Russian investigators (Luria, 1966; Pavlov, 1941) have suggested that visual processing is carried out on two separate levels, termed *primary* and *secondary analyzers*. While not specifically localized, the functions ascribed to the primary visual analyzer imply a posterior (calcarine area and surrounding unimodal association cortex) site, while the functions of the secondary analyzer (recognition activities resembling heteromodal association) were located at a distance from the primary visual area. This theory is fully consistent with the processing model presented here.

Initial visual processing (reception/discrimination/unimodal association) is performed by a series of interrelated neurons located in and around the calcarine fissure. Hubel and Wiesel (1968, 1979) demonstrated columns of cells (modules) in the visual association cortex through which increasingly complex analysis of visual signals is performed. The interconnections of these columns to additional processing columns in the same and the opposite hemisphere provide a rich latticework for the formation of visual percepts. Visual percepts are formulated by the occipital and selected posterior parietal cortices and their connecting pathways, a relatively hard-wired network dedicated to unimodal visual association.

Visual imagery, however, demands additional processing of visual signals, carried out at sites distant from the primary visual processing area and dependent on pathways to conduct the visual percept. Some pathways that carry this visual information are known. Rich connections to the homologous cortex of the opposite hemisphere, primarily traversing the splenium of the corpus callosum, subserve unimodal activities. A small midline connection in the juxtastriate cortex (Geschwind, 1965; Pandya and Seltzer, 1986) allows the two hemispheres to visualize a single image, not the two separate images that are processed by the two hemispheric visual reception systems.

A series of white matter tracts, the superior and inferior occipital frontal fasciculi and the superior longitudinal fasciculus, connect the parietal–occipital visual cortex to the frontal association cortex. These tracts provide pure visual information to prefrontal cortical areas and, probably even more importantly, exert frontal control over the primary visual processing system. A stable visual image is created from an almost constantly mobile visual input (e.g., when one's head and eyes move, the image of the visualized background remains stable), a function at least partially based on frontal control input.

Of considerable importance for visual processing is the inferior longitudinal fasciculus, a white matter tract that courses from visual association cortex through the fusiform and lingual gyri into the posterior-inferior portion of the temporal lobe, the so-called inferotemporal cortex. Primate studies (Desimone and Ungerleider, 1989; Gross, 1973; Herel, Keating, and Misantine, 1975; Mishkin, 1982) demonstrate that this area is active in visual form discrimination, and pathology in the inferotemporal cortex or its connections to primary visual cortex is said to produce visual agnosia (Levine, 1978) and/or prosopagnosia (Benson, Segarra, and Albert, 1974). This connection appears to subserve unimodal associations alone.

Finally, multiple short tracts connect the occipital–parietal visual association cortex (Brodmann areas 18 and 19) with the adjacent angular gyrus. Clinical evidence indicates that cross-modal association, the mixture of images from multiple sensory channels, depends on intermodality connections through the angular gyrus (Butters, Barton, and Brody, 1970; Geschwind, 1965).

Information from other areas of the brain is used to develop a full visual image, most data being processed through the angular gyrus. A visual percept can be formed without heteromodal associations, but a full visual image demands them. The angular gyri (both right and left) carry out cross-modal associations but act only as a central point with connections to many areas of cortex. Through the intermediary of the angular gyrus, purely visual percepts can be associated with the vast body of data available from other sensory modalities, from language and emotion, and from previously learned experiences. A visual image involves much of the cortex via a rich neural network that depends on connections in the angular gyrus.

THE NEURAL BASIS OF VISUAL–SPATIAL FUNCTION

As we have seen, *reception* of visual information in the cortex follows transmission from the retina to Brodmann area 17. Visual stimuli become organized, but categorization remains rudimentary. Reception merely provides the raw data needed to form a visual image. *Discrimination* can be divided into separate categories. Nielsen (1936/1948) proposed five types of visual discrimination: color, light intensity, direction of movement, dimension of visual stimulus, and form. Clinical evidence (see Cases 7.1 and 7.5) implies that different combinations of unimodal association neurons process these attributes (Damasio, 1985; Grüsser and Landis, 1991).

Unimodal association, in which discriminated visual data undergo further categorization, is more clearly defined functionally. Case studies suggest that unimodal association is an activity of areas 18 and 19 but occurs, at least partially, in separate cell aggregates. Studies of achromatopsia (Damasio, 1985; Damasio, Damasio, and Chui, 1980) indicate that color appreciation (and discrimination) is carried out by the unimodal visual association cortex located in the medial occipital area inferior to the calcarine cortex. Disturbed pattern discrimination follows destruction of bilateral posterior inferior temporal cortex (Gross, 1973; Keating and Horel, 1972; Levine, 1978; Mishkin, 1982). Bilateral damage to a relatively discrete portion of dorsal parietal convexity (area 19) apparently interferes with an animal's ability to discriminate the direction of a visualized moving object (Zihl, von Cramon, and Mai, 1983), and this area shows increased metabolic activity in subjects observing movement in their visual environment.

Discrimination and unimodal association apparently represent distinct activities carried out by different neuronal systems in the visual association cortex of the posterior hemispheres. Figure 7.8 outlines the steps in the initial analysis of visual signals; additional elements might be considered, but the unimodal association aspects of Figure 7.8, and the clinical observations upon which they are based, provide a basic conception of the neural structure for the initial processing of visual information. When combined, the three increasingly complex steps in visual processing produce a unimodal percept.

Essential to unimodal association is referral to previously experienced

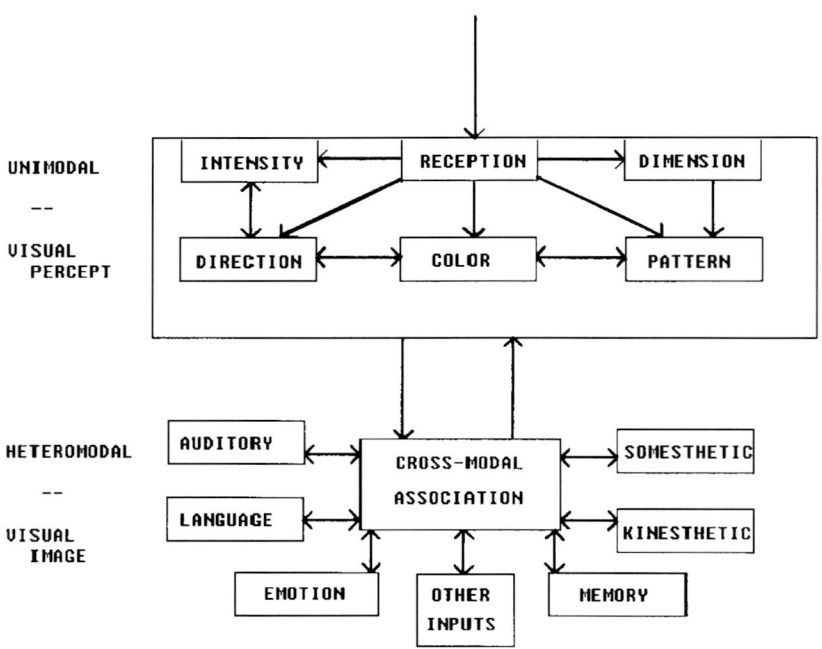

Fig. 7.8. Graphic presentation of the complex interactions necessary for visual image formation. Note the division into unimodal and heteromodal associations. The input to the unimodal processing area may be a visual stimulus (*upper area*), but similar activation can follow input from any of the processing units that interact in heteromodal associations.

information (memory) that has been processed and stored. A vast amount of previously learned, purely visual information must be available for categorization and single modality identification. To date, there is no firm knowledge of the neural mechanisms underlying this process, but that unimodal memory function is not the same as the memory function performed by limbic memory channels (see Chapter 9) is obvious—formation of visual percepts is fully normal in individuals with severe limbic memory disorders. The incomprehensibly large system needed to store visual information for comparison purposes represents a major aspect of elementary visual processing and a major memory resource. The same must be true for the other sensory modalities.

Heteromodal association, the fourth step in the formation of a visual image, links relevant information from stores of auditory and somesthetic modalities, emotion, frontal executive control, and other cerebral activities to identify and further categorize the visual percept. The enriched visual image formed in this step becomes an integral part of the thinking process. When the visual percept is linked with other information, an identified awareness is possible, which is called *recognition*.

A related visual activity, discrimination of position in space through the use of visual data, is of immense functional significance. Not only is relative placement of objects in extracorporeal space mediated primarily through visual processing, but visual–spatial discrimination plays an important role in our sense of body placement in space (body scheme). Visual–spatial gnosis is not readily assigned to a single neural network. From clinical observations we know that damage to a number of anatomical sites can interfere with visual–spatial discrimination. To a considerable degree, the nature of the visual–spatial disturbance depends on the site involved. For instance, environmental agnosia (Case 7.5) is consistently associated with damage to medial occipital cortex, whereas topographagnosia (Case 7.6) is associated with parietal convexity damage. Similar distinctions can be made for many higher level visual gnostic functions such as face or object recognition, constructional skills, and dressing ability, and case studies demonstrate that disorders of any one of these functions can occur without the others. No single cerebral site underlies visual–spatial discrimination. The even more complex function of visually oriented construction can be disrupted by damage to either hemisphere (Case 7.9) (Warrington, 1969), probably because any problem more complicated than the most elementary construction task demands both visual–spatial discrimination (right hemisphere) and motor execution (left hemisphere) activity.

Clinical experience strongly indicates that the right posterior hemisphere is more important for visual–spatial discrimination than other cerebral areas (Arrigoni and De Renzi, 1964) and can be considered dominant for visual–spatial competency in the way that the left hemisphere is dominant for language (Benson and Barton, 1970; Benton, 1967). In the hierarchy of visual sensory processing presented here, visual–spatial localization represents one aspect of the total information package necessary for the transmodal determination of the position of one object in reference to other objects in space.

The final stage, heteromodal processing, produces a visual image. For a visual image to be identified, information must be obtained from multiple sources that include but are not limited to visual memory stores. Moreover, a visual image can be triggered without stimulation of the primary visual sensory system. Auditory, emotional, and kinesthetic stimuli easily trigger cross-modal associations that lead to a visual image and visual identification. The palinopsia of Case 7.7 illustrates a visual phenomenon that can occur with brain pathology, but all normal humans experience visual images regularly in day-dreaming and imagination; the heteromodal association process provides a rational explanation for this phenomenon.

The steps of visual processing are performed rapidly, to the point of apparent simultaneity. Visual stimulation almost immediately produces a broad array of associations with multiple identifications. Most heteromodal associations remain subconscious; in fact, most visual stimuli entering the cortex do not reach the level of conscious awareness. Without attention to the stimulus, rapid degradation occurs. Only selected stimuli receive ongoing attention, but, as experiments in subliminal stimulation (Dixon, 1971; Hilgard, 1977) indicate, cross-modal processing of visually presented material can occur without conscious awareness and still lead to long-term retention. The range and limits of subliminal awareness (as exemplified by the use of hypnosis to extract subconscious information) remain unknown, but most processed sensory information goes unheeded and disappears.

Although visual processing is a distinct operation, its product is rapidly assimilated into the complex totality of mental processing, the stuff of thought. Conversely, stimuli from other sources, both external and internal, can trigger associations that produce visual imagery. Thinking may be possible without imagery (Humphrey, 1963), but most thought includes sensory input and, of these, visual images are of greatest consequence.

8

The Neurology of Communication Disorders

> The relation between thought and word is a living process: Thought is born through words. A word devoid of thought is a dead thing, and a thought unembodied in words remains a shadow. The connection between them, however, is not a preformed and constant one. It emerges in the course of development and itself evolves.
> —L. S. VYGOTSKY, 1934/1962

> Let it be admitted, then, that language is not the essence of thought. But this conclusion must be carefully limited. Apart from language, the retention of thought, the easy recall of thought, the interweaving of thought into higher complexity, the communication of thought, are all gravely limited.
> —ALFRED NORTH WHITEHEAD
> (QUOTED IN CRITCHLEY, 1970A)

AXIOMS/POSTULATES

Speech, language, and thought are distinct functions.

Language, the most widely recognized element of human thought, is not essential for thinking.

Language processing is intimately interrelated with many other mental functions that produce the material of thought.

Discrete neuroanatomical systems perform specific communication activities, but a single anatomical site may function in several different operations.

Despite long-standing acceptance of the fact that the brain controls speech, language, and thought, the neural correlates of language have a rather short and tumultuous history. At the beginning of the nineteenth century, Gall argued that mental attributes, including language, are the products of circumscribed areas of the brain, contradicting the established teaching that all mental functions, including language, were performed by the entire brain (Gall, 1825; Gall and Spurzheim, 1809). The holistic view prevailed until Broca's demonstration (1861) of language loss following damage to frontal brain regions and his later recognition (Broca, 1865) that only left hemisphere pathology (now called *aphasia*) caused language loss.

Following Broca, many observers reported cases of language loss due to focal brain damage and often embellished them with personal theories about the brain's role in language. Most notable was Wernicke (1874), who demonstrated the difference between a sensory, posteriorly localized aphasia and a motor, anteriorly localized aphasia. Wernicke's observation was elaborated (Lichtheim, 1885; Wernicke, 1881), and various neural theories of language were proposed (Bastian, 1887; Charcot, 1889; Dejerine, 1914/1977; Henschen, 1922; Kleist, 1934a; Nielsen, 1936/1948). Most of these theories correlated disturbance of an aspect of language function (e.g., reading) with damage to a given brain "center." Many were based on a single observation that could not be replicated. The process was called *diagram making* by Head (1926), who described the result as chaos.

The excesses of theorizing led, inevitably, to a countermovement. A more psychological, whole-brain approach to language rapidly gained ground (Freud, 1891/1953; Head, 1926; Isserlin, 1932; Jackson, 1868; Marie, 1906; Pick, 1931/1973; Schuell, Jenkins, and Jimenez-Pabon, 1964; Weisenburg and McBride, 1933/1964; Wepman and Jones, 1964; Wilson, 1926). Scientific data to support a unitary language function came from von Monakow and Mourque (1928), Lashley (1929), and others. Again, the pendulum swing became extreme; all impairment of language associated with brain damage was explained by the same mechanism—damage to a "central language processor"—augmented by focal motor or sensory dysfunction to explain the variations of language loss so obvious to the clinician.

Another shift, again sharp, occurred during the 1960s after Geschwind (1965) presented the disconnection theory. The localization approach to language study was resurrected. Numerous clinical–anatomical correlations were reported by such investigators as Benson (1979b), Goodglass (1978), Hécaen and Albert (1978), Kertesz (1979, 1983), Lhermitte and Gautier (1969), Luria (1947/1970), Penfield and Roberts (1959), and Poeck (1982), based on improved methods of language interpretation and anatomical correlation.

Concurrent with this increased interest in aphasia, a revolution was occurring in linguistics, often attributed to a single individual, Noam Chomsky (1957, 1975), who stressed the generative and transformational qualities of grammar. To Chomsky, the core process of language is syntax, the uniquely human capability of combining verbal symbols in a specific order to create a grammatically meaningful sentence. His approach challenged established linguistic theories and considerably broadened the scope of language/thought theorizing.

Language has been considered a royal road to the contemplation of thought and an essential element of thinking. While the relationship between language and thought has been approached from many directions, few would dispute that the neurological investigation of aphasia represents one of the most enlightening ways to correlate human language and the brain. It offers an obvious approach to the neurology of thinking.

VARIETIES OF COMMUNICATION DISORDERS

Communication embraces a complex variety of functions by which individuals share information. Some of the terms used to denote aspects of communication require discussion.

Definitions

Three functions—speech, language, and thought—are major components of human communication. Failure to distinguish these functions leaves a muddy field for inquiry. While absolute separation is not possible, common sense and everyday observation indicate that the differences are strong.

Speech refers to the output of meaningful communication produced by motor effectors. Verbalization, writing, gesture, facial grimacing, body posture, and other motor output aspects of communication all represent speech, broadly defined, and each is the product of specific neuromuscular components. Clinical observations readily isolate speech from other communication activities. A patient with bulbar paralysis or severe Parkinsonian rigidity has the knowledge to be communicated, but the output is hampered, to a greater or lesser degree, by mechanical disturbances. Speech disorders, by affecting the neuromuscular systems necessary for speech production, distort what would be an otherwise adequate verbal output.

Language is the encoding and decoding of semantic and syntactic elements used in some aspects of the production and comprehension of a thought or idea. While operationally related to the neuromuscular mechanisms of speech, language represents a different set of psychological functions.

Thought represents the ideas, not necessarily verbal, that will be put into the symbols and grammatical organization of language expressed through speech. That thought can occur without engaging linguistic or speech mechanisms is probable but difficult to prove (McGinn, 1982). Disordered thought, however, is a hallmark of some psychiatric disorders (see Chapter 12) and can occur with neither speech nor language malfunction (Benson, 1973).

As the terms representing the major elements of communication remain vague, many investigators (Binet, 1903; Critchley, 1967; Piaget, 1926; Sokolov, 1972; Vygotsky, 1934/1962) have proposed additional steps under labels such as *inner speech, internal speech, endophasia,* and *preverbiculum* (Critchley, 1967). "Inner speech" is more amorphous than an articulated utterance. It dispenses with some of the niceties of grammar and omits "empty" words; meaning-rich words constitute most of inner speech. Word order is logical, not conventional, as inner speech exists for the speaker, not the listener. Early developmental psychologists (Piaget, 1926; Vygotsky, 1934/1962) suggested that inner speech is a remnant of the child's initial egocentric speech that has survived as an incomplete language form existing between thought and the stylization of formal language.

Vygotsky (1934/1962) distinguished three forms of speech: inner speech, social speech, and written speech. Inner speech, speaking to oneself, is the least formal and omits most modifiers. Social speech is more complete but is routinely simplified, aided by the speaker's ability to communicate with gesture and vocal inflection plus information gathered by monitoring the listener's comprehension. Written speech must be considerably more formal with grammatically complete sentences, well-considered modifiers, and adequate background explanation as the speaker has no means of communication other than the written word. Inner speech, in this model, is a way-station in language formulation. Figure 8.1 presents a scheme of communication activities.

Brain damage often involves several aspects of communication simultaneously, but disorders that involve only one aspect are well known. For

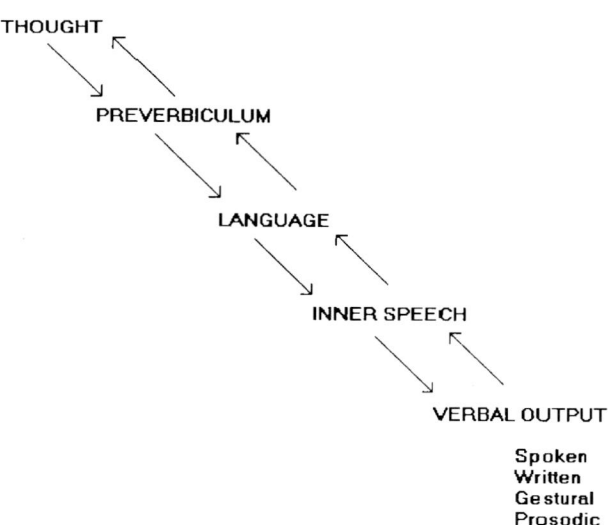

Fig. 8.1. Graphic conception of the flow of communication within the brain. The flow is bidirectional. Thought, language, and verbal output are clearly separated; preverbiculum and inner speech, while not readily defined, represent logical intermediate steps in the processing of communication.

Table 8.1. Four Types of Language

Language Function	Left Hemisphere	Right Hemisphere
Gestural (motor) language	Participates	Participates
Prosodic (vocal) language		
Rhythm	Dominates	
Inflection	Participates	Participates
Timbre	Participates	Participates
Melody		Dominates
Semantic (meaningful) language		
Verbal meaning	Dominates	
Concept formation	Participates	Particpates
Visual imagery		Dominates
Syntactic (relational) language		
Sequencing	Dominates	
Relationships	Dominates	

Adapted from Benson, 1986.

instance, the output disorder following laryngectomy involves speech alone. Such individuals have neither thought nor language disorder but cannot communicate their ideas through vocal speech. Similarly, some aphasic patients have only a single disordered language attribute. Pure word-finding, reading, and comprehension disorders may be unrelated to either speech or thought abnormality. Finally, in the early stages of some types of dementia and in some psychotic disturbances, ideation alone may be disordered. Although these three aspects of communication are intimately associated, recognition of their differences helps toward understanding communication disorders.

Language can be further characterized by dividing it into four varieties—gestural, prosodic, semantic, and syntactic (Ross, et al. 1981) (Table 8.1). *Gestural* language refers to alterations of body position and facial expression used to convey meaning. Smiling, frowning, or grimacing, shaking a fist or waving a hand, stooping or twisting the body, and many other gestures convey meaning and are routinely monitored as aids to communication. Gestures can be considered a language of body movements (Birdwhistell, 1952; Critchley, 1975; Hall, 1959).

Closely related to gestural language is a form of motor expression called *prosody*. Unfortunately, prosody has been broadly and variously defined (Darkins et al., 1988; Monrad-Krohn, 1947; Ross, 1981). For this chapter, four elements of prosody will be stressed: melody, inflection, rhythm, and timbre. All four are present in normal vocalization, but in clinical practice one or more may be disordered while the others are not. As noted in Chapter 6, melody may be seriously disturbed following right frontal damage, whereas the other aspects of prosody are affected little or not at all (Alexander, Benson, and Stuss, 1989; Ross, 1981; Ross and Mesulam, 1979). Conversely, rhythm appears to depend on an intact left frontal control system. Most higher mammals communicate freely with both gestural and prosodic language. Thus the elevated ruff, bared teeth, and body tension of an angry dog obviously have different meaning than the happy, jumping, tail-wagging postures seen under other circumstances. Similarly, the tonal differences of the snarl, the warning bark, and the happy, excited bark are readily appreciated. These two forms of language—gesture and prosody—are not uniquely human and can be disturbed by damage in either hemisphere.

The other two language types are predominantly or exclusively human. *Semantic language* refers to substantive words and their symbolic meaning (Goodglass et al., 1966; Katz and Fodor, 1963; Osgood, Suci, and Tannenbaum, 1957). Words represent (symbolize) actions, objects, emotional states, and so forth. Individual words often have different meanings (e.g., pen as a writing instrument or an abridgement of *penitentiary*). Conversely, single ideas or meanings are often represented by multiple words. Different languages have strikingly different semantic contents (e.g., Navaho and Bantu vs. English and French) (Pei, 1949; Sapir, 1921). Animal studies have shown that a few higher primates can learn a limited lexicon of semantically significant symbols (Gardner and Gardner, 1969; Premack, 1971). In contrast, the human lexicon is monumental and apparently demands participation by much of the brain. Words represent a shorthand, allowing a myriad of information to be coded, interchanged, and stored efficiently. Table 8.1 indicates that both hemispheres function in some aspects of semantics.

Syntax refers to the organizational, relational aspects of language. It includes both a corpus of terms used to portray relationships (e.g., prepositions, many adjectives, and adverbs) and the serial ordering of individual words to produce grammatically proper, meaningful utterances (e.g., the difference between mother's brother and brother's mother). Comparative linguistics suggests that syntax represents the most highly developed of language faculties (Chomsky, 1957; Goodglass, 1968), a competency that is virtually absent in animals.

Various combinations of normal and disordered language elements comprise the structure of aphasic syndromes (Hécaen and Angelergues, 1964), and some of the disordered elements and their terminology must be defined in order to discuss the case examples. The basic clinical disorders include *aphasia,* defined as the loss or impairment of language function due to brain damage; *alexia,* the loss or impairment of the ability to comprehend written or printed language; and *agraphia,* the loss or impairment of the ability to produce written language (Benson, 1979b). Several fundamental elements of language that are disrupted by brain damage deserve description.

Fundamental Language Functions

Spontaneous Speech. Spontaneous speech comprises the quality of conversational speech and is characterized by rate, articulatory competency, degree of effort, phrase length, prosodic quality, paraphasia, content, and grammatical sufficiency of the verbal output. By tradition, spontaneous speech is divided into two categories—fluent and nonfluent (Benson, 1967; Jackson, 1864; Poeck, Kerchensteiner, and Hartje, 1972; Wagenaar, Snow, and Prins, 1975; Wernicke, 1881). Table 8.2 presents the eight characteristics that distinguish nonfluent from fluent aphasic outputs. Nonfluent aphasic output most often occurs when the language-dominant hemisphere is damaged anterior to the central sulcus; fluent aphasia is most often associated with lesions posterior to this area (Fig. 8.2). Unfortunately, the terms *fluent* and *nonfluent* imply flow, and interpretations of spontaneous speech based on the characteristic of flow alone will not provide the information needed to characterize verbal output.

Repetition of Spoken Language. A valuable, straightforward language function concerns the ability to repeat verbal material, ranging from single digits to complex sentences. In general, inability to repeat spoken language in an aphasic patient indicates an abnormality involving the perisylvian language structures, whereas significant aphasia with intact repetition suggests involvement of the vascular border zone areas (Fig. 8.3).

Comprehension of Spoken Language. The ability to comprehend spoken language is disturbed to some degree following damage to many parts of the language area of the brain. Differences in comprehension disability reflect the involvement of different neural systems needed for full understanding of spoken language (Benson, 1979b). Inability to comprehend semantically specific names (e.g., point to a named object), to comprehend grammatically pertinent structures (e.g., the difference between *in* the house and *on* the house), or to comprehend and maintain sequences of

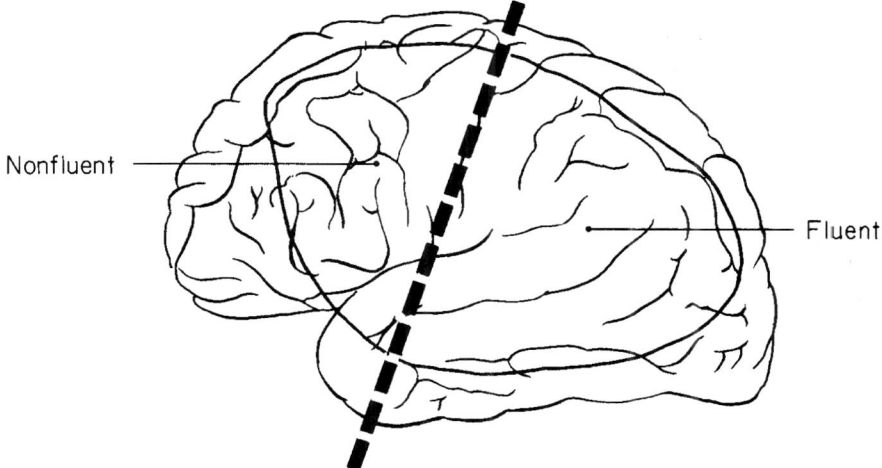

Fig. 8.2. Simple diagram of the left hemisphere outlining the language area divided by a *broad broken line* that separates anterior (nonfluent) and posterior (fluent) language areas.

Table 8.2. Fluent/Nonfluent Aphasic Output Characteristics

Characteristic	Nonfluent	Fluent
Quantity of output	Sparse	Normal (or excessive)
Effort in Production	Considerable	Normal (easy)
Articulation	Dysarthric	Normal
Phrase length	Short (1 or 2 words)	Normal (5–8 words)
Prosody	Abnormal (dysprosodic)	Normal
Grammatical structures	Often omitted (agrammatism)	Normal
Content words	Normal or higher in frequency	Often omitted
Paraphasia	Uncommon (mainly literal)	Common (both literal and semantic)

related material (e.g., maintain multiple items in sequential order) (De Renzi and Vignolo, 1962) are among the variations in disordered comprehension noted by clinicians. Although most commonly associated with temporoparietal pathology, the comprehension of spoken language is so complex that some abnormality of this function is present in most individuals with acquired language disorder, irrespective of the locus of pathology.

Naming. The ability to present a name when shown an object, action, color, and so forth is a standard test for language competency but often proves difficult to interpret. Distinct variations of word-finding defect (anomia) are recognized (Geschwind, 1967a; Luria, 1966), and neuroanatomical correlations based on the characteristics of the naming disorder have been proposed (Benson, 1979b, 1988b).

Reading. In testing reading disorders, the ability to comprehend written material (a language function) must be distinguished from the ability to read out loud (a motor speech function). Some patients with impaired language function can comprehend written material but cannot read aloud; the opposite, inability to comprehend written material that can be correctly read out loud, is also seen (Benson, 1985; Dejerine, 1892).

Writing. Competency in writing is limited in most humans, particularly compared with competency in oral output. Writing disorder (agraphia) is the language dysfunction most frequently seen with brain damage. Two varieties of agraphia—aphasic and mechanical—are easily recognized, a distinction that mirrors the differences between language and speech disorders (Benson and Cummings, 1985).

CLINICAL EXAMPLES

Disorders of communication are rarely pure or precise. Mixtures of speech, language, and thought disorders are common, as are mixtures of

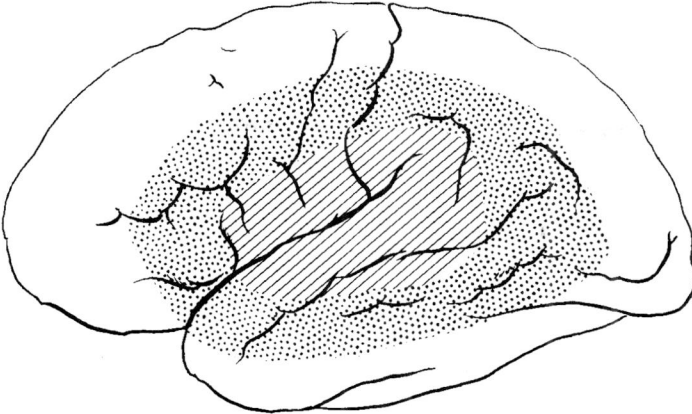

Fig. 8.3. Outline of the left hemisphere with the overall language area divided into two clinically distinct areas—a central peri-Sylvian area (*parallel lines*) and an outer border zone area (*stippled*). Structural lesions involving the peri-Sylvian area produce repetition defects. Pathology involving border zone area produces aphasia with retained repetition ability.

the varieties of aphasia. The picture is confusing, but the clinical cases described over the past century reveal that certain clusters of disordered language tend to recur. In some instances only a single aspect of communication function is involved.

Case 8.1

A 20-year-old student was a passenger in a motor vehicle involved in a head-on collision. He was rendered unconscious and remained in coma for nine days. When he regained consciousness a bilateral ptosis, more pronounced on the right than the left, and irregular, dysconjugate eye movements were noted, as were a partial right third nerve paresis and limb clumsiness, greater on the left than on the right. The movement disorder had components of both spastic paresis and cerebellar ataxia. When the patient regained conversational ability, there was a striking alteration in his verbal output. He had a full vocabulary, comprehended spoken language in a normal manner, and could repeat, name, read and write, but communication was hampered by a prolongation of verbal output. Almost all words and even some syllables of multisyllabic words were pronounced individually and with almost uniform inflection. The output was mechanical (it resembled electronic verbalization)—a disturbance called *scanning speech*. Imaging techniques showed enlargement of the aqueduct of Sylvius in the midbrain. (DFB)

The clinical findings in Case 8.1 suggest that damage to the upper brain stem produced coma and partial third nerve paresis greater on the right than on the left. In their review of this disorder, Kremer, Russell, and Smyth (1947) suggested that damage to the ascending dentato-rubro-thalamic tract and the descending motor tract of the cerebral peduncle just above the red nucleus (where these paths abut each other) produced the unusual combination of cerebellar ataxia and upper motor neuron paralysis of the same limbs. An accompaniment of this sharply focal neurological pattern was the scanning speech, a motor disturbance that involved neither language nor thought.

Case 8.2
A 32-year-old, left-handed man arrived at a hospital in an alert, mobile, but mute status. Phonation was limited to the production of gutteral sounds. A right arm weakness had been reported, but by the time of hospitalization both physical and neurological examinations were within normal limits. There was no evidence of primary laryngeal pathology, but a buccofacial apraxia was noted. Thus, when asked to whistle, stick out his tongue, wrinkle his nose, and so on, the patient failed, whereas similar requests for limb or whole-body movements were readily carried out. He could not express himself spontaneously, repeat spoken language, or name objects. On the other hand, he expressed himself in full and correct sentences with pencil and paper, could write the names of all objects presented, and wrote to dictation without difficulty. His comprehension of spoken language appeared to be intact. The clinical picture was termed *aphemia*. The patient's verbal output slowly improved but remained difficult to understand because of breathiness, lack of inflection, low volume, and slow, hesitant verbalization. This gradually improved, but the cadence and inflection remained altered, suggesting a foreign accent. Figure 8.4 shows a small lesion in the left frontal opercular area undercutting Broca's area in the left hemisphere of this patient. (DFB)

Case 8.2 illustrates another pure disorder of motor expression but with different features. The original mutism without laryngeal or language disorder (called *aphemia* or *pure word dumbness*) developed into an

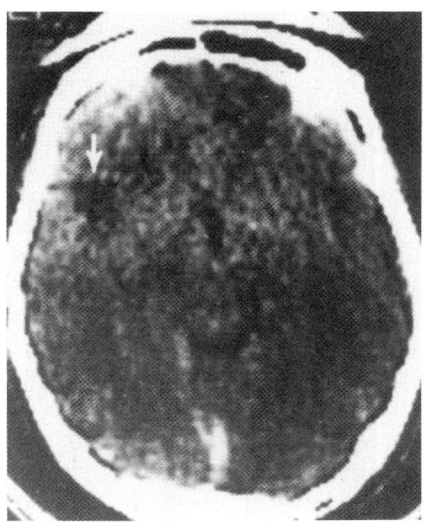

Fig. 8.4. X-ray CT scan of Case 8.2 demonstrating a small lucency (*arrow*) undercutting Broca's area in the left hemisphere. From Stuss and Benson, 1986.

expressive abnormality characterized by a purely prosodic disturbance in which rhythm and inflection were sufficiently altered that the patient seemed to be speaking English as a second language (called the *foreign accent syndrome*). Well described by Bastian (1898), this clinical syndrome has also been called *cortical anarthria*. Both cortical (Bastian, 1898; Mohr, 1973, 1976) and immediate subcortical (Souques, 1928; Mohr, 1973) loci of pathology involving the dominant hemisphere operculum (Broca's area) have been reported. Monrad-Krohn (1947) noted the persistent dysprosody that follows improvement and described the foreign accent residual. The motor output dysfunctions of Cases 8.1 and 8.2 represent two of the many forms of motor speech disorder in which neither language nor thought is involved.

Many other sites of pure speech disturbance can be localized in the subcortex, diencephalon, and brain stem (Darley, Aronson, and Brown, 1975), and some evidence suggests a purely cortical dysarthria (Tonkonogy and Goodglass, 1981). While speech and language disorder are often combined, the mechanical aspects of speech have their own neural basis (Darley, Aronson, and Brown, 1975; Metter, 1985).

Case 8.3

A 47-year-old man was hospitalized for treatment of purulent drainage from both ears. Antibiotic treatment proved ineffective, and he suffered a grand mal seizure followed by a lethargic state. A mass lesion was found in the left temporal lobe and an abscess involving the midportion of the left second temporal gyrus was surgically drained. Subsequent recovery was comparatively uneventful.

For the first few days after the operation the patient was unable to comprehend spoken language, and his verbal output was a jargon. This cleared rapidly. His conversational speech was fluent and effortless until a substantive word, particularly a noun that indicated a specific and imageable item, was necessary. Sometimes he would say "I can't think of that word," but more often he described the function of the object. Thus his attempt to say pencil was "Oh, I can't think of the name, it's the thing I pick up to write with." If the name was spoken by the examiner, the patient immediately identified the correct item. He had no problem with comprehension or repetition of spoken language, and he read adequately, both aloud and for comprehension. He had great difficulty with tests of naming ability, rarely producing the correct name for an item but almost always describing the item and its function. At times the description would include the desired name. Thus, when asked to name a comb, he said "That's the thing I use to comb my hair. Hey, that's the word—that's a comb." In speaking he sometimes used the correct word but did not realize it. When shown a hammer, he said "That's the thing I use to hammer in a nail, but I can't remember what it's called." The ease with which he pointed to a named object was in dramatic contrast to his inability to name the same object. (DFB)

The major problem in Case 8.3 was impaired presentation of names of imageable items. That the patient recognized objects that he could not name was affirmed by his lucid descriptions of their function. Called *amnesic aphasia* (Goldstein, 1924; Weisenburg and McBride, 1933/1964),

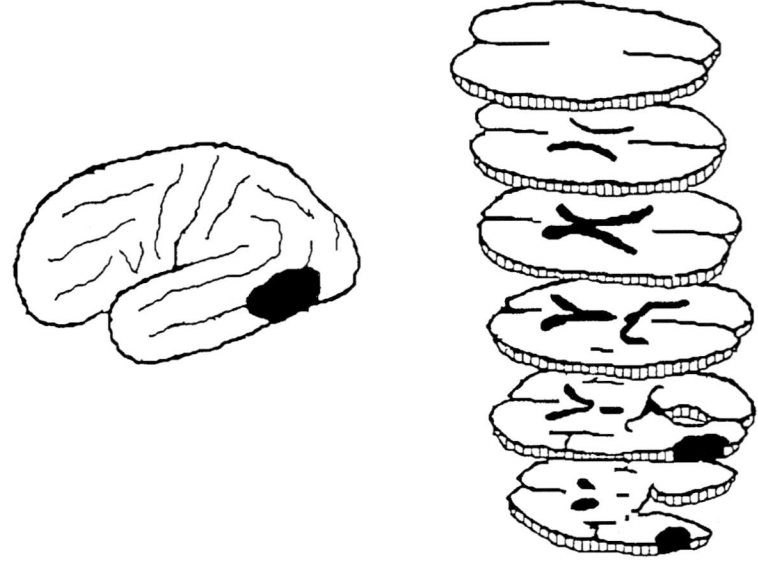

Fig. 8.5. Schematic conception of a left hemisphere lesion involving Brodmann area 37. From Alexander and Benson, 1991.

anomic aphasia (Goodglass and Kaplan, 1972), *verbal aphasia* (Head, 1926), and *word selection anomia* (Benson, 1979a), this disorder most often is associated with damage to the left posterior-inferior temporal lobe. In Case 8.3 the lesion involved the posterior aspects of the second temporal gyrus and the superior portion of area 37 (Nielsen, 1936/1948), the junction of the inferior temporal lobe with the occipital lobe. Figure 8.5 illustrates the location of area 37.

Case 8.4

A 52-year-old, right-handed man was admitted to the hospital for treatment of seizures and cardiac arrhythmia. He was in atrial fibrillation and was said to have "an obvious right hemiparesis with aphasia." The paresis quickly improved, and he was transferred to the neurology service for evaluation and treatment of the language disorder. His verbal output was fluent but loud, with exaggerated melody and inflection. Paraphasias (language substitutions) were rare. Repetition was impossible, though, in contrast, the patient easily named objects. His comprehension of spoken language was severely impaired but he recognized and named nonverbal sounds (e.g., telephone ring, hand clapping, dog barking). He could read aloud and showed normal comprehension. He expressed his own thoughts in writing without difficulty but could not write to dictation. (DFB)

In Case 8.4, the problem was an inability to comprehend orally presented language that contrasted sharply with the patient's full competency in using written language. A diagnosis of word deafness was made, and over the next few months he improved sufficiently to warrant a diagnosis of "pure" word deafness. Again, only a single function, the reception of spoken language, was involved.

Case 8.5

A 53-year-old postal employee was admitted directly to the hospital from his workplace following the onset of a rapidly progressive right hemiparesis. An initial confusional state cleared rapidly. Conversational speech became fluent but with evidence of some word-finding problems (emptiness). Comprehension of spoken language was fully normal, and repetition was intact. The patient had difficulty naming objects, even common ones, on confrontation, but always showed that he recognized the object by manually or verbally demonstrating its use. He could spell out loud and immediately recognized words that were spelled aloud. He could write, both to command and to dictation, but he *completely failed to interpret written language*. He could name a few individual letters but recognized no written words, not even his own name. In contrast, he read numbers aloud and even performed simple arithmetic problems. The disorder was called *alexia without agraphia*.

Both the paresis and the sensory loss improved, though right homonymous hemianopia and the reading disturbance remained. Figure 8.6 shows an infarction involving the medial aspect of the left occipital lobe; it can be surmised that the splenium of the corpus callosum was also damaged. (Benson and Tomlinson, 1971)

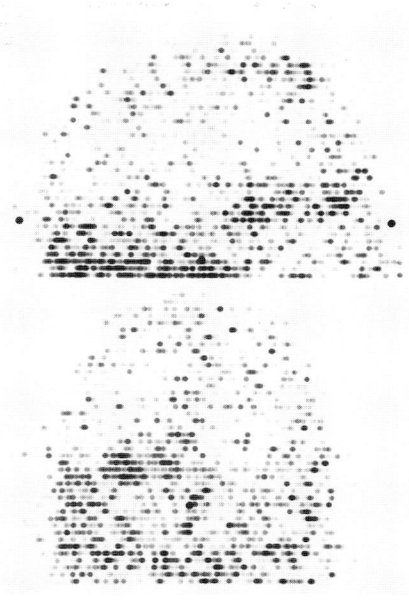

Fig. 8.6. A radioisotope brain scan of Case 8.5 showing increased radioactivity in the left occipital region in the territory of the left posterior cerebral artery. From Benson and Tomlinson, 1971.

In Case 8.5, an extensive left posterior cerebral artery infarction produced alexia (impairment of reading) without agraphia, a dramatic disorder first described a century ago by Dejerine (1892). All aspects of language function were intact except for the transmission of visual language symbols from the right visual cortex to the appropriate heteromodal association area for interpretation and recognition.

In each of these clinical examples a single aspect of communication was significantly involved, leaving other communication functions relatively intact. In Case 8.1, a focal brain stem lesion produced disordered verbal output but did not affect language or thought. Case 8.2 demonstrates a different and more complicated speech disturbance, one in which a lesion located just inferior to the motor speech cortex first produced mutism, then a breathy, hypophonic, and slow output with eventual recovery to a status of altered prosody. Language was not altered. Case 8.3 suffered a language disorder, loss of the ability to retrieve names, but no other language disorder.

The pure word deafness syndrome of Case 8.4 is a well-known clinical entity, familiar to most aphasiologists. In this case, as in other disorders that can be called "pure," the ability to handle language was not disturbed; the disturbance involved only the reception of auditory signals. Two distinctly different neuropathological patterns of pure word deafness have been recorded (Barrett, 1910; Schuster and Taterka, 1926; Weisenburg and McBride, 1933/1964). In one pattern, pathology involves the medial aspect of the left posterior temporal lobe, affecting the primary auditory cortex (Heschl's gyrus) and/or fibers carrying auditory sensory stimuli into Heschl's gyrus. It is assumed that auditory language signals are not received, that they never reach the dominant hemisphere auditory association cortex for interpretation as language. In the other neuropathological pattern, pure word deafness stems from bilateral damage to the medial aspects of the temporal lobes (Goldstein, 1974). Auerbach et al. (1982) postulated that the bilateral lesions interfered with auditory span, obstructing the ability to maintain the sequence of auditory signals characterizing spoken language.

Case 8.5 represents another well-known disturbance, alexia without agraphia (Ajax, 1964; Dejerine, 1892), also called *posterior alexia* (Benson, 1985) and many other names. The dramatic discrepancy between the ability to write and the inability to read written material has been closely studied. Since Dejerine's original description (1892) of the syndrome, a fairly consistent pathology has been reported: involvement of the dominant posterior cerebral artery territory plus damage to the splenium of the corpus callosum (Damasio, 1985b; Gloning et al., 1955; Greenblatt, 1983). A similar clinical picture is associated with structural damage, usually from neoplasm or hematoma, that undercuts the angular gyrus (subangular alexia) (Greenblatt, 1973, 1977). In all instances, visual language signals cannot reach the dominant hemisphere language area for processing. There is little disturbance of language except for the inability to interpret writing.

Each case (8.1 to 8.5) features a relatively pure processing disturbance, but only one (the pure anomia of Case 8.3) involved language function. The others involved sensory input or motor output.

Case 8.6

A 69-year-old woman was examined nine years after suffering a cerebrovascular accident. Her verbal output was effortful, hesitant, and lacking in grammatical function words. Articulation was seriously disturbed and repetition was involved although not as severely as spontaneous speech. Object naming was poor but improved considerably with phonetic cues. The patient produced some written language, but her writing was effortful, clumsy, and agrammatic. Her comprehension of spoken language was relatively intact for short, simple material. She easily pointed to objects named singly but failed if the same object names were presented as a sequence of three of four. Similarly, she could recognize a few written words but could not understand a sentence. She consistently failed to recognize grammatical words (prepositions, articles), whether written or spoken. A CT scan revealed a sizable lesion involving much of the left posterior inferior frontal lobe (Fig. 8.7). A diagnosis of a persistent Broca's aphasia was made. (Stuss and Benson, 1986)

The aphasia of Case 8.6 features disturbed language output and has been called *expressive* or *motor aphasia*. The problem goes beyond pure motor speech disorder, however, as demonstrated by the written language dysfunction and the persistent inability to comprehend grammatical (syntactical) words in either spoken or written discourse. The term *Broca's aphasia* is most commonly used for this disorder characterized by nonfluent output, relatively preserved comprehension, poor repetition,

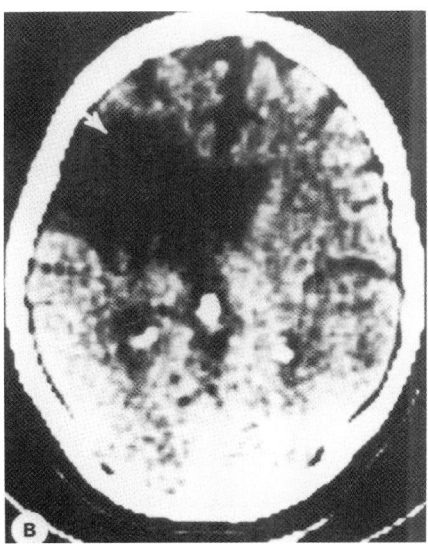

Fig. 8.7. X-ray CT scan demonstrating a large lesion in the anterior portion of the left hemisphere of Case 8.6. From Stuss and Benson, 1986.

poor naming, and limited ability to read or write with particular difficulties interpreting syntactical language.

Case 8.7

A 47-year-old man suffered an acute cerebrovascular accident, presumably due to an embolus. At the onset he was mute with striking buccofacial apraxia, limb apraxia, and agraphia but only a mild right-sided motor weakness. Comprehension of spoken language was preserved except for sentence-length material dependent on passive tense or possessives. The patient made a rapid recovery. In the early stages his speech was effortful, and he tended to omit syntactical structures. Within four months there was no paresis, his verbal output contained appropriate grammatical structures, and he produced complex sentences. Hesitations were frequent, with prolonged transition from one word to the next or from one phoneme to the next, producing an arrhythmic, dysprosodic verbal output. He had problems with some grammatical structures such as verb tense, a mild visual confrontation naming defect, and limited ability to generate word lists (names in a specified category); even so, his ability to communicate was functional. A diagnosis of "recovered" Broca's aphasia or "little Broca" aphasia was suggested. A relatively small lesion involved the posterior inferior frontal lobe and the underlying white matter tissues (Fig. 8.8). (Stuss and Benson, 1986)

The original language problem of Case 8.7 was a language disorder with the characteristics of Broca's aphasia, but this rapidly improved to a state that might be called *aphemia plus,* the aphemia of Case 8.2 plus persistence of agrammatism. The terms *little Broca* and *big Broca* have been

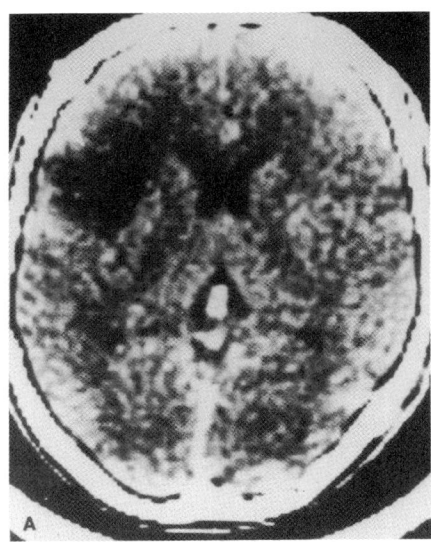

Fig. 8.8. X-ray CT scan of the left hemisphere of Case 8.7 demonstrating a radiolucency involving the opercular region of the left hemisphere but not extending deep to the ventricle or basal ganglia. Compare with Figure 8.7. From Stuss and Benson, 1986.

suggested to delineate the difference (Mohr et al., 1978; Stuss and Benson, 1986). Big Broca usually starts as a global aphasia, but with time comprehension improves more than expression, leaving a Broca-type aphasia. Little Broca starts with nonfluent aphasia but relatively normal comprehension and improves to a mild motor speech disorder with some degree of agrammatism.

Case 8.8

A 76-year-old physician had an acute onset of confusion while at work. His verbal output was rapid but contaminated by many paraphasic substitutions of phonemes and words (neologistic jargon). In addition, his comprehension of spoken language and his ability to repeat it were severely impaired. He could not comprehend written language. His attempts to write produced real letters in meaningless combinations. He could not name, always making paraphasic substitutions that he often augmented with additional jargon to define the use of the object. There was no weakness, sensory loss, or visual field defect. Over the next few months the quantity of jargon decreased, particularly the semantic substitutions. Comprehension and repetition improved only slightly, however. An isotope brain scan revealed a focal lesion in the left posterior superior temporal region, and a diagnosis of Wernicke's aphasia was made. (Kertesz and Benson, 1970)

Wernicke's aphasia is the most commonly used name for an aphasic disorder in which verbal output is fluent but comprehension of both spoken and written language is severely disordered. Sometimes called *receptive* or *sensory aphasia,* the disorder goes beyond the pure sensory/reception problem seen in Case 8.4, as language is not comprehended, paraphasias are prominent, and naming ability is deficient. Both sensory processing (reception, discrimination) and language processing (heteromodal associations) are involved.

Case 8.9

A 73-year-old retired businessman was admitted to the hospital for treatment of a language disturbance. The neurological examination was normal except for a right visual field defect, most pronounced in the upper quadrant, a mild right facial paresis, and a minimal sensory impairment. Conversational speech was fluent but interrupted by frequent word-finding pauses. Three- to five-word phrases were produced with normal inflection and rhythm. Literal and verbal paraphasias were evident. Comprehension appeared intact through a series of demanding tests. Repetition of spoken language was severely disturbed. While the patient could repeat single digits and occasional single syllable words, double digits, multisyllabic words, phrases, or sentences were contaminated with multiple paraphasic substitutions. When asked to name on confrontation, he was often incorrect because of literal paraphasic substitutions. Reading aloud produced paraphasic jargon, but he fully comprehended the written material. He was unable to write. Prominent buccofacial and limb apraxia persisted. A diagnosis of conduction aphasia with ideomotor apraxia was made.

The patient died several years later after a second cerebrovascular accident. At postmortem a large, recent infarction was found in the right hemisphere. The left hemisphere showed several small, old infarcts, the most striking of which involved both the cortical surface and the underlying white matter of the left supramarginal gyrus. (Benson et al., 1973)

Conduction aphasia refers to an aphasic abnormality in which comprehension is intact (or nearly so), verbal output is fluent, but repetition is severely disturbed by paraphasias (Benson et al., 1973). While written language is comprehended, it cannot be read out loud. Ideomotor apraxia and naming disturbances are seen in some but not all cases. The most common site of pathology is the supramarginal gyrus of the dominant hemisphere (Damasio and Damasio, 1980) but other sites have been reported (Kleist, 1934a), and the disconnection of auditory comprehension areas from motor speech areas is considered crucial to the syndrome (Mendez and Benson, 1985). Figure 8.9 shows the CT scan of a patient with conduction aphasia.

Case 8.10
A 64-year-old man was referred for evaluation of persistent aphasia secondary to a cerebrovascular accident approximately three months earlier. A nonfluent output with sparse, dysarthric, and effortful verbalization and a right hemiparesis had been present. The paresis cleared over several weeks, leaving only slight clumsiness plus hyperactive reflexes on the right. The patient's verbal output, however, remained limited, effortful, hypophonic, and poorly articulated. Most verbalizations consisted of a single significant word; rarely was there a preposition or modifier. Comprehension was relatively intact, failing only when complex sequences of material were presented. Repetition was excellent, standing in stark contrast to the limited, nonfluent spontaneous output. The patient could name most objects but often needed prompting. He could read, both out loud and for comprehension. He did not write spontaneously but could write to dictation. A diagnosis of transcortical motor aphasia was made. (DFB)

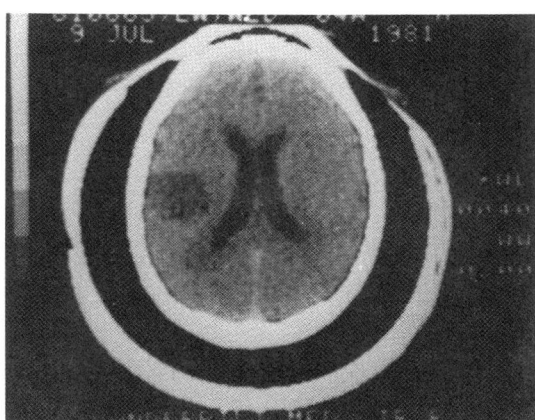

Fig. 8.9. X-ray CT scan demonstrating a well-demarcated radiolucency in the region of the arcuate fasciculus of the left hemisphere in a patient with conduction aphasia. From Kirshner, 1986.

The term *transcortical aphasia* has long been used to designate a disorder in which repetition is intact but one or more other language parameters are abnormal. Transcortical motor aphasia resembles Broca's aphasia except for the intact repetition. Luria and Tsvetkova (1967) suggested the term *dynamic aphasia* to highlight the patient's difficulty in initiating verbal output. Pathology involving the frontal tissues anterior and/or superior to Broca's area is present in transcortical motor aphasia (Freedman, Alexander, and Naeser, 1984; Rubens, 1976).

Case 8.11

A 47-year-old professional piano player was admitted for language therapy. He was unable to give a history. The neurological examination showed a mild right hyperreflexia, and sensory testing revealed astereognosis, defective two-point discrimination, and difficulty with position sense in the right upper extremity, but his appreciation of pain was intact and no visual field defect could be demonstrated.

Language testing showed a limited but fluent output, consisting mostly of phrases such as "You know" and "Oh boy" plus neologistic and semantic paraphasias. Almost no information was conveyed by the patient's conversational speech. He regularly failed tests of comprehension but appeared to gather some meaning from conversational speech (probably by interpreting verbal inflection and gesture). He was unable to name, most often producing generalizations (e.g., "one of those things") or a semantic substitution. Both reading and writing were severely disturbed. In marked contrast, his repetition of spoken language was flawless to the level of long, complex sentences. He even reproduced spoken nonsense material without difficulty. A diagnosis of transcortical sensory aphasia was made, and an isotope brain scan demonstrated a large parietal disturbance located above and slightly posterior to the Sylvian fissure. (DFB)

Case 8.11 exemplifies transcortical sensory aphasia with fluent output, severe comprehension disorder, but good repetition. In this case, like most others in the literature, the pathology involved the posterior vascular border zone area but spared Wernicke's area (Alexander, Hiltbrunner, and Fischer, 1989). If both anterior and posterior border zones are damaged, a mixed transcortical aphasia—a global aphasia with good repetition—is the result.

Case 8.12

A 74-year-old male suffered acute right hemiplegia and aphasia while participating in a St. Patrick's Day Parade. At the hospital he was alert and oriented but mute and had a right hemiplegia, right hemisensory loss, and right homonymous hemianopia. CT scan showed a sizable hematoma deep in the left hemisphere involving thalamus and internal capsule.

Over a course of several weeks the patient developed a soft, slow, throaty verbal output with many literal paraphasias. His comprehension was adequate to limited complexity levels, but naming produced paraphasias. In contrast, he could repeat four- to five-word sentences without paraphasias. He improved consistently, and by two months after onset his verbal output was only mildly hypophonic, slightly slow, and without paraphasia. The hemiplegia, hemisensory loss, and visual field disturbance, on the other hand, remained dense, and a repeat CT examination showed a residual area of lucency in the site of the hematoma. The diagnosis was subcortical (thalamic) aphasia following an intracerebral hemorrhage. Figure 8.10 shows both the acute and the follow-up CT scans. (DFB)

Case 8.12 also had aphasia with intact comprehension, but the pathology was deep in the dominant hemisphere tissues. Recovery of language functions was relatively rapid despite the remaining structural defect.

Table 8.3 presents one of the many classifications of aphasia based on clusters of salient features. This scheme correlates the six basic language functions discussed earlier plus characteristic neurological dysfunctions and the locus of pathology characteristic for each syndrome.

No two aphasic patients perform exactly the same on a series of language tests, but a sizable majority of aphasics are better placed in one feature cluster than in any other (Benson, 1979b; Howes, 1964; Kertesz, 1979). The syndromes listed in Table 8.3 were developed over decades and should not be considered rigid or precise. Modifications in clinical features and improved techniques for clinicopathological correlation continue to refine the categorization. For instance, Cases 8.6 and 8.7 are both diagnosed as Broca's aphasia, but they are quite different. Modifying terms such as big Broca/little Broca or recovered/persistent Broca's aphasia, while unsatisfactory, help to demarcate variations. Classification remains a problem.

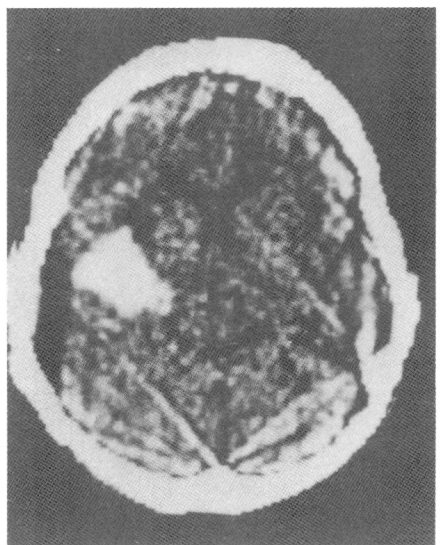 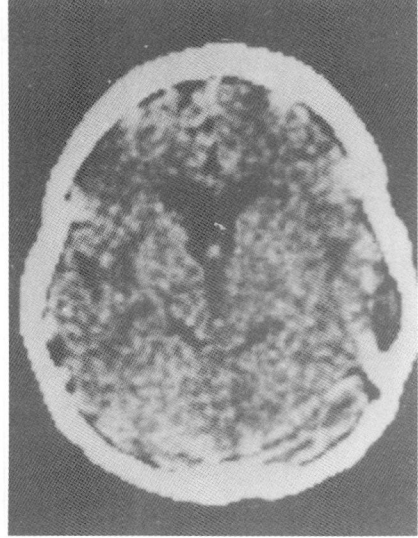

Fig. 8.10. X-ray CT scans, exposed acutely (*left*) and several months later (*right*), illustrating the site of the left hemisphere intracerebral hemorrhage in Case 8.12. Note the area of lucency in the later scan demonstrating persistent damage. While originally aphasic, there was no aphasia at the time of the second CT scan.

Table 8.3. Classification of Aphasia

Type of Aphasia	Spontaneous Speech	Repetition	Comprehension	Naming	Reading	Writing	Motor	Sensory	Visual Field	Anatomical Locus (Dominant Hemisphere)
Broca's aphasia	NF	−	+	−	−	−	−	+	+	Posterior inferior frontal
Wernicke's aphasia	F,P	−	−	−	−	−	+	±	±	Posterior superior temporal
Conduction aphasia	F,P	−	+	−	+	−	+	−	+	Supramarginal gyrus
Global aphasia	NF	−	−	−	−	−	−	−	−	Perisylvian language area
Transcortical motor	NF	+	+	−	+	−	±	+	+	Frontal, anterior, and/or superior to broca's area
Transcortical sensory	F,P	+	−	−	−	−	+	−	−	Parietal–temporal border zone
Transcortical mixed	NF	+	−	−	−	−	−	−	−	Arterial border zone area
Anomic aphasia	F	+	+	−	+	+	+	+	+	—
Subcortical aphasia	F,P	+	+	+	+	+	−	−	−	Subcortical nuclei or tracts

Adapted from Benson, 1981.

NF, nonfluent; F, fluent; P, paraphasia; +, normal; −, abnormal; ±, either normal or abnormal.

Table 8.4. Frontal Language Disorders

Aphemia	Lower motor cortex and posterior operculum
Broca's asphasia	
Little	Lower motor cortex and full operculum
Big	Lower motor cortex and full operculum plus deep extension
Transcortical motor aphasia	Dorsolateral frontal (cortex or deep white matter)
Supplementary motor area aphasia	Medial (sagittal) frontal lobe superior to corpus callosum

Adapted from Alexander, Benson, and Stuss, 1989.

Table 8.4 presents a subclassification of frontal language disturbances including the area of frontal lobe damage most often associated with them (Alexander, Benson, and Stuss, 1989). Aphemia (Case 8.2) is primarily a disturbance of motor speech while transcortical motor aphasia (Case 8.10) appears to be a disturbance of activation. Formal language is largely intact in both disorders. In contrast, both types of Broca's aphasia show disordered language function. Mixtures of features from several of the frontal aphasic disorders is common, in fact almost routine. Alexander, Benson, and Stuss (1989) described four frontal activities crucial for communication and indicated how each is affected by damage in the right or left frontal lobes (Table 8.5). The motor and cognitive aspects appear rather strongly lateralized as the dysfunction varies considerably, depending on whether the right or the left frontal lobe is involved. Activation and formulation seem to be less strongly lateralized since disturbances of these functions occur when either hemisphere is involved.

A relatively recently described language disorder, subcortical aphasia (Case 8.12), is paradoxical and controversial. Acute lesions (hemorrhage or infarction) limited to subcortical structures can cause a language disturbance correctly termed *aphasia,* but the disturbance tends to be transient. Even though the subcortical lesion remains, the aphasic features disappear. Apparently the activation necessary to produce language can eventually be provided by other brain regions.

Case 8.13

A 63-year-old, right-handed man suffered an abrupt onset of weakness in the left hand along with dysarthria. Alert and cooperative, he had a moderate left-sided hemiplegia involving the arm more than the face or leg, decreased response to pain over the left face, and decreased sensitivity to pain, position, and vibration in the distal left upper extremity.

Language examination revealed no abnormalities except a verbal output that was flat and monotonous. Almost no emotionality could be detected in the patient's voice, even when he discussed experiences of considerable emotional content. He was unable to sing, producing only a monotonic delivery of the lyrics. In addition, there was a notable lack of gesture and facial expression. CT scan showed a single infarct that involved the right inferior frontal lobe and the anterior parietal operculum. Amelodia (motor aprosodia) was diagnosed. Figure 8.11

Table 8.5. Frontal Communication Activities

Activity	Localization	Lateralization	Left Activity	Right Activity
Motor	Posterolateral frontal and subcortical	Strong	Articulation and linguistic prosody	Affective and pragmatic prosody
Cognitive	Lateral frontal	Strong	Grammatical usage, word-finding	Affective reasoning, inferential, capacity visual–spatial factors
Activation	Medial frontal	Moderate	Initiation of verbal communication, maintenance of verbal content	Initation of affective communication, maintenance of affective content
Formulation	Anterior frontal	Moderate	Narrative capacity, abstract verbal skills, paralinguistic functions	Critical self-assessment, attention/intention, suprasegmental contention structure

Adapted from Alexander, Benson, and Stuss, 1989.

diagrams the general location of the pathology recorded in several such cases. (DFB)

In Case 8.13 a serious disturbance of communication followed a relatively small infarction of the right frontal and parietal operculum areas. Disturbance of the production of melody, needed to communicate emotion, was described in an earlier case (6.4).

Case 8.14

A 37-year-old man suffered infarction of the medial aspect of the right frontal lobe following surgical clipping of an anterior communicating artery aneurysm. This resulted in paresis of the left lower extremity and shoulder. While the patient was never mute, his verbal output remained sparse and laconic; the language examination was normal. Melody in his verbal output was diminished but not absent, and he produced excellent melody when singing. His verbal discourse was tangential and disorganized, easily distracted from the train of conversation by trivial associations. In addition, the responses often lacked monitoring; he tended to produce statements that were insulting or degrading to himself and others or that could appear threatening, embarrassing, distasteful, or otherwise inappropriate. At times he made statements that could not be substantiated (confabulation). He was apathetic, showed little or no interest in anything, and found it difficult to maintain social relationships. Even family members tended to avoid him. Figure 8.12 shows that the infarction involved the right medial frontal region. (DFB)

Case 8.14 represents a different communication problem that can follow right frontal damage, one that has been called *verbal dysdecorum*

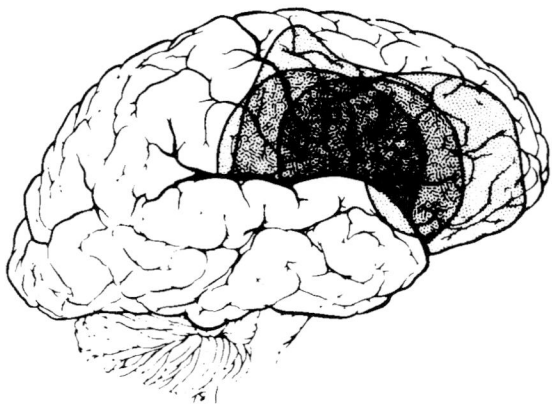

Fig. 8.11. Representation of the right cerebral hemisphere outlining the location of lesions in three cases of amelodia. From Ross, 1981.

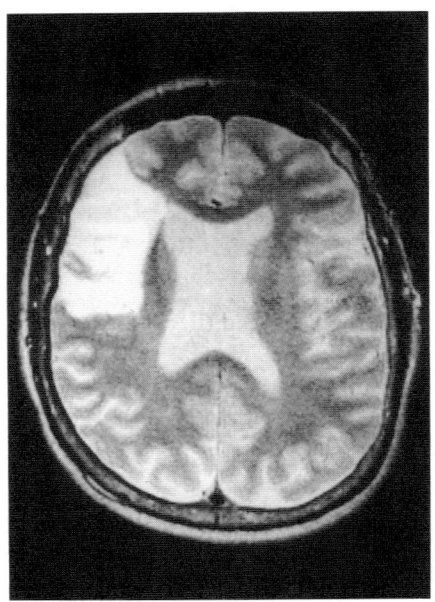

Fig. 8.12. Magnetic resonance scan of a patient with a large right frontal lesion that produced a clinical state that included verbal dysdecorum.

(Alexander, Benson, and Stuss, 1989). Along with other behavioral manifestations of frontal malfunction such as apathy, slowness, and decreased melodic output, the verbal output is notable for a lack of self-monitoring. While his use of language was full, this patient said things that should have been censored (monitored) for optimal social relationships. Confabulations, tangentiality, distractibility, and embarrassing, disinhibited statements are notable characteristics of verbal dysdecorum.

The right hemisphere has additional functions in communication. Gazzaniga (1970), Sperry and Gazzaniga (1967), and especially Zaidel (1976, 1978, 1985) have demonstrated language functions in the right hemispheres of patients following section of the corpus callosum. Most language comprehension by the right hemisphere of split-brain patients involves picturable words, either spoken or written, but it also includes expressions denoting strong emotional states (Campbell, Landis, and Regard, 1986; Landis, Assal, and Perret, 1979), and in one unique case stenographic shorthand was fully understood by the right hemisphere (Regard, Landis, and Hess, 1985). The isolated right hemisphere has little ability to use spoken or written language for expressing ideas but when other means of communication are provided, some language processing can be demonstrated. Table 8.6 outlines Zaidel's view (1985) of the language capacity of the right hemisphere of the split-brain patient.

Clinical studies demonstrate that some communication is performed best by one or the other of the hemispheres, as outlined in Table 8.1. The right hemisphere appears dominant for the melodic portion of prosody, while the left hemisphere is dominant for several aspects of communication, most notably syntactic language. Both hemispheres participate in language function to some degree, but the division of labor is uneven. The left hemisphere strongly dominates the most complex levels—semantics and syntax.

Case 8.15

Following an acute epileptic seizure, a 42-year-old man had right hemiplegia, right hemisensory loss, right homonymous hemianopia, fluent aphasia, and total loss of the ability to read and write. Motor function recovered fully, the sensory loss diminished to insignificance, but the right homonymous hemianopia remained. The aphasia cleared so that the patient could name, comprehend,

Table 8.6. Right Hemisphere Language Characteristics

Language comprehension is better than language expression
Auditory language comprehension is better than written language comprehension
Reading is ideological—pictographic/semantic—without intermediate phonological representation
Lexical semantic competency is relatively rich
Syntax and phonology are seriously deficient
Short term verbal memory is limited

Adapted from Zaidel, 1985.

repeat, and speak without significant abnormality. Reading and writing, however, did not return; he had an acquired illiteracy. This state persisted, and regular evaluations showed no improvement in either reading or writing. Postmortem study, some 10 years after the initial episode, revealed an old, scarred infarct in the area of the left angular gyrus extending to the ventricle, completely destroying the left geniculocalcarine tract, about two-thirds of the angular gyrus, and much of the white matter underlying this structure. (Dejerine, 1891)

This classic case was termed *alexia with agraphia,* an acquired illiteracy that follows dominant parietal infarction, particularly when the angular gyrus is damaged. Written language disorders often coexist with aphasia but, as Case 8.15 reveals, alexia/agraphia can occur as an almost separate problem. The combined loss of both reading and writing in this case contrasts with the retained writing ability of Case 8.5.

Case 8.16
A 53-year-old, college-educated man was admitted for additional speech therapy approximately one year after the onset of an acute right hemiparesis and aphasia. He still had a mild but distinct spastic hemiparesis affecting his face, arm, and leg on the right side. Sensation was normal to routine testing, and no visual field defect was demonstrated. His verbal output was sparse and effortful, with articulatory problems and agrammatism. Repetition was also limited, but his comprehension of spoken language was intact except for complex grammatical constructions. He could name most objects on presentation but occasionally needed phonetic cues. He could only write his own name and a few words to dictation, but he could copy without difficulty. All writing was performed with the left hand. Spelling aloud and comprehension of spelled words were both poor. He comprehended simple written commands, could match a word with a picture, and correctly performed sentence completion tests. While extremely slow, he eventually interpreted written paragraph-length stories. He was unable to read aloud except for some nouns, all of which were imageable. He could not identify written letters. While he could recite the alphabet and write individual letters when dictated, he could not read individual letters. He easily read single-digit numbers aloud. When attempting to read a sentence, he would read aloud the semantically specific words, omitting all grammatical words such as "the" or "at" and often misreading or omitting final syllables such as "en" or "er." Most dramatic was his ability to read aloud a word such as "pea" although he could not identify (i.e., name, read) the letter "p." A diagnosis of recovered Broca's aphasia with literal alexia was made. (DFB)

Though as profound and disabling as the problem in Cases 8.5 and 8.15, the alexia in Case 8.16 had different characteristics. The profound problem in reading individual letters of the alphabet (literal alexia) and the strong tendency to omit syntactically significant words resembles anterior (Broca's) aphasia. This disorder has been called *anterior alexia* (Benson, 1977, 1985).

Case 8.17
A 34-year-old woman was evaluated for a long-standing language problem. Ten years earlier, while delivering a baby, she had suffered a hemorrhage in the left

parietal region. She had been hemiplegic with right sensory loss, visual field defect, and a global aphasia, but with time and therapy she had recovered many functions. Mild right paresis, cortical sensory loss, and a right inferior quadrant visual field defect persisted. Her language output was fluent despite word-finding problems; she could present her personal history and respond to questions with acceptable detail. Her greatest difficulty was in reading. She had been completely unable to read or write since the stroke. Certain words that recurred commonly in her household duties (e.g., *milk* on the appropriate carton) were seen so often that she could now recognize this symbol when seen out of context. When this aspect was probed, she could "read" (aloud) a sizable number of individual words but often made semantic substitutions. Thus, when the word *infant* was written, she read it as *baby*. She substituted *car* for the written word *automobile*, *gun* for *rifle*, *rug* for *carpet*, and so forth. When *living room* was written she hesitated, then said, "Oh, I know what that is, that's the place my husband and I go after supper to have a cup of coffee and talk." This patient had a posterior aphasia with fluent paraphasic output; some limitations of comprehension, naming, and repeating; and alexia and agraphia except for the reading of some picturable words. Her reading was often contaminated by semantic paralexias, a condition called *deep dyslexia*. (Benson and Geschwind, 1969)

The neurological basis of alexia has been clarified in recent years but suffers maximum terminological confusion. Based on the syndrome approach, Table 8.7 presents four types of alexia, listing the reading abnormalities and locations of brain damage. *Posterior (occipital) alexia* (Case 8.5) seems a classic example of disconnection (Geschwind, 1965) in which the visualized material has been properly perceived (unimodal association) but cannot be recognized (heteromodal association) because the competent visual area and the equally competent language area have been separated by damage to connecting pathways (Benson, 1985; Dejerine, 1891; Geschwind, 1962). *Central (parietal) alexia* (Cases 8.15 and 8.17) is associated with damage to the angular gyrus area of the dominant hemisphere. Written symbols no longer have meaning, and the patient is rendered illiterate (Benson and Geschwind, 1969; Dejerine, 1891; Kirshner, 1986). *Anterior (frontal) alexia* (Case 8.16) occurs when the ability to decipher syntactical material, both to use grammatical structures and to maintain relationship (sequence) in spoken language, is disordered. The problem in deciphering written syntax closely matches the frontal aphasic patient's disordered comprehension of syntactical aspects of spoken language (Samuels and Benson, 1979; Zurif, Caramazza, and Myerson, 1972). Originally called the *third alexia* (Benson, 1977; Kirshner and Webb, 1982), anterior alexia almost always accompanies Broca's aphasia. The fourth variety, *deep dyslexia* (Case 8.17), features semantic paralexia (Marshall and Newcombe, 1966). First described as a separate variety of reading disturbance by linguists (Coltheart, 1980; Marshall and Newcombe, 1980), deep dyslexia appears to be a stage in recovery from total alexia (Marin, 1980). Benson and Geschwind (1969) suggested that semantic paralexia, the key clinical feature of deep dyslexia, occurred when a visual image was produced in the right hemisphere in response to

Table 8.7. Types of Alexia

	Written Language	Neighborhood Characteristics	Locus of Pathology
Posterior alexia (alexia without agraphia, occipital alexia)	Verbal > literal alexia, comprehends spelled words, normal writing to dictation and command, slavish copy of written language	Normal spoken language, no paresis or hemisensory loss, right homonymous hemianopsia, color agnosia	Dominant medial occipital plus splenium of corpus callosum
Central alexia (alexia with agraphia, parietal alexia)	Verbal plus literal alexia, cannot comprehend spelled words, agraphia, slavish copy of written material	Fluent aphasia, paresis may or may not be present, field defect may or may not be present, hemisensory loss	Dominant parietal lobe (angular gyrus)
Anterior alexia (frontal alexia)	Literal > verbal alexia; comprehends many spelled words; mechanically poor writing, with agrammatism; copy better than writing to dictation	Nonfluent aphasia, hemiparesis sensation and visual fields usually intact, Naming often needs prompting	Dominant frontal lobe (Broca's area and adjacent deep structures)
Deep dyslexia	Global alexia and agraphia except for limited (mostly imageable) words, semantic paralexia	Aphasia (fluent or nonfluent); hemiparesis; hemisensory loss; and hemianopia common	Large dominant hemisphere language area lesion

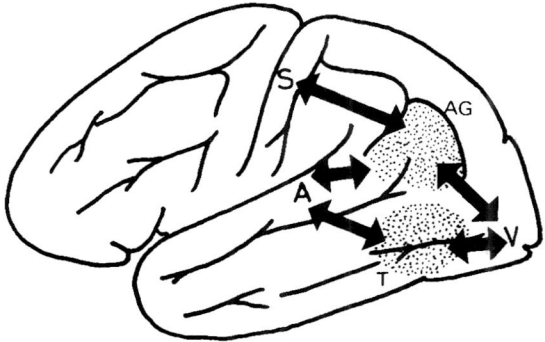

Fig. 8.13. Representation of the left cortex suggesting areas of consequence for reading competence in the Japanese. V, visual area; A, auditory cortex; S, somesthetic cortex; AG, angular gyrus; and T, posterior temporal lobe. From Iwata, 1986.

a written word and an attempt is then made to name the visual image. A word that is different from the written word but that correctly identifies the visual image may be produced.

Studies of the neural basis of reading in Oriental languages offer some insights into these problems. Contemporary written Japanese contains a mixture of pictographic and phonetic characters that allow disassociation of visual and verbal language symbols (Sasanuma et al., 1977; Yamadori, 1975). Bilingual competency (e.g., Chinese plus English) can produce the same dissociative potential (Lyman, Kwan, and Chao, 1938). In Japanese the reading of pictographic (Kanji) characters is more severely disturbed by lesions involving the posterior part of the dominant hemisphere, while the phonetic characters (Kana) are more disturbed by dominant hemisphere temporal or anterior parietal lesions (Sasanuma and Fujimura, 1971; Yamadori, 1975, 1980). Iwata (1986) and others (Mochizuki and Ohtomo, 1988) have demonstrated an additional disassociation in Japanese alexics; lesions affecting the temporal–occipital junction produce a greater disturbance in Kanji reading, whereas temporal–parietal lesions produce greater disturbance in Kana reading. Iwata hypothesized that two visual-language circuits for reading exist within the left hemisphere; one deals with visual imagery while the second interprets auditory signals (see Fig. 8.13).

NEUROANATOMICAL SUBSTRATE

Two basic clinical observations, fluency–nonfluency and repetition, have clear anatomical correlations. Nonfluent verbal output is noted (almost exclusively) when brain damage involves language territory anterior to the fissure of Rolando. In contrast, fluent aphasic output most often signals pathology involving structures located posterior to the fissure of Rolando. Figure 8.2 illustrates this simple but important dichotomy.

Some aphasic patients repeat readily (Cases 8.3, 8.10, 8.11, and 8.12), but in others repetition is seriously disturbed (Cases 8.6, 8.7, 8.8, 8.9, 8.16, and 8.17). Almost invariably, aphasics with repetition difficulty have lesions in the peri-Sylvian region (Benson and Geschwind, 1985; Damasio and Damasio, 1980). In contrast, aphasic patients who repeat well have damage in other areas sparing the peri-Sylvian structures (Kertesz and McCabe, 1977; Rubens, 1976). Figure 8.3 illustrates this distinction.

Other major language functions are not accurately defined by simple anatomical dichotomies. The anatomical basis for facets of the comprehension of spoken language, naming ability, reading, and writing will be discussed below.

Comprehension of Spoken Language

Neuroanatomical correlates can be suggested for four aspects of comprehension—reception, perception, recognition, syntactic relationships—each illustrated by a clinically distinct disorder of comprehension of spoken language. Disordered *reception* is illustrated by the pure word deafness of Case 8.4. The anatomical site of damage producing this disorder lies deep in the posterior, medial aspects of the dominant temporal lobe, disrupting auditory pathways and/or the primary auditory cortex, interfering with the reception of auditory signals, and precluding connection with the language-processing cortex.

Disordered *perception* is illustrated by Case 8.8. Auditory signals are received by the left hemisphere auditory association cortex, but either they cannot reach the dominant hemisphere auditory association cortex or this area itself is damaged, preventing discrimination and unimodal association (perception) of the auditory signals. Lesions that produce perceptive disturbance often involve receptive functions and vice versa; mixtures are the rule, but many cases of pure disturbance have been reported (Albert and Bear, 1974; Auerbach et al., 1982; Goldstein, 1948a; Goldstein, Brown, and Hollander, 1975; Kertesz, Sheppard, and MacKenzie, 1982) (Case 8.8).

A third, distinctly different comprehension disturbance involves *semantic recognition* (Case 8.11). In this disorder, the patient receives and perceives the auditory signal sufficiently well to allow accurate repetition of the spoken phrase but fails to interpret the meaning. Spoken language can be repeated accurately but not comprehended (transcortical sensory aphasia). The word no longer has symbolic meaning, much as a foreign word might be pronounced correctly but not understood. The anatomical substrate of this disorder is variable but always involves posterior dominant hemisphere border zone tissues, never the immediate peri-Sylvian structures. While often centering on the angular gyrus of the parietal lobe, transcortical sensory aphasia can occur with pathology in the border zone of the posterior temporal lobe as well. Combinations of this disturbance with perception problems (Wernicke's aphasia) are common, but pure transcortical sensory aphasia is well recorded (Alexander, Hiltbrunner, Fischer, 1989; Hier et al., 1980; Kertesz and McCabe, 1977) and is com-

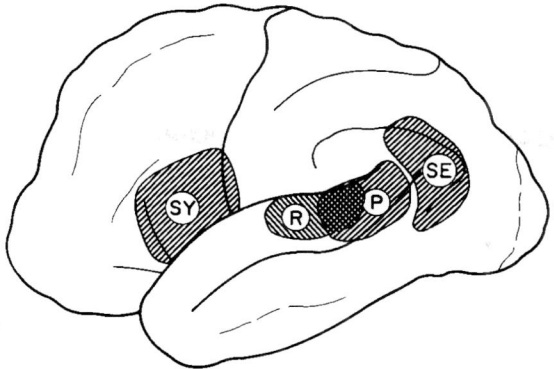

Fig. 8.14. Representation of the left hemisphere illustrating four areas that participate in clinically distinct comprehension tasks. Note the overlap between the areas for reception (R) and perception (P) in the temporal lobe. SE, Semantic area; SY, anterior region influential in syntactical and sequencing activities. From Benson, 1979b.

mon in degenerative dementia, particularly Alzheimer's disease (Cummings et al., 1985; Dejerine, 1914/1977).

A fourth comprehension disturbance involves *syntactic* functions. The patient receives, perceives, and comprehends individual bits of language but fails to understand syntactical structures or maintain sequences of information. Cases 8.6, 8.7, and 8.10, all with pathology in the anterior dominant hemisphere, suffered agrammatism and disturbances in sequencing. Dominant hemisphere operculum and/or adjacent prefrontal area are involved.

Comprehension of spoken language is a complex mental activity, and full capability demands proper function of many brain regions, but the four discussed here can be viewed as a basic neuroanatomical network for language comprehension. Figure 8.14 outlines this network.

Naming

The verbal presentation of a name for an object, a seemingly simple but uniquely human language function, also demands a complex anatomical network (Benson, 1979a). Four variations of anomia (the acquired impairment of naming) associated with aphasia can be defined and given anatomical localizations. *Word production anomia,* a failure to name based on disturbed production of verbal output, has two variations. One, *articulatory initiation* disturbance, occurs in patients with anterior (Broca's) aphasia (Case 8.6). Failure to produce a name on confrontation testing is often overcome when the initial phoneme is whispered or otherwise presented by the examiner. The patient is adamant, and experience supports, that the name is known; it is initiation of the appropriate verbal output that is inordinately difficult. A second variation of word production anomia can be called *paraphasic* and occurs most clearly in patients with conduction aphasia (Case 8.9). These patients also claim knowledge of the correct name but, when attempting to produce the name, substitute so many phonemes that the response is incorrect.

A different word-finding problem can be called *word-selection anomia*. The patient cannot present the name of the object but can describe its function and can point to the object when the name is given by the examiner. Case 8.3 illustrates pure anomia without comprehension disorder. Pathology in cases of word-selection anomia involves the posterior inferior temporal lobe.

Semantic (word recognition) anomia, a third variation, is characterized by inability to name on confrontation or to point to the appropriate object when the name is offered. The word has lost its symbolic meaning. Patients with this disorder may repeat the name but fail to interpret what they have said. Case 8.10 illustrates this disorder. The pathology is located in the posterior border zone area, usually including the angular gyrus.

Finally, a fourth anomia, *disconnection anomia*, has three recognized subdivisions. One, *callosal disconnection anomia*, is characterized by an inability to name objects palpated by the left (nondominant) hand even though the correct object can be selected later from a group of objects. The tactile information entering the right hemisphere cannot be transferred to the left hemisphere because of the callosal separation—unilateral tactile anomia (Geschwind and Kaplan, 1962; Patel, 1969). A second subdivision has been called *category-specific anomia* and is best characterized by color agnosia (see Case 7.2). In this situation a correctly perceived color stimulus (demonstrated by correctly matching colors) is separated

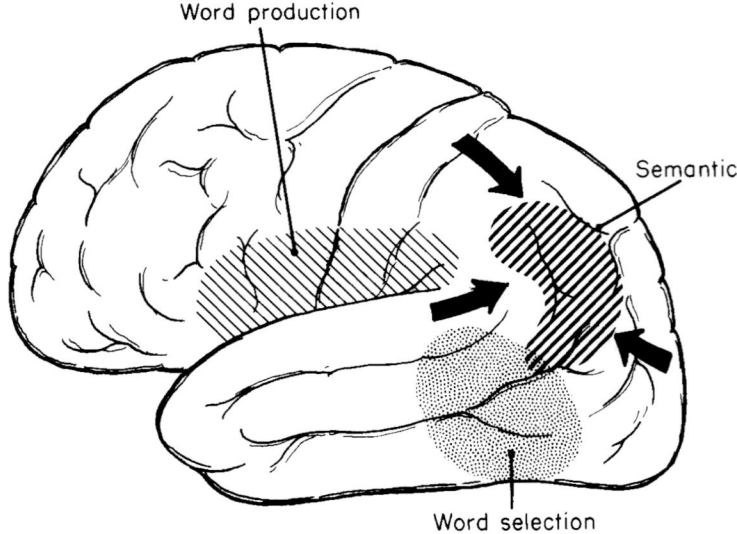

Fig. 8.15. Representation of the left hemisphere showing three areas of pertinence for naming and the direction of input of primary sensory information needed for naming tasks.

from the language area by either callosal or deep white matter pathology (sometimes both), disrupting the ability to produce the name. Other category-specific naming problems can involve body parts or room objects (Benson, 1979a; McKenna and Warrington, 1978; Warrington and Shallice, 1984). Although pure examples are rare, tendencies toward greater difficulty in naming in one or the other category occur with brain damage separating the language area (primarily the angular gyrus) from the appropriate unimodal association area. The third subdivision of disconnection anomia is called *modality-specific anomia* (Brown, 1972). In cases of visual agnosia (Case 7.3) and auditory agnosia (Case 4.3), stimuli in a given sensory modality are successfully received but cannot be interpreted. In each disconnection anomia the primary pathology separates a functioning sensory reception/perception area from the equally intact language processing area. Figure 8.15 diagrams the relative localizations of pathology underlying the types of anomia. An extensive neuroanatomical network, not a single center, is needed for naming.

Reading

Cases 8.15, 8.16, and 8.17 represent varieties of alexia with distinct anatomical correlations (see Table 8.7). *Posterior alexia* (alexia without agraphia) is invariably associated with pathology of the dominant hemisphere occipital lobe. Infarction in the territory of the left posterior cerebral artery damages geniculocalcarine pathways and produces a right homonymous hemianopia; if the splenium of the corpus callosum is also damaged, the intact right visual area is separated from the intact left hemisphere language area (see Case 8.5). A variation, subangular alexia (Greenblatt, 1973, 1977, 1983), follows neoplasm or acute hematoma in dominant posterior parietal tissues that undercut the dominant angular gyrus. In either variation the dominant language cortex is isolated from visualized verbal information.

Central alexia (alexia with agraphia) is an acquired illiteracy (both reading and writing are disordered). Pathology involves the inferior aspect of the dominant parietal lobe, particularly the angular gyrus. Central alexia is consistently present in cases of transcortical sensory aphasia and Wernicke's aphasia.

Anterior (frontal) alexia (Case 8.16) accompanies Broca's aphasia. The patient cannot read grammatically significant words and individual letters. Pathology involves the dominant frontal lobe, particularly the operculum and tissues surrounding this area.

Deep dyslexia (Case 8.17) features semantic substitutions in reading and occurs during recovery from global language disturbance caused by left posterior hemisphere damage. It has been suggested that the semantic substitutions indicate right hemisphere interpretation of the written material. Deep dyslexia and central alexia share the same regions of structural damage (Marin, 1980). Figure 8.16 diagrams the major sensorimotor activities that underlie reading.

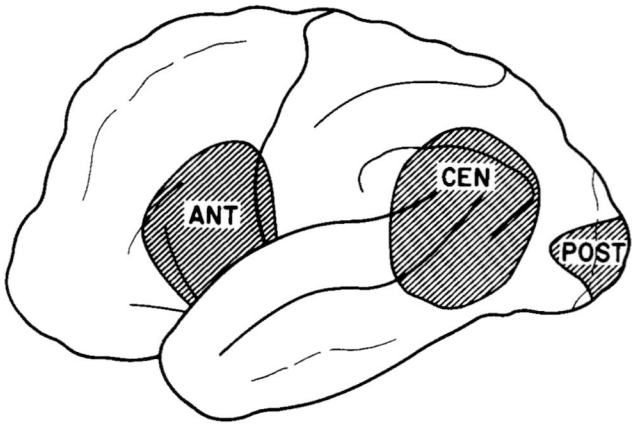

Fig. 8.16. Representation of the left hemisphere showing the three areas of brain damaged in the production of anterior, central, and posterior alexia.

Writing

Writing disorders can also be subdivided (Leischner, 1957). Benson and Cummings (1985) proposed two categories of agraphia—mechanical and aphasic—and further classified the aphasic agraphias as fluent and nonfluent. *Mechanical agraphia* refers to writing problems based on motor defects (paralysis, basal ganglia or cerebellar disturbance) that interfere with the smooth digital coordination necessary to produce written language. *Aphasic agraphia* refers to an abnormal written output that reflects language disturbance. In nonfluent aphasic agraphia the patient produces semantically meaningful words but omits the functional, relational words. In contrast, patients with fluent aphasic agraphia use real letters in combinations that resemble words; some combinations are correct, and others make no sense (Case 8.8). The fluent and nonfluent writing disturbances share the anterior/posterior anatomical correlations of fluent and nonfluent verbal outputs. Admixtures of mechanical and aphasic graphic disturbances (particularly nonfluent aphasic agraphia) are common, and, to add to the confusion, multiple variations of mechanical agraphia and of the fluent and nonfluent aphasic agraphias are recognized (Benson and Cummings, 1985; Marcie and Hécaen, 1979). Details necessary to delineate clearly the variations are often lost in the mixture of defects.

In summary, there are distinct neuroanatomical correlates for many specific language dysfunctions, but none can be explained simply on the basis of a language center. Rather, disturbances affect portions of a complex, organized, and integrated but anatomically fixed network (Mesulam, 1990; Stuss and Benson, 1986). Damage localized to one part of this network will produce one cluster of language defects (a syndrome).

THE NEURAL BASIS OF COMMUNICATION

Based on the study of aphasia, a neural network underlying communication functions can be proposed. The divisions in Figure 8.17 are artificial, highly abridged, and possibly misleading. Many steps occur simultaneously, and feedback and feedforward components within the reverberating circuitry of this neural network considerably complicate the process. Interconnections with other mental processes (e.g., memory, emotion, attention) influence many of these steps. With these essential caveats, each step in the proposed hierarchy of language processing can be discussed separately.

Reception is the initial step of the sensory processing scheme presented in Chapters 3 and 7. Input from auditory, visual, somesthetic, and other sensory systems (autonomic, visceral, kinesthetic) provides material for the next two steps—*perception* and *unimodal association*. Each type of sensory input carries out this process in a separate, dedicated neural unit.

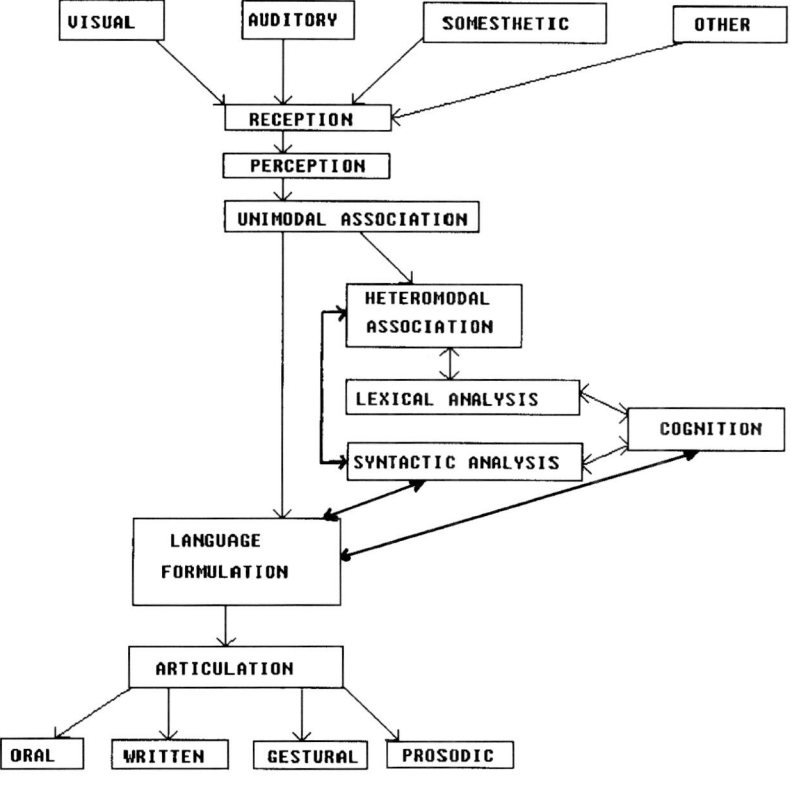

Fig. 8.17. A graphic illustration of the individual steps involved in language processing. While functionally separate, most of these activities are bidirectional, and most have numerous connections with other mental processing units.

Each of these three steps plays a significant role, but one or more of the steps in any single modality can be removed from the overall process (Figure 8.17) and the resulting clinical abnormality will be recognized only as a disorder of auditory, visual, or other sensory processing. No single step of percept formation is essential for language function; loss of input from any sensory system decreases the material available for language processing but does not preclude language function. Raw material for language is available from many sensory systems.

The fourth step, *heteromodal association,* does appear to be essential for language (Geschwind, 1965). In this step, the percepts received from the unimodal sensory systems are compared with information from other sensory deposits (both current and old) via a broad associative network, and appropriate information is gathered and amalgamated. This cross-modal association step is crucial for language. To illustrate, a single-modality stimulus such as the written word *elephant* rapidly produces multiple associations in a variety of sensory formats. One can "hear" the word, picture the animal, visualize a circus or zoo, image the movements of the trunk, the presence of tusks, and the size of the animal, recall films of the animal, and remember the smells associated with elephants and the toughness and scratchiness of their hide. Multiple simple and complex associations occur immediately upon visualizing the combination of letters that spell *elephant.* Heteromodal association provides the full range of stored memories that are key to human language.

Cross-modal association is not sufficient, however, to explain all language functions; the information must be processed further. A significant process concerns *syntax,* the relationship of the stimulus word to other words in the sentence or phrase. Incoming language signals must be properly parsed to realize the logical structure and to provide full meaning. Such parsing is also necessary for language production.

Three additional steps are apparent. First, if the original stimulus requires a verbal response based on interpretation of information, this may involve *cognition* (see Chapter 10). Second, after verbal information is processed, it enters a *formulation* process with several different steps. Material from the lexicon (the individual's storehouse of words) and appropriate syntatic elements are synthesized to compose a correct linguistic response. Communication, however, has various routes. The third step, *articulation,* can take such forms as gesture, vocalization, verbalization, and written language. Different neural systems under different influences are available for communicative response.

9

The Neurology of Memory Disorders

> Memory is the diary that we all carry about with us.
> —OSCAR WILDE
> *THE IMPORTANCE OF BEING EARNEST, 1895/1941*

> Memories (engrams) are distributed and interactive cortical networks of infinite variety that in themselves contain the experience of the individual and of the species.
> —J. M. FUSTER (1989)

AXIOMS/POSTULATES

Memory, an essential element for thinking, consists of several different functional processes.

The various processes of memory have different neuroanatomical bases—some anatomical sites are shared, but the networks underlying the memory functions are discrete.

Each memory function participates in thought but one or more may be fully or partially inoperable without impairing other aspects of memory.

In the usual sense, memory refers to the experiences and information that we remember. Each of us has a vast supply of memories that constitute an important aspect of our individuality. Personal as the contents of memory are, however, they also have a general element, derived from formal and informal education, parental and religious teaching, and common social experiences. This memory bank supplies much of the material that is processed in human thought.

Psychoanalysts revealed that alteration of the factual detail stored in memory is a common, although largely unrecognized, process (Freud, 1938; Rosenzweig and Mason, 1934). Memories are selectively retained (or abandoned) and are subject to distortion and repression.

At the other end of the clinical spectrum, Wilder Penfield (Penfield and Mathieson, 1974; Milner, 1966) stimulated cerebral tissue during neurosurgery. In some individuals, personal memories could be elicited by electrical stimulation of the cortex of the temporal lobe (Penfield and Perot, 1963). Based on these observations, Penfield and his colleagues suggested that memories were stored in the temporal lobe. This theory was contested (Walshe, 1957), but their work supported the idea of an anatomical site for memory storage.

Most studies of memory have been conducted by psychologists through a variety of approaches. Experimental psychologists, primarily through the investigation of learning ability in normal subjects, have explored the effect of retention interval, interference, encoding specificity, and other aspects of memory formation (McGeogh, 1932; Underwood, 1957). Cognitive psychologists and information theorists have demonstrated that ultra-short memory is an essential component of both verbal and nonverbal information processing (Baddeley, 1966, 1992; Gardner, 1985; Saffran and Marin, 1975). Physiological psychologists have stressed reverberating neural circuits in memory formation and have proposed that a reverbatory trace might become a stored memory following structural change (Bailey and Chen, 1983; Gibbs and Ng, 1977). The time following stimulation before a memory becomes "fixed," particularly in the case of retrograde amnesia (loss of previously learned material or behavior) in laboratory animals, has been widely studied (McGaugh and Gold, 1976; Squire and Spanis, 1984). Neuropsychologists have probed memory function in individuals suffering amnesias of various causes such as trauma (Russell and Nathan, 1946), electroshock (Squire and Chace, 1975), infectious diseases (Cermak and O'Connor, 1983; Rose and Symonds, 1960), and Korsakoff's psychosis (Butters and Grady, 1977; Victor, 1969). Against this background neurologists have taken the approach of correlating behavior and neuroanatomy in the effort to provide a consistent structure against which theoretical models of memory can be tested (Brierly, 1966; Damasio et al., 1985).

VARIETIES OF MEMORY DISORDER

The diversity of approaches to memory research has generated diverse terminology: storage, retrieval, consolidation, learning, retention, interference, encoding, decoding, reverberating channels, retrograde and anterograde memory, immediate, short-, intermediate-, and long-term memory, declarative and procedural memory, episodic and semantic memory, primary and working memory, and many more terms are in current use. Overviews have been written (Benson and McDaniel, 1990; Squire, 1982; Squire and Zola-Morgan, 1991; Tulving and Donaldson, 1972), and some consistency can be seen. All current theories divide memory into different psychological or neurophysiological processes. Signoret (1985) suggested five such processes:

1. A holding process in which information is retained momentarily until other memory processing can take place
2. An acquiring process that encodes material that has been selected for placement in general memory; the acquiring process can be subdivided

into chunking (the efficient gathering of information) and linking (the correlation of bits of information)
3. A storing process (often called *consolidation*), which places the bits of information into a permanent or semipermanent storage that includes the reception of new memory traces, rehearsal, and maintenance
4. A retrieval process in which bits of information learned previously are recaptured for use
5. A scanning process that allows items relevant to the current situation to be selected from an array of memory traces

Most fundamental memory processes are not mirrored precisely by clinical disorders; partial disruption of one or several memory processes is usually mixed with breakdown of other essential mental processes. Caution is needed in the interpretation of clinical studies of memory.

BASIC MEMORY FUNCTIONS

Three types of memory function will be discussed here, but this division is only one of many classifications of memory function appearing in the literature. Table 9.1 presents some of these proposed classifications.

Immediate Recall

Immediate recall is the ability to reproduce accurately information just received. Although early psychotherapists (Bergson, 1911; Bumke, 1919) suggested that every bit of information ever received is permanently stored, it has been demonstrated that most of the material processed in early phases does not enter permanent storage (Baddeley and Warrington, 1973). Immediate recall refers to information received and retained only for a short interval, usually measured in seconds unless additional mental processing is carried out (Brown, 1964).

George Talland and colleagues outlined several features that characterize immediate recall (they called it *primary memory*), including (1) complete accuracy of recall, (2) limited number of bits of information handled, (3) short duration of retention, and (4) deterioration with distraction (Talland, 1965; Waugh and Norman, 1972). In normal subjects John Brown (1964) carefully measured these parameters and demonstrated that factors such as recency, distraction, and quantity affect immediate recall of information.

Learning

Learning, simply defined as the act of putting information into storage (Hilgard and Bower, 1966), has been given many names—*recent memory, secondary memory, short-term memory* (a term also applied to immediate recall)—and represents both the acquiring and the storing processes of the

Table 9.1. Proposed Divisions of Memory

Three memories
Primary, secondary, tertiary
Short term, long term, intermediate term
Registration, consolidation, retrieval
Encoding, storage, retrieval
Imprinting, imaging, coding (categorization)
Immediate recall, learning, retrieval
Immediate, recent, remote

Two memories
Memory, habit
Memory with record, memory without record
Generic, contextual
Hippocampal (temporal), diencephalic
Retrograde, anterograde
Episodic, semantic
Verbal, nonverbal
Bodily, mental
Conscious recollection, skill
Reference, working memory
Fact, skill
Explicit, implicit
Declarative, procedural
Knowing what, knowing how
Locale, taxon
Cognitive, semantic
Elaboration, integration
Autobiographical, perceptual
Representational, dispositional
Vertical association, horizontal association

Signoret framework. While the first two aspects described by Signoret can be separated in theory and experiment, the distinction is not readily demonstrated in clinical testing; only the overall function—learning—will be discussed here.

Among the characteristics of learning are the following: (1) large quantities of material can be accumulated, (2) the material is stored in a less-than-fully accurate fashion, (3) material remains available for relatively long periods of time, and (4) the material is likely to be distorted during this process (Waugh and Norman, 1972). Although large quantities of information can be "learned," only a small portion of the stimuli continually entering the nervous system and temporarily held for immediate recall enter this stage. Learning, the active memory-forming process, is crucial to education, and a vast literature deals with both normal and disordered learning (Graf and Schacter, 1985; Jacoby, 1978; Posner, 1967; Zangwill, 1969).

Retrieval

Retrieval is the ability to bring forth information learned previously. Many different terms—*tertiary memory, remote memory, long-term memory*—relate to this process. There is an obvious overlap between learning new material and retrieving learned material; it is impossible to test learning without challenging the ability to retrieve. Nonetheless, clinical experience convincingly demonstrates disability in the learning process of individuals whose ability to retrieve previously learned material remains intact. To the retrieval process, Signoret (1985) added scanning, the ability to peruse an array of information and select pertinent bits. Others (Waugh and Norman, 1972) characterized tertiary memory as follows: (1) a vast amount of information is more or less readily available; (2) this information is maintained for a long time (in many instances for a lifetime); (3) retrieved material has only limited accuracy; and (4) the information may be disorted through sublimation, repression, and substitution of other information. Extraction of information from storage (retrieval) is obviously distinct from the process of putting information into storage (learning).

CLINICAL EXAMPLES

The three aspects of memory function that serve as subheadings below (immediate recall, learning, retrieval) can each be represented by case studies.

Immediate Recall

Case 9.1

A 41-year-old man (*Case 5.2 with a different emphasis here*) was hospitalized with acutely altered mental status due to food poisoning. A 36 hour episode of vomiting and diarrhea left him in a debilitated, confused state. Blood tests revealed a low serum sodium level, and treatment was initiated. The patient was weak but without paralysis, sensory loss, or visual field loss. Language was intact, but attention was disordered. He could not maintain a coherent line of thought, would initiate a response appropriately but soon be distracted, and discuss unrelated topics. He often failed attempts to repeat two digits and totally failed reversing the order of digits. Attempts to have him learn new information failed. When offered one or two names to remember, he could not retain them. The examiner's name was frequently presented for the patient to learn. While he occasionally repeated the single name, he never maintained it for even ten or fifteen seconds.

With treatment the patient rapidly recovered from the confusional state. Three days later he next saw the examiner in a hallway, distant from the surroundings of the original meeting; he stopped what he was doing, stared at the examiner and said, "I know who you are—you are Dr. Benson" but could not remember where he had met the examiner or under what circumstances. (DFB)

This patient suffered an acute confusional state as discussed in Chapter 5. His ability to retain information (immediate recall) was severely compromised. That he could learn during this period was demonstrated by his recall of the examiner's name three days after it had been taught. That his learning potential had been severely limited was obvious from his inability to recall where or under what circumstances he had learned the examiner's name.

Case 9.2
A 74-year-old widower, retired and living with his son and daughter-in-law, became agitated, anxious, and paranoid one night. He stormed about the house giving directions for barricading rooms, mentioned names and situations unknown to the family, demonstrated concern over voices and visual images not perceived by the family members, and misinterpreted the headlights of passing cars and other noises from the environment. At a hospital emergency room it was discovered that he had a low-grade fever. Although generally in good health, coherent, and self-caring, he had suffered an upper respiratory infection several weeks earlier with a residual, productive cough.

During the examination in the emergency room, he was unable to maintain coherency of thought and his verbal output rambled as he proposed plans, shouted warnings, and expressed suspicions but maintained none for more than a few seconds. He could not even perform simple mental tests such as digit span because of the distractibility. Laboratory studies confirmed bacterial pneumonitis, which responded to antibiotic therapy. The mental problems disappeared completely after the fever subsided. (DFB)

This patient experienced an acute confused state, a disturbance of awareness that affects many mental functions including memory. Reduced awareness is accompanied by decreased attention span and a general dulling of intellectual processes (often called *clouding of consciousness* [Engel and Romano, 1959; Weinstein and Kahn, 1955]) that makes the individual appear perplexed or bewildered (Strub, 1982). Inability to maintain a coherent line of thought manifests as difficulty in maintaining verbal sequences and entering into, maintaining, or shifting mental sets. The result is a distractible, inattentive, inintentive patient (Heilman et al., 1985b; Mesulam 1981, 1985a).

The acute confusional state disrupts memory function. The confused patient cannot maintain new information sufficiently long for rehearsal, and learning and retrieval of material learned in the past is hampered.

The memory disorder of acute confusion has defining characteristics. The inability to maintain a sequence is demonstrated by limited digit span (often 2 or less) that severely restricts the material available for learning; in addition, both distractibility and inattention limit retrieval. While memory functions are severely disordered, they are not totally inactivated during the period of acute confusion. If a stimulus is repeated with sufficient frequency (as in Case 9.1), the material may be rehearsed sufficiently to be learned and become available for retrieval after the confusion has cleared. Following recovery from trauma, many patients report vague memories (lacunes) of occurrences during periods of apparent unconsciousness. The lacunes are often associated with a novel stimulus (e.g., being prepared for an x-ray) or a painful experience (e.g., the setting of a fracture) (Russell, 1959). Following recovery from a confusional state, a patient may "know" that a friend or relative has been present, even though denying memory of what occurred during the period of confusion. With recovery from confusion, the abilities to maintain a span of information, to learn new material, and to retrieve old information are rapidly recovered.

Learning

Case 9.3

A 53-year-old attorney was hospitalized for the consequences of long-standing alcoholism. A significant mental disorder and severe peripheral neuropathy were present in a physically debilitated patient. For over three months he was unable to learn any information such as the examiner's name, the name of the hospital, the month and year, or his medical problem despite being fully attentive (a digit span of 8 forward) and possessing a full vocabulary. He told of cross-country journeys completed "yesterday" and always gave confabulatory responses to orientation questions. Although unable to retrieve any information about the ten to fifteen years before hospitalization, he related, with accuracy, details of his activities as a naval officer during World War II. A Wechsler Adult Intelligence Scale (WAIS) (Wechsler, 1958) administered during the period of total amnesia showed a Full Scale IQ of 133. His tendency to confabulate eventually decreased, he began to learn small amounts of new information (e.g., the examiner's name), and the peripheral neuropathy improved, but on discharge he needed custodial care because of ongoing learning disorder. (DFB)

Case 9-3 is a classic example of Korsakoff's disease, an amnesia most often resulting from long-term alcohol abuse. The learning disability was highlighted by the patient's normal digit span, superior results on IQ testing, and accurate retrieval of information learned in the distant past. Figure 9.1 shows the gliotic lesions of the mamillary bodies seen in Korsakoff's disease.

Case 9.4

A 36-year-old man was evaluated for possible treatment of a long-standing memory disorder. In his mid-20s, while in the armed forces, he had sustained a serious closed head injury in a traffic accident. He eventually regained normal physical and neurological status except for an inability to learn. He was eventually discharged from the service and went to live with his mother.

On examination he was a healthy, cooperative, but inordinately passive person with no basic neurological disturbance. Language function was intact, and his WAIS Full Scale IQ was 126, not only above average but close to his premorbid

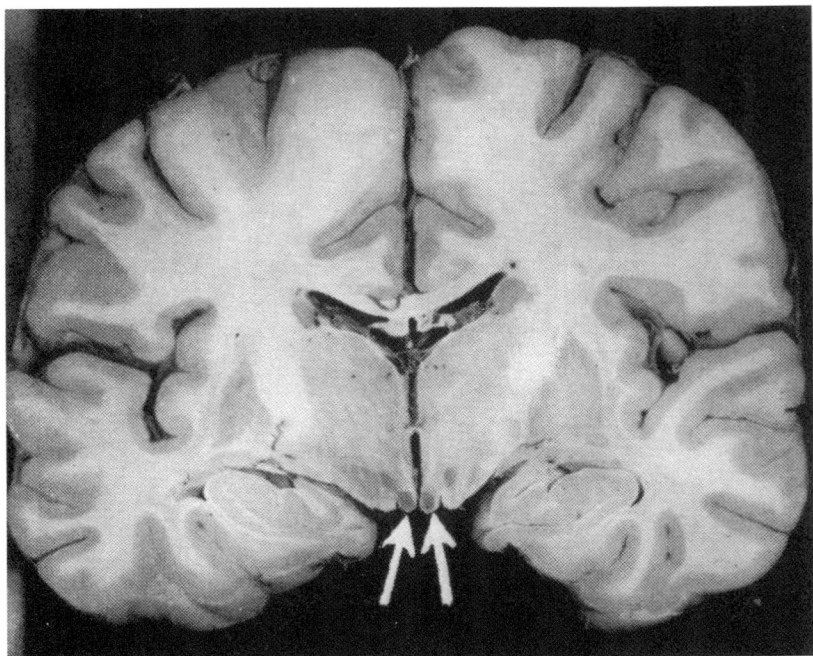

Fig. 9.1. Coronal section of whole brain through the mamillary bodies in a case of Korsakoff's disease. The *arrows* point to the pigmented, gliotic mamillary bodies. From Malamud, 1957.

IQ. His Wechsler Memory Quotient (MQ) (Wechsler, 1945) was only 106, but the difference between IQ and MQ did not reflect the severity of the memory disorder. Tests of immediate recall (digit span, letter span, word span) were fully normal, but he failed to learn verbal material unless given extensive rehearsal. Thus, over a period of several weeks he was taught a doggerel verse containing orientation information (the name of the hospital, the names of his doctors, the name of the President, and so forth) set to a simple melody. When prompted with the melody, he could recite the entire piece of doggerel; however, if asked specific questions from this verse such as "What is the name of this hospital?" or "What is the name of the President of the United States?" he could not retrieve the information. He learned some new motor skills and could find his way about the hospital and locate his ward bed, but he never learned the names of the doctors, nurses, or other patients. He carried out daily activities, both physical and social, gave modestly detailed descriptions of his early life, and even recognized and named individuals known to him when he was a youth. Intensive efforts to retrain memory functions were unsuccessful. (DFB)

Case 9.4 represents the most common cause of amnesia, head trauma, but is exceptional in that learning function remained permanently disordered. Almost everyone who suffers brain trauma has some degree of amnesia but in the vast majority it is transient.

Case 9.5

A 66-year-old man was seen for mental disturbances that followed acute bilateral occlusion of the posterior cerebral arteries. Angiography had demonstrated total obstruction to flow in both posterior cerebral arteries, with collateral circulation around the occipital poles from branches of the medial cerebral artery. The patient was alert, attentive, and provided details of his earlier life. Neurological examination was negative except for markedly decreased visual fields. Formal perimetry revealed that his field of vision was limited to a few degrees in each eye. He could not read but wrote easily and otherwise used language normally. He had significant trouble learning new information, eventually learning the examiner's name though he usually needed a cue. On hearing the examiner's voice or footsteps he would (unconsciously) tap his package of cigarettes (Benson and Hedges) and then state the examiner's name. Although he acted as though both blind and amnesic, features of Anton's syndrome (see Case 5.7), neither condition was complete nor did he deny his visual problem. (Benson, Marsden, and Meadows, 1974)

Another recognized cause of amnesia, posterior cerebral artery occlusion, is well illustrated in Case 9.5. Again, it was the inability to learn, not immediate recall or retrieval problems, that characterized this amnesic stroke.

Case 9.6

A 50-year-old engineer survived severe encephalitis with initial coma that improved to a state of right hemiparesis, aphasia, and dementia. Herpes encephalitis was confirmed by laboratory studies (Adams and Miller, 1973), and the more severe neurological deficits slowly cleared; the paresis disappeared completely, and his aphasia improved to an anomia that also eventually disappeared. Basic cognitive functions returned, but a severe memory disorder persisted. Repeated evaluations over the next ten years showed a Full Scale IQ of 133 but a Wechsler Memory Quotient of only 90.

The patient was cooperative, expressed himself well, and was pleased to participate in testing activities. He was utterly disoriented for time and place unless in his own home. Despite a retrograde amnesia that obliterated memories for several years prior to onset, he did recall incidents from his early life. Extensive testing demonstrated severe (almost total) inability to retain newly presented verbal material and an even more severe disturbance in the retention of new nonverbal material. In contrast, the patient learned new motor skills and when retested after some months, while needing prompting, relearned the task more easily. (Cermak and O'Connor, 1983)

In Case 9.6 encephalitis caused a permanent disorder of learning with little effect on other mental functions. Cases 9.3, 9.4, 9.5, and 9.6 all suffered amnesia, a clinical syndrome with distinct features including normal immediate recall, severely disturbed ability to learn new material, relatively well-preserved retrieval of old information (except for a retrograde amnesia measured in years), and nearly intact cognitive and personality functions (Barbizet, 1963; Benson and Blumer, 1982; Lishman, 1971a; Symonds, 1966). Table 9.2 outlines the major clinical features that characterize amnesia.

Table 9.2. Clinical Definition of Amnesia

Amnesia is a persistent disorder of memory occurring in a clear state of consciousness with the following characteristics:

1. Immediate recall is normal
2. Learning ability is significantly decreased
3. Retrieval of previously learned information is normal (except for a period of retrograde amnesia)
4. Cognitive functions, language, and personality are normal

Although the number of causes of relatively pure amnesia is limited (Table 9.3), the major problem, difficulty in learning, is present in many neurological disorders. Stroke patients, head injury victims, and demented patients often show some degree of amnesia mixed with other mental disturbances. Although not pure amnesia as defined in Table 9.2, the inability to learn new material betrays a memory disorder. To highlight the learning problem, several disorders causing pure amnesia will be discussed below.

Korsakoff's Disease. In 1883 a Russian physician, S. S. Korsakoff, described a syndrome that featured serious mental alterations (Victor and Yakovlev, 1955). By 1904 Bonhoeffer had defined four cardinal findings of the Korsakoff syndrome: (1) defective memory for recent events, (2) retrograde amnesia, (3) disorientation, and (4) confabulation.

The onset is acute, often during the course of a prolonged alcoholic binge in which almost all caloric intake comes from alcohol. Acute withdrawal from drinking, often because of the onset of gastric hemorrhage or head injury, can produce Wernicke's encephalopathy (acute onset of ataxia, ophthalmoplegia, and confusion) (Victor, Adams, and Collins, 1971). Wernicke's encephalopathy is devastating, often fatal, but, if immediately treated with injections of thiamine, the ataxia and ophthalmoplegia improve rapidly (24 hours) with a slower improvement (2 to 5 days) in the confusional state. When the latter has cleared, a striking memory disturbance may be present, the chronic amnesia known as Korsakoff's disease or psychosis.

Patients with Korsakoff's disease, severely limited in learning new information, may present bizarre, untrue answers in response to simple questions (confabulation). The tendency to confabulate characteristically decreases concomitant with increasing awareness of the memory disturbance. Neither the severity of the learning disability nor a premorbid tendency toward suggestibility relate to the degree of confabulation; rather, confabulation appears to be related to decreased self-criticism, a prefrontal dysfunction that will be discussed in Chapter 11 (Mercer et al., 1977; Shapiro et al., 1981).

The exact site of pathology causing Korsakoff's disease remains controversial (Parkin, 1984). Gliosis (sclerosis) of the mamillary bodies of the posterior hypothalamus was recognized early as a feature of Korsakoff's

Table 9.3. Etiologies of Amnesia

Disorder	Site of Major Pathology
Korsakoff's disease	Diencephalon (mamillary bodies)
Traumatic brain injury	Widespread, predominantly medial temporal
Cerebral vascular disease (most often posterior artery occlusion)	Medial temporal
Cerebral infection (most often herpes encephalitis)	Limbic, medial temporal
Surgical lobectomy (removal of the temporal lobe)	Medial temporal
Neoplasm	Medial temporal, fornix, thalamus
Epilepsy/electroconvulsive therapy	
Anoxia	
Transient global amnesia	
Psychogenic amnesia	

disease (DeLay, Brion, and Elissalde, 1958a,b; Gamper, 1928) and is often considered pathognomonic. Some pathologists have demonstrated cell loss in the medial dorsal and anterior nuclei of the thalamus (Malamud and Skillicorn, 1956; Victor, Adams, and Collins, 1971). There is no cortical damage, and most other brain stem and diencephalic structures are not involved. A similar, if not identical, memory syndrome follows disconnection of the mamillary bodies from input through the fornix (Brion et al., 1969) or outflow through the mamillothalamic tract (Guberman and Stuss, 1983). The inability to learn in Korsakoff's disease appears to result from bilateral damage to limbic structures or pathways.

Post-traumatic Amnesia. Head trauma is by far the most common cause of amnesia, but the condition often goes unrecognized in the face of other serious medical problems (Russell, 1951). Following brain injury, the recovery from coma and confusional state is so gratifying to the family and medical caregivers that an ongoing inability to learn may be temporarily overlooked.

Retrograde amnesia, one feature of ongoing amnesia (Seltzer and Benson, 1974), may be seen during posttraumatic amnesia (PTA). The patient fails to remember not only the accident but also all information learned for several years before the brain injury (long retrograde amnesia). With recovery from PTA, a much shorter retrograde amnesia, often measured in seconds or minutes before the injury, may remain. A period of shrinkage of the long retrograde amnesia has been noted (Benson and Geschwind, 1967; Russell and Nathan, 1946). Most investigators agree that damage in the medial temporal region underlies PTA (Jennett, 1969; Symonds, 1962) and that frontal dysfunction is necessary for confabulation (Kapur and Coughlan, 1980; Stuss et al., 1978).

Amnesic Stroke. When amnesia occurs after cerebrovascular accident, the posterior cerebral arteries (PCA) are almost invariably involved, usually bilaterally (Benson, Marsden, and Meadows, 1974; Victor et al., 1961). Amnesic stroke is frequently associated with Anton's syndrome, the denial of blindness, a disorder so dramatic that the amnesia is often overlooked (Anton, 1896). While most reported cases of amnesic stroke follow bilateral occlusion in the PCA territory, amnesia may occur after unilateral (always left) infarction alone (Benson, Marsden, and Meadows, 1974; Mohr et al., 1971). In amnesic stroke some degree of visual field disturbance (cortical blindness, homonymous hemianopsia, or quadrantopia) is present, as the PCA also feeds the calcarine (primary visual) cortex. In most cases of amnesic stroke the pathology is bilateral, but in several cases that went to autopsy there was unilateral posterior cerebral artery infarction alone (Geschwind and Fusillo, 1966; Mohr et al., 1971).

Anoxic Amnesia. Classic amnesia may result from the anoxia caused by acute cardiopulmonary arrest. With CPR and reinstatement of oxygenated blood flow, many patients now survive short periods of total brain anoxia. If the period of anoxia is sufficiently short, recovery may be complete, but if somewhat longer, recovery may be accompanied by a persistent amnesia (Hirst and Volpe, 1982; McNiell, Tidmarsh, and Rastall, 1965). At postmortem, the most prominent finding is cell loss in the hippocampus (Cummings et al., 1984; Zola-Morgan, Squire, and Amaral, 1986).

Psychogenic Amnesia. A common lay view of amnesia is that it involves inability to remember one's own name or other highly personal information. One psychodynamic view is that this form of amnesia represents an attempt to escape an overwhelming psychic trauma, a selective forgetting (American Psychiatric Association, 1957; Janet, 1920/1965).

Psychogenic amnesia has a unique clinical picture, and the clinician should have little problem with diagnosis. What is lost from memory is highly overlearned, personal information. Patients with psychogenic amnesia cannot remember their own name, the names of family members, current home address, or recent personal events, but they easily recall the names of Presidents, newsworthy events, and sports results of recent vintage and they retain vocabulary, social graces, and other learned behaviors. In addition, they learn new information such as the names of the hospital and their doctors and nurses, can remember three words over five minutes, and so on. Testing shows that only personal information is unavailable.

Psychogenic amnesia is a rare clinical phenomenon. When it is suspected, evidence of acute mental stress such as depression, threat of arrest, recent business or personal reversals, or family breakdown should be sought. The disorder is usually short lived, but the underlying psychiatric problems may be difficult to manage.

Retrieval

Case 9.7

A 47-year-old man was hospitalized because of deteriorating social competency. He had never married but had worked steadily as a clerk until four years before admission, leaving the job because of increasing motor clumsiness and mental deterioration. Examination revealed chorea, and a family history of Huntington's disease (HD) was eventually established.

The patient was mobile but made multiple irregular jerking movements that involved the limbs and trunk, grimaced, and had an uneven, dancing quality to his gait. He routinely sat on his hands to keep them from flinging about. His verbal output was dysprosodic and hypophonic, with irregular tone and cadence but adequate lexicon and normal use of grammatical structures. He could perform simple cognitive tasks (calculations and idioms) but failed more complex tasks. His digit span was normal and old information such as names of Presidents or events during World War II was available, but he had difficulty handling new information. If a short series of words was repeated until retained and then requested ten or fifteen minutes later, he usually stated that he had forgotten and could remember none. If given a cue such as the category of one of the words (e.g., color), he often recited not only the correct word but most of the other words also. The word list had been learned, but retrieval could not be initiated unless prompted. In addition, questions concerning current events such as baseball scores, political events, and disasters were correctly answered. He was learning new information, albeit with less than normal efficiency. (DFB)

This patient had Huntington's disease, a genetically determined, late-onset movement disorder with progressive dementia. Whether memory dysfunction is present in HD has been controversial, and the problem is well illustrated by Case 9.7. The patient could learn but often had difficulty demonstrating it. Memory tests in which prompting was given indicated that his problem concerned initiation of retrieval. He could place new information in memory but had difficulty gaining access to it.

Case 9.8

A 32-year-old mailman complained of a severe headache and soon lapsed into a coma. A large hematoma had formed in the anterior fossa as a result of a ruptured anterior communicating artery aneurysm. Surgical treatment was successful. Postoperatively, language and sensorimotor functions were intact, and there was no disorder of visual imagery. Cognitive tasks were performed adequately despite a memory disorder that, while variable, had consistent features. The patient's immediate recall was intact, but he had retrograde amnesia. For instance, he could not remember that he was married or that he had two children. With prompting, however, he named his wife and both children, gave the children's approximate ages, his home address, and his former living status. Formal psychometric tests produced similar results. He routinely failed tests of verbal learning, but when prompted he scored within the normal range. (Damasio et al., 1985)

In this well-documented case, Damasio and colleagues demonstrated that, although the memory disorder appeared to be general in that it affected many parameters of memory, careful testing could show a retrieval disturbance that was considerably more severe than the inability to learn new material.

Disorders of retrieval are not as clearly demarcated as disorders of learning and may be difficult to distinguish from a normal state. Retrieval disorders resemble forgetting, a ubiquitous and probably essential characteristic of human mental functioning. Vast quantities of information enter both conscious and unconscious memory channels, but only selected pieces are maintained in long-term storage. For instance, while one can usually recall what one had for lunch yesterday, very few lunches consumed in past years are maintained in memory.

Forgetting may be a pathological disturbance, however. "Forgetting to remember" refers to an inability to remember, with ease, information that remains in storage (Hécaen and Albert, 1978). Forgetting to remember also occurs normally (e.g., inability to remember the name of a friend when introducing him), a trait that appears to increase with advancing age (Kahn et al., 1975). Forgetting can become a serious problem and separating the inability to retrieve information from attention and/or learning disorders often proves difficult. Several pathological states in which temporary inability to retrieve well-learned information is prominent deserve discussion.

Senescence. With advancing age, a slowing of all mental activities occurs, including memory functions (Birren, 1974; Clark, 1979; Cummings and Benson, 1992; Welford, 1977). Forgetfulness is a common complaint of the elderly, but when given formal memory tests most functionally competent elderly subjects score in the normal range. Immediate recall remains normal, and elderly individuals can both retrieve information from long-term storage and learn large amounts of new and unrelated material (Cummings and Benson, 1983). While it may take the elderly a bit longer to learn, tests show that they retain as much information as younger subjects (Craik, 1977). The memory complaint of the elderly appears to stem from inefficient processing.

The most prominent change in memory function with aging concerns retrieval. Memory function in the elderly improves appreciably when semantic clues are offered; younger subjects require fewer such aids for recall (Smith, 1977). When provided with an appropriate cue, the elderly person often produces quantities of information from both old and recent stores. The information was always available but not readily accessed. Buschke and Grober (1986) demonstrated that most normal elderly subjects could learn as efficiently as younger adults, but many needed hints for recall. When the problem becomes sufficiently intense, a subgroup of the aged population warrants the classification of "benign senescent forgetfulness," also known as "age-associated memory impairment" (Crook et al., 1986). Whether the disorder represents a normal aging function or should be considered pathological remains unsettled. It differs from normal forgetfulness in degree only.

Dementia. A division of dementia into two major types—cortical and subcortical—has been proposed (Albert, Feldman, and Willis, 1974; Cummings, 1990; Cummings and Benson, 1984). The traditional example of cortical dementia is Alzheimer's disease, which features progressive impairment of many mental functions. The memory problem seen in the early stages of Alzheimer's disease resembles the classic amnesia outlined in Table 9.2. As the disorder relentlessly progresses, patients have difficulty with the retrieval of old information and eventually with immediate recall. The ability to learn is impaired early and represents a key defining feature of Alzheimer's disease (Damasio and Van Hoesen, 1986; McKhann et al., 1984).

In contrast, classic examples of subcortical dementia (e.g., Parkinson's disease, Huntington's disease (HD), Wilson's disease, progressive supranuclear palsy) feature memory impairment that is best described as a retrieval disturbance. Albert, Feldman, and Willis (1974) noted that forgetfulness is a significant finding in progressive supranuclear palsy. Others (McHugh and Folstein, 1975; Caine, Ebert, and Weingartner, 1977) demonstrated a similar problem in HD, and many Parkinson's disease patients have a retrieval difficulty (Albert, 1978; Wilson et al., 1980). The memory disorder of subcortical dementia is intermixed with other problems such as impaired cognition, psychomotor slowing, and, in most instances, a significant motor disorder. Each additional problem interferes with the clear demonstration of memory dysfunction, but retrieval difficulty is prominent.

Many other causes of dementia produce retrieval problems. For instance, lacunar vascular dementia (Hachinski, Lassen, and Marshall, 1974), Binswanger's disease (Caplan and Schoene, 1978), systemic disorders such as cardiac and pulmonary insufficiency (Benson and Blumer, 1982), chemical intoxications and medication overdoses (Cummings, 1985b), increased intracranial pressure, and hydrocephalus (Katzman, 1977) all produce memory disorders with retrieval deficit greater than disturbance of new learning. Unlike the memory disorders of cortical dementia, faulty retrieval of learned information is the most prominent memory difficulty in subcortical dementia.

Frontal Brain Damage. Whether damage to the frontal lobe produces a memory disturbance has been debated for years (Hécaen, 1964; Hécaen and Albert, 1978; Luria, 1973; Stuss and Benson, 1986). Significant memory disorder has been reported following frontal damage (Alexander and Freedman, 1984; Damasio et al., 1985; Lindquist and Norlen, 1966) but may be absent even in cases with massive frontal pathology (Ackerly and Benton, 1947; Black, 1976). Part of the confusion stems from failure to separate retrieval from learning.

Frontal damage can impair control of many mental functions, including memory (Stuss and Benson, 1986). The ability to maintain directed attention and to ignore interfering stimuli is disturbed, seriously decreasing immediate recall. Information may be received but not maintained sufficiently to be learned. Patients with frontal brain damage often have trouble maintaining sequences of information (Fuster, 1980), limiting their ability to retain information for learning. Memory tests that use an interference task (e.g., the Peterson and Peterson [1959] paradigm) routinely demonstrate significant memory problems in patients with frontal damage. Inability to control distractions and inadequate maintenance of sequences are significant limiting factors. A third source of frontal memory dysfunction concerns retrieval. Memory retrieval demands initiation of drive, a function linked to midline frontal structures (Damasio and Van Hoesen, 1983; Stuss and Benson, 1986), and most published studies documenting frontal memory disorder show involvement of midline structures (Alexander and Freedman, 1984; Damasio et al., 1985). Thus, the activation of memory retrieval appears to depend on intact function of midline frontal structures.

NEUROANATOMICAL SUBSTRATE

In the past three decades clear correlations between focal areas of brain damage and memory disturbances have been established. Damage to any portion of the brain may impair memory to some degree, but the primary processing disturbances have specific anatomical correlations.

Immediate Recall

The ability to maintain a limited quantity of information (in digit tests, the magical number seven, plus or minus two) with complete accuracy for a limited period of time is a significant step in memory function (Miller, 1956). Few of the disorders that impair immediate recall (e.g., confusional state) are based on focal anatomical damage; more common are disorders of other body systems that affect the brain as well. Some features of the confusional state, however, suggest tentative anatomical correlations.

One common feature of confusion—decreased level of awakeness—can be localized. Moruzzi and Magoun (1949) and subsequent investigators (Hobson, 1974; Magoun, 1963; Rossi and Zanchetti, 1957) demonstrated that bilateral damage to the reticular substance and its connections (the reticular activating system) produces somnolence; lesions elsewhere in the brain do not. The drowsiness, lethargy, decreased alertness, and clouded consciousness that are present in some acute confusional states strongly suggest abnormality of the mesencephalic reticular substance and/or its connections (see Chapter 5).

A second aspect of the confusional state, disturbance of attention, suggests a different anatomical focus. The inability to attain or maintain a mental sequence of information in the face of interference, or the tendency to abandon it once established, may reflect frontal dysfunction (Fuster, 1989; Stuss and Benson, 1986). Similarly, perceptual misinterpretations (hallucinations, delusions) suggest deficient frontal control (Benson and Stuss, 1990; Miller et al., 1986), as do other manifestations of the confusional state—distractibility, agitated restlessness, hallucinatory experiences, and poor hold on reality. The locus of frontal dysfunction leading to these malfunctions remains unsettled, but interference with immediate recall is one result.

Learning

Most diseases or injuries that impair learning (causing true amnesia) involve focal neuroanatomical damage. The list of causes of amnesia in Table 9.3 includes the locus of neuroanatomical damage underlying each disorder. An interconnected anatomical substrate can be noted. One key area, the medial temporal region, encompasses the hippocampus and such parahippocampal structures as the subiculum, entorhinal area, and hippocampal cortex (Damasio and Van Hoesen, 1986; Milner and Penfield, 1955; Scoville and Milner, 1957). A second area includes midline diencephalic structures, particularly the rostral hypothalamus (mamillary bodies) and medial thalamus. Both areas—the medial temporal and the midline diencephalic—are part of the limbic system. Figure 9.2 illustrates the major limbic structures involved in learning. A large body of clinical and

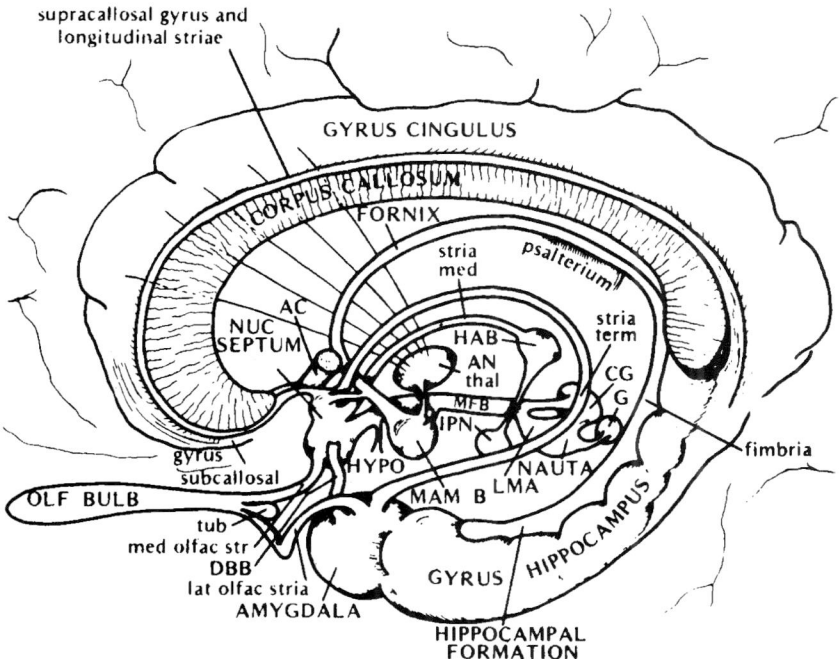

Fig. 9.2. Schematic illustration of the hippocampal–limbic system. Of proved significance for learning are the hippocampal formation, fimbria, fornix and mamillary bodies; these structures represent an inner core of the limbic system. From Heilman et al., 1985a.

experimental work demonstrates that bilateral damage to segments of the temporal and/or diencephalic limbic system impairs learning.

Other anatomical structures deserve consideration. The fornix connects the medial temporal limbic structures with the mamillary bodies; evidence indicates that bilateral fornix separation produces a typical amnesia (Grafman et al., 1985; Heilman and Sypert, 1977; Sweet, Talland, and Ervin, 1959). Bilateral damage to other limbic areas such as the anterior thalamic nucleus or cingulate cortex may interfere with memory processing (Damasio et al., 1985), but the clinical findings are sufficiently obscured by other symptomatology that firm evidence is lacking.

The only neuroanatomical areas involved in pure amnesia (Table 9.3) are limbic structures (Benson and McDaniel, 1990; Squire, 1987). Structural damage to other brain regions does not cause amnesia.

Is the anatomical substrate for learning lateralized? In most reported cases of pure amnesia, the pathology has been bilateral. Unilateral lesions may produce amnesia (Benson, Marsden, and Meadows, 1974), but the memory disturbance tends to be transient and/or demands sophisticated neuropsychological testing for detection. Appropriate testing demonstrates that right hemisphere temporal/limbic damage interferes with nonverbal memory and left temporal/limbic damage primarily affects verbal memory but that both types of learning can be accomplished after either of the temporal lobes has been removed (Milner, 1966; Rausch, 1985).

Retrieval

Though retrieval disturbances are usually accompanied by other behavioral abnormalities, a specific anatomical substrate can be suggested for them. In particular, damage to selected mesencephalic or diencephalic nuclei and/or their connections to the medial frontal lobe is probably essential. We know that the mesencephalic/diencephalic nuclei involved in information retrieval are distinct from those involved in the alertness aspect of immediate recall, since disorders with significant mesencephalic pathology (e.g., progressive supranuclear palsy, Parkinson's disease) cause no problem with wakefulness but do interfere with retrieval (Case 9.7). Some of the mesencephalic/diencephalic nuclei utilize dopamine as a neurotransmitter, which indicates that retrieval disturbance may warrant consideration as a disorder of dopamine metabolism (Graybiel, 1990; Kety, 1972; Martin et al., 1984). Bachman and Albert (1984) suggested that the rate of information processing slows when disease causes dopamine deficiency.

Retrieval of already learned information is closely associated with drive and motivation and is governed by two closely related neuroanatomical regions—the mesencephalic/diencephalic areas controlling arousal and the midline frontal lobe structures involved in attention. Damage to any area in this continuum can disrupt retrieval of learned information, but accompanying signs and symptoms differ with the site of pathology.

THE NEURAL BASIS OF MEMORY

The neural theory of memory proposed here will follow the three divisions of memory outlined earlier (see pages 179–181) and will posit an additional element, unimodal memory, underlying information storage.

Unimodal and Heteromodal Association

The process that achieves identification or recognition in a single sensory modality (unimodal association) requires the availability of previously processed information in that modality for comparison and the ability to retrieve this information from storage. It follows that previously learned information in the single modality is stored in the appropriate unimodal association area. Thus the site of much memory storage is the unimodal association areas.

Heteromodal association brings together stored information from many unimodal systems, a process independent of the limbic memory circuit. Intermodal association of basic sensory and motor information occurs through networks including angular gyrus and other heteromodal association areas.

Two anatomically and functionally distinct memory systems—unimodal and heteromodal—are proposed here. Most modern discussions of memory concern the processing that follows heteromodal activity, but a basic memory store is essential to form the sensory percept. Most memories are stored in the unimodal and heteromodal association cortices; their interconnecting circuitries are the crucial sites of memory storage.

Immediate Recall

Newly acquired information is processed through the networks of unimodal and heteromodal association neurons described above, but, unless the limbic circuit is activated, this material rapidly degrades and disappears (Brown, 1964; Vallar and Shallice, 1990). Multiple associations utilize the same pathways, and many of the originally activated circuits are blocked by competing patterns. Most information produced by higher level associations is lost within moments. Even when conscious attempts to learn are made, accurate retention of information is short lived—the limitation of immediate recall.

Learning

Learning seems to depend on the limbic system, but what precise role does limbic circuitry play in memory processing? One theory holds that most declarative material placed in long-term memory storage is processed through the inner limbic system during rehearsal. As proposed by Damasio and colleagues (Damasio and Van Hoesen, 1986; Hyman et al., 1984), the entorhinal area acts as a gathering site for sensory information from the entire brain and the subiculum acts as a staging area for information outflow from the medial temporal limbic structures. Between them lies the hippocampus, which receives most of the entorhinal output and sends most of its efferents through the subiculum. Pathological studies support this theory; severe neural degeneration is noted in both the entorhinal area and the subiculum in Alzheimer's disease, a disorder in which declarative memory disturbance is prominent (Hyman et al., 1984).

Another theory holds that the limbic system provides a nonspecific output that enables cortical circuits to rehearse and maintain newly received information (Benson and McDaniel, 1990; Squire, 1987). The nature of the limbic activity is uncertain but so few direct connections exist between the limbic system and the sensorimotor association areas that the limbic action must be indirect.

Despite the uncertainties, a number of solid points about the neural basis of learning can be made. First, the inner limbic circuit is essential for most verbal and much nonverbal learning. Second, each hemispheric limbic circuit is capable of performing most of the activity necessary for learning; memory impairment caused by unilateral limbic disorder is usually so mild that only sophisticated neuropsychological testing can demonstrate it (Milner, 1966; Rausch, 1985). Third, memory is not stored in the medial temporal region; large amounts of medial temporal tissues can be removed without significantly diminishing memory. Fourth, for a relatively long time after information is placed into memory storage, limbic activity is necessary for its retrieval; but information learned many years previously can be retrieved when the limbic circuitry is no longer functioning (Alberts, Butters, and Levin, 1979; Seltzer and Benson, 1974). Fifth, motor skills can be learned despite damage to limbic core structures. Sixth, unimodal learning is not affected by limbic disorder.

Retrieval

An incredibly vast quantity of information is held in long-term storage, but little is known about the storage structures. It may be that information is maintained in cortical–cortical and cortical–subcortical networks, similar to the networks initially activated during the unimodal and heteromodal association phases. Most of the information placed in storage presumably is spread through an extensive network of neural structures in both hemispheres. The many areas involved may explain why complex individual memories are rarely lost following focal brain damage. If a brain-damaged patient is sufficiently intact to respond, much of the store of old knowledge can be activated. On the other hand, following focal brain damage, retrieval through one association modality may be far more difficult than through another (e.g., a patient with alexia has severely limited memory retrieval on viewing a written word but no problem when the same word is spoken). Retrieval disturbance is eased when additional stimuli (prompts, cues) activate additional inputs to the neuronal network.

The retrieval process requires priming—some stimulus, either internal or external—to activate the appropriate network. The many associations noted by Galton (1879a,b) on his Pall Mall walk (Chapter 2) provide a good example of sensory priming. After priming, however, other brain circuits must also participate in retrieval. Thus inner limbic circuitry is needed for access to recent memory stores and midline mesencephalic and frontal circuits activate (drive) their retrieval. Even if recently stored memories are intact, the ability to retrieve them depends on both limbic and frontal system activation.

10

The Neurology of Cognitive Disorders

> But well-connected meaning-structures let you turn ideas around in your mind, to consider alternatives and envision things from many perspectives until you find one that works. And that's what we mean by thinking!
> —M. MINSKY, 1985

> The mental features discoursed of as analytical are, in themselves, but little susceptible of analysis.
> –EDGAR ALLEN POE, 1841/1980

AXIOMS/POSTULATES

Cognition produces novel constructs by synthesis and manipulation of available information.

Cognition utilizes both newly processed sensations and previously accumulated information.

Cognition is performed by posterior and basal neural systems.

Depending on one's perspective, *cognition* can refer to either a broad, multistep processing of information (Ellis and Young, 1988) or a relatively precise step in the thinking process (Chapter 1). Almost every conceivable mental activity is relevant to cognition, but in this chapter the term will be used in the restricted sense.

VARIETIES OF COGNITIVE ACTIVITY

As narrowly defined in Chapter 1, *cognition* refers to the manipulation of mental data. Cognition combines information already analyzed and synthesized through the various unimodal and transmodal processing steps with information stored in memory to form new compositions of data. Input comes from numerous sources including sensory pathways, cortical memory stores, the emotions, linguistic processing activities, and advanced visual–spatial imagery, but cognition goes beyond the basic unimodal and transmodal associations of sensory processing.

An elementary example from arithmetic helps to illustrate this limited definition of cognition. When one is asked the sum of 2 + 3, the answer is based on rote memory. The answer was learned in school and has become part of the individual's fund of knowledge. In contrast, if one is asked the sum of 42 + 93, the answer does not come directly from memory because the sum has not been learned. Instead, bits of information taken from memory stores (2 + 3, 4 + 9) and a learned computational process (carrying) are combined. Previously learned material is manipulated to provide the correct answer. This is cognition in its most elementary form.

A more subtle manipulation of knowledge occurs in the interpretation of a proverb. If the saying "One shouldn't cry over spilled milk" is to be interpreted, the statement must be altered through analysis of linguistic metaphors. "Spilled milk" becomes an action or social situation, broad or specific, and "shouldn't cry" represents the futility of reliving irremediable events from the past. Proverbs are deciphered by substituting stored (realistic) information for their metaphorical elements. Competency in both arithmetic and proverb interpretation varies with intelligence, formal education, and familiarity with the problem. In the testing situation, appropriate levels of difficulty must be determined to challenge an individual's ability to interpret proverbs (Gorham, 1956) or perform mathematics. Mere restatement of the elements of the proverb without any attempt at metaphorical analysis indicates disordered cognition (concrete thinking), and an acquired inability to manipulate numbers is called *acalculia*.

CLINICAL EXAMPLES

Although mental manipulation tasks are routine elements of the mental status examination, cognitive dysfunction is often obscured, partially or fully, by disturbances in other mental activities, a problem to be noted in all of the clinical cases presented below.

Case 10.1

A 53-year-old, right-handed man was examined after partial removal of a low-grade glioma from the left posterior parietal convexity. Following his recovery from surgery, a full neurological evaluation revealed no basic defects; there was no paralysis, sensory loss, visual field loss, or aphasia. However, all four elements of the Gerstmann syndrome were present—difficulty in distinguishing right from left; considerable difficulty in naming or identifying fingers (despite excellent naming ability for other body parts and no problem in recognizing the name of any body parts except fingers); agraphia (he could write a few words to dictation but spelling errors were common; he could not formulate a sentence); and acalculia. The calculating problem was new; he had worked with numbers most of his life, both as a cashier in a restaurant and, in an even more demanding situation, as an independent bookie handling bets. A variety of errors impeded his attempts to calculate, including substitution of one number for another when repeating or writing a dictated problem, misnaming written numbers, and miswriting numbers as parts of the problem or as the answer and then misnaming the incorrect number he had just written. In both written and orally presented addition, subtraction, and multiplication problems, paraphasic substitution of one number for another (a language disorder) was frequent. In addition, however, the patient tended to make errors in the computational process. Thus, when given a modestly complex multiplication problem (e.g., 326 × 54 = ____), he would multiply the first line of numerals, add the second group, multiply the third, and so forth. (Benson and Denckla, 1969)

The calculating disorder of Case 10.1 included paraphasic substitutions, perseveration, and difficulty in using the correct computational process. The first two difficulties relate to language formulation and the ability to handle sequences, respectively. The third problem, inability to manipulate numbers (compute), represents a disorder of cognition. The patient's acalculia combined language, sequencing, and cognition disturbances.

Case 10.2
A 58-year-old, right-handed army sergeant was hospitalized following the acute onset of right-sided weakness and aphasia. The paresis and a right visual inattention defect cleared rapidly; within one week there was no evidence of weakness or visual field defect, but a mild cortical sensory loss (disturbed position sense, graphesthesia, and stereognosis) persisted. The aphasia also changed rapidly so that one week after onset the patient's verbal output was fluent but contaminated with literal paraphasias; his comprehension of spoken language was excellent, but he had serious difficulty in repeating or naming. These are the hallmarks of conduction aphasia. Written language was easily comprehended, but reading aloud was impossible because of paraphasias; written output was filled with paragraphic substitutions not unlike the paraphasic substitutions noted in repetition. All four components of the Gerstmann syndrome (finger agnosia, right–left disorientation, agraphia, and acalculia) were present.

Analysis of the patient's acalculia was hindered by his aphasia. He could count only to ten before making paraphasic substitutions, and when presented with a written number he often substituted an incorrect number in his oral response. In contrast, if a number was written and then either an oral number or a series of dots presented, he always matched correctly. When given written problems he often misread the numbers (paraphasia), and when numbers were dictated he frequently wrote them incorrectly (paragraphia). When asked to solve problems with multiple numbers he not only stated the numbers incorrectly but also, in doing the calculations, stated incorrect numbers for the intermediate sums as well as the answer. If he simultaneously wrote and recited numbers, the paragraphic output was often different from the paraphasic spoken number. Despite these errors, he followed the rules of computation and always respected place-holding values. If a multiple choice of answers for a written problem was offered, he was almost invariably correct in his choice. For example, given the problem 4 + 5, he answered "8," wrote the number 5, and confidently selected the number 9 from a multiple choice list. In more difficult problems his oral and written responses were invariably wrong, but he almost always picked the correct response from a multiple choice. A diagnosis of conduction aphasia with posterior extension of the lesion to produce the Gerstmann syndrome was suggested. (Benson and Denckla, 1969)

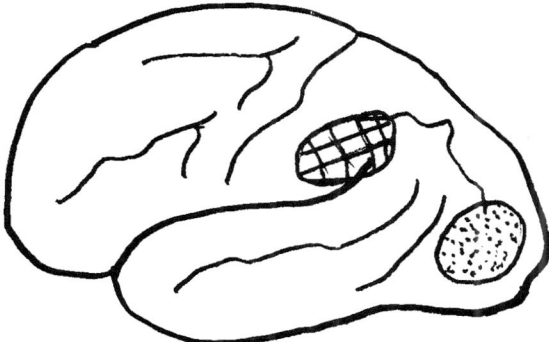

Fig. 10.1. Lateral view of the left hemisphere showing the suspected sites of pathology in Cases 10.1 and 10.2. The *stippled area* of pathology located in the occipital–posterior parietal area represents the location of the tumor in Case 10.1; the *cross-hatched area* in the supramarginal gyrus represents an area of suspected infarction in Case 10.2.

In this case, unlike Case 10.1, errors in calculations were not accompanied by errors in computational strategy. In both cases, a language-processing disorder was manifested by the paraphasic substitutions, but only Case 10.1 appeared to have lost the ability to manipulate numbers, a cognitive disorder. Figure 10.1 illustrates the location of the lesions in the two cases.

Case 10.3

A 42-year-old, college-educated industrial relations executive was involved in a minor traffic accident in which he sustained a blow to the left skull. He did not lose consciousness. Mild right-sided neurological findings and a fluent aphasia were present. These problems cleared within a few days, but the patient then discovered that he could not read or write or perform even simple arithmetic. Many tests, including EEG, lumbar puncture, carotid angiography, and pneumoencephalography, failed to reveal distinct pathology, but an isotope brain scan demonstrated a small area of increased uptake in the posterior parietal region of the left brain.

A neurobehavioral evaluation performed several years later revealed mild residual dysfunctions in neurological and mental activities. A slight asymmetry of optokinetic nystagmus, a homonymous, partial right lower quadrant visual field defect, a slight clumsiness of the right limbs, and a mild decrease in stereognosis and two-point discrimination in the right hand were found. The patient could read, but at a slow and laborious pace and only at an upper-grade-school level, well below his premorbid capability. His writing was also slow and below premorbid competency. He had learned to monitor and correct his difficulty in right–left orientation. Similarly, he had learned to compensate for his difficulty in naming and/or identifying fingers. The most profound residual disorder involved calculation.

The calculation problem varied with the difficulty and type of computation to be performed. The patient insisted that before the injury he had been remarkably adept at mathematics, mentally performing percentages when discussing salary and benefits with potential employees. On examination he was fully competent in number language and could perform all rote addition, subtraction, and multiplication problems (e.g., 7 + 4; 9 − 6; 8 × 7) presented orally or in written form. He wrote dictated problems correctly and retained the methods of computation. While he could add, subtract, and multiply, he failed if carrying or borrowing was needed, and he tended to change computational mode in the midst of a problem (e.g., adding one portion, multiplying another). Periodic reevaluation over the next five years demonstrated that the calculation disorder remained fixed, although reading and writing abilities and the other aspects of the Gerstmann syndrome improved. (Benson and Weir, 1972)

In this case, the patient's basic rote memory stores and ability to handle number language appeared intact, but his ability to manipulate the data was compromised. The acalculia was based on a focal brain lesion.

Arithmetical calculation provides a clear example of the manipulation of knowledge (Binet, 1894), and acalculia, the acquired impairment of calculation, is readily noted in the clinic. Henschen (1922) documented over 100 published cases of acalculia in his review of the aphasia literature. Despite this frequency, clinical investigation of calculation disorders remains limited (Hécaen, Angelergues, and Houillier, 1961; Spiers, 1987), and most formal studies of calculation are based only on written problems and record only success or failure.

To study calculating ability adequately requires analysis of competency with number language and number concepts (e.g., that three dots are equivalent to the written number 3), visual–spatial ordering (place-holding value) of numbers, the individual's understanding of computational signs, and the mechanics of the computational processes themselves. There are three major variations of calculating disorder: (1) aphasic acalculia in which the patient is unable to handle number language; (2) visual–spatial acalculia in which the patient cannot maintain appropriate place-holding values; and (3) anarithmetria in which the processes of computation are disturbed (Hécaen, 1962). Aphasic acalculia occurs primarily with dominant (left) hemisphere damage. Posterior nondominant hemisphere pathology can result in an inability to place numbers in space (e.g., when a column is added, single digits, tens, and hundreds are not placed in appropriate columns). The individual steps of computation may be performed correctly, but the final product is wrong (Cohn, 1961). Although clearly described, anarithmetria is more difficult to demonstrate and to correlate with neuropathology. Some authors have noted that anarithmetria is most prominently seen in brain disorders with diffuse pathology such as Alzheimer's disease and have suggested that computational ability depends on widespread cerebral function (Critchley, 1953; Grewel, 1952).

In Cases 10.1 and 10.2 aphasic acalculia was clearly demonstrated by the patients' inconsistency in handling spoken or written number language. Each retained computational function, but Case 10.2 performed better than Case 10.1, a person who had used basic arithmetic frequently in his occupation. It must be assumed that Case 10.1 suffered at least some degree of anarithmetria.

Case 10.3 is one of the few reported cases in which focal brain damage produced a relatively pure disturbance of computational skill. Of four potential causes of the patient's acalculia—inability to remember (retrieve) the multiplication tables; inability to add the initial products; inability to carry digits forward as needed; and confusion of the processes of multiplication, addition, or carrying—all but the fourth were excluded by specific tests. His anarithmetria apparently resulted from posterior parietal damage in the dominant hemisphere.

Cases 10.1, 10.2, and 10.3 all manifested the combination of four abnormalities called the Gerstmann syndrome (right–left disorientation, finger agnosia, agraphia, and acalculia). Each individual component can result from other abnormalities (e.g., aphasia, visual–spatial defect, unilateral neglect). No single component provides localizing information, but, when all four findings are present, a specific site of damage is probable (Benson and Geschwind, 1970; Gerstmann, 1924, 1927, 1931). Gerstmann (1924) originally suggested that the co-occurrence of all four findings indicated dominant hemisphere parietal lobe damage, a premise accepted by many of his peers (Poeck and Orgass, 1966; Schilder, 1931; Stengel, 1944). The validity of the syndrome has been strongly challenged by Benton (1959, 1961, 1977, 1992), whose views are supported by studies that have failed to demonstrate consistent grouping of the four findings in brain-damaged patients (Benton, 1959; Critchley, 1966; Heimburger, Demyer, and Reitan, 1961). Nonetheless, the Gerstmann syndrome remains a useful localizing syndrome in behavioral neurology. Although each part of the syndrome can be produced by damage elsewhere in the brain, when all four are present with few other abnormalities, dominant parietal dysfunction is probable (Benson and Geschwind, 1975; Nielsen, 1938; Roeltgen, Sevush, and Heilman, 1983). Each element of the Gerstmann syndrome is related to disordered manipulation of mental data, a cognitive disturbance.

Case 10.4

A 56-year-old man (same as Case 12.9) was evaluated for a second opinion regarding the diagnosis of Alzheimer's disease. The patient was a successful general surgeon who had continued active surgical practice until a few months before the examination. For several years, however, his wife, office personnel, and colleagues had noted increasing forgetfulness. Despite his difficulty in remembering names of patients, times of appointments, and so on, his surgical skills apparently remained intact. He was finally advised to withdraw from his practice, and a diagnosis of Alzheimer's disease was proposed.

When examined, the patient was happy, healthy, and alert, with no signs of physical disease. His basic neurological status was normal, and he appeared younger and more vigorous than anticipated for his age. Mental status examination, however, showed that he was only vaguely oriented, had tremendous problems learning new information (e.g., the examiner's name), and expressed himself poorly because his speech lacked specific, semantically significant words. He produced only a few words in categories suggested by the examiner (e.g., animals, American cities). His ability to calculate was severely hampered even though he could recite numbers and correctly answer rote addition and multiplication problems; he completely failed to formulate or perform even slightly complex problems. Proverb interpretation was rigidly concrete. He interpreted the proverb "one shouldn't cry over spilled milk" as meaning that "the milk can't be used anymore anyhow." He interpreted the proverb "people who live in glass houses shouldn't throw stones" as "everyone knows that stones will break the glass." He failed to recognize how a boat and an airplane were similar and flatly denied any similarity between a coat and a dress, an apple and an orange, and so forth. Over the next several years the dementia gradually worsened; serial CT scans showed progressive enlargement of the ventricles and increasing cortical atrophy. Postmortem examination of his brain some eight years after the initial clinical evaluation showed multiple senile plaques and neurofibrillary tangles, confirming the diagnosis of Alzheimer's disease. (courtesy of Bruce L. Miller, M.D.)

This patient had problems with many higher level mental functions, including language, memory, and visual–spatial responses. Defective cognition was demonstrated by his inability to perform complex calculations at a time when his ability to perform rote calculations and use number language was intact. The concrete responses to relatively simple proverbs by a well-educated individual also suggest cognitive dysfunction, although the presence of aphasia complicates this interpretation. It must be acknowledged that his failures in calculation and in the interpretation of proverbs and similarities and differences were matched by many other mental impairments including amnesia, aphasia, and constructional disturbance. Nonetheless, when he was first evaluated, his difficulty in manipulating knowledge was considerably more severe than his problems with language, memory, and physical function. No focal neuroanatomical lesion is found in Alzheimer's disease; rather, there is widespread cortical pathology that is most profound in parietal/temporal association areas (Cummings and Benson, 1992; Greenfield et al., 1958). Cognitive abnormality is an early and progressively troublesome problem in Alzheimer's disease, but the findings are easily overshadowed by the presence of other mental dysfunctions.

Case 10.5
A 53-year-old man (reported in more detail as Case 11.2) with bifrontal traumatic brain damage was admitted for rehabilitation of persistent behavioral impairment. He was apathetic, disinterested, and unconcerned, but careful testing revealed no problems in language, memory, visual–spatial functions, or cognition. He readily and accurately performed multiple digit calculations, both with and without paper and pencil. He was superb at interpreting proverbs (far better than his attending physicians) and performed well above normal in discerning similarities and differences. Thus, despite a gross personality alteration and disabling psychomotor retardation caused by frontal damage, there was no evidence to suggest problems in the manipulation of previously learned knowledge. (DFB)

Despite a persistent, disabling mental disorder based on bifrontal brain damage, this patient had no difficulty utilizing and manipulating his knowledge base to perform calculations, interpret proverbs, and recognize

Case 10.6

A 61-year-old man was admitted to the Boston VA hospital to probe the influence of bifrontal leucotomy on his psychological functions. Twenty-seven years earlier, at age 34 years, he had undergone bifrontal leucotomy to treat schizophrenia. His postoperative course included some days of mutism and many weeks of psychomotor retardation, but he improved, was discharged to the care of his family, eventually maintained himself in his own living quarters, and worked steadily at menial jobs. He had been without evidence of psychotic behavior for over 20 years when examined at the Boston VA. Figure 10-2, a CT scan performed as part of the evaluation, demonstrates the bifrontal damage produced by the leucotomy procedure.

An extensive neuropsychological battery included four tests selected to probe cognitive function (Stuss and Benson, 1983). The Wechsler Adult Intelligence Scale showed average intelligence (full scale, 104; verbal, 106; performance, 101). A Visual–Metaphor Test (Winner and Gardner, 1977) probed the patient's ability to understand metaphors (e.g., a heavy heart) by selecting an appropriately descriptive picture. He had little difficulty with this test. The Visual–Verbal Test (Feldman and Drasgow, 1960) also required interpretation of an abstract concept. The patient had to tell how three of four figures on a card were alike in some way;

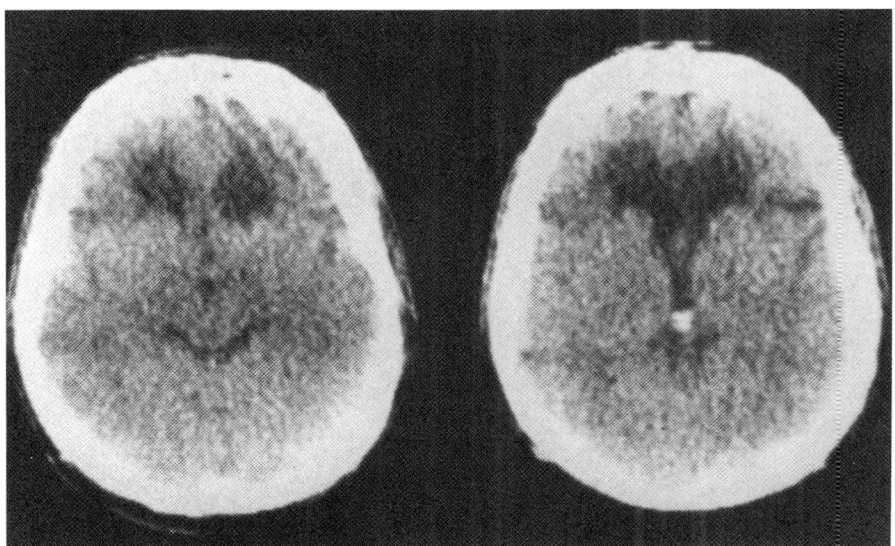

Fig. 10.2. X-ray CT scans of Case 10.6 demonstrating the area of leucotomy damage. The lower cut *(left)* shows two large, deep prefrontal lesions. The somewhat higher cut *(right)* shows the relationship of these lesions with the frontal horns of the ventricles. From Naeser et al., 1981.

then, how three of the four figures were alike in some different way. He had no difficulty with the initial abstraction but could make the shift to the second abstraction in only a few of the problems. The fourth test, the Wisconsin Card Sort Test (Grant and Berg, 1948; Milner, 1963), in which he had to select a correct response (e.g., color), maintain this choice for ten steps, and then select and maintain another response, all without verbal instruction, proved very difficult. He attained only three correct responses (six to eight would have been anticipated) because he failed to maintain the mental set. He became disinterested, responded randomly, and perseverated. (Naeser et al., 1981)

Although the frontal lesions in Case 10.6 were sizable, the patient readily performed tasks that required considerable cognitive skill in discovering metaphorical meanings for words and phrases. He did poorly on the Wisconsin Card Sort Test, however, a task requiring maintenance as well as manipulation of sequentially presented material. His failure involved the maintenance of sequential material (serial order preservation), but not the basic manipulations of cognition.

NEUROANATOMICAL SUBSTRATE

Little information points to specific neuroanatomical sites or pathways dedicated to cognitive functions. Clinical data, however, do provide several indications of the scope of these activities and the anatomical substrates involved.

First, cognition demands recognition and integration of pertinent information from multiple sources, a synthesis based on cross-modal associations. Following the premise advanced in Chapter 2, the angular gyrus of the parietal lobe appears to be crucial for cross-modal integration. Thus the angular gyrus, the surrounding cortical association areas, and their interconnections may be of particular importance in cognition.

The best support for this view of the role of posterior parietal cortex in the manipulation of information comes from cases of acalculia like those presented above. Three distinct disturbances affecting calculating ability were presented, along with clinical evidence indicating that different cerebral areas were involved. The process of calculation most dependent on cognition—computation—appears most sensitive to posterior dominant hemisphere parietal damage (Cases 10.1 and 10.3). While the quantity of clinical data supporting this statement is limited, a number of reports of the Gerstmann syndrome and several reported cases of pure anarithmetria (Benson and Weir, 1972; Roeltgen, Sevush, and Heilman, 1983) are in agreement. Computation, however, is a complex act dependent on number language and visual–spatial and computational competency. It draws on many brain areas in both hemispheres.

Negative findings provide additional clues to the localization of cognition within the brain. Cases 10.5 and 10.6 show that prefrontal damage does not interfere with the ability to perform cognitive tasks. In Cases 10.5 and 10.6 cognitive processing was successful despite significant prefrontal damage. In contrast, Case 10.4 with Alzheimer's disease, a disorder often described as beginning with parietal/temporal cortex dysfunction (Lishman, 1987), lost the ability to perform calculations and interpret proverbs early in the disease course.

This chapter has stressed the verbal dimensions of cognition but the manipulation of visual–spatial information should be recognized as a cognitive function and also depends on parietal/occipital activity, primarily in the right or nondominant hemisphere. The discussion of topographagnosia in Chapter 7 provides a clinical description of the disorder affecting the ability to perform tasks involving spatial analysis (Hécaen et al., 1956). Psychological tests such as route-finding and maze-learning require the manipulation of visual–spatial information; performance of both tasks is most affected by right hemisphere, posterior lesions (Corkin, 1968; Hécaen and Albert, 1978; Milner, 1964). Similarly, tests of the ability to perform an abstract 180 degree rotation of a complex scene is most difficult for individuals with right posterior hemisphere damage (Butters, Barton, and Brody, 1970).

The posterior hemispheric localization in these cases does not indicate a center for cognition. Rather, this area appears to serve as a blender, fusing information from many other sources. Cognition requires more than just the transmodal capability of the posterior parietal region.

NEURAL BASIS OF COGNITION

The narrow definition of cognition excludes processes such as the reception and processing of information, the retrieval of previously stored information, the influence of emotion, the executive control functions, and the establishment of responses. Cognition builds on and alters available information that can be placed in storage, acted on, verbalized, or used to initiate a gesture or an emotional response. The output of cognition accounts for much of an individual's memory stores.

Manipulation of information is pivotal in such aspects of thinking as concept formation (Bruner, Goodnow, and Austin, 1956; Nelson, 1973; Piaget, 1950) and problem solving (Bolton, 1972; Gilhooly, 1982; Sanford, 1987). Yet serious disorders of thought processing may be coupled with excellent ability to manipulate information, as in Cases 10.5 and 10.6. Cognition is not the equivalent of thinking; rather, it is one important step in the overall process.

11

The Neurology of Higher Mental Control Disorders

> What is the function of that large and excitable mass of brain situated in front of the motor zone?
> —BIANCHI, 1922

> The entire period of human evolutionary existence can be viewed as the age of the frontal lobe.
> —TILNEY, 1928

AXIOMS/POSTULATES

Higher mental control functions influence most brain operations, including thought processing.

Higher mental control functions operate upon and through the basic mental functions.

Five higher mental control functions can be proposed: drive, sequencing, executive (cognitive) control, future memory, and self-awareness.

Higher mental control is a function of the prefrontal neural systems.

It is widely recognized, if not fully accepted, that the prefrontal cortex, that portion of the frontal lobe lying anterior to the unimodal motor association cortex, plays a major role in the control of human mental functions (Goldman-Rakic, 1987; Stuss and Benson, 1986). Exactly what the prefrontal cortex does has proved unexpectedly difficult to ascertain, however. This chapter will explore the neurology of prefrontal disorders and attempt to place prefrontal activities in the overall pattern of brain function. These activities are termed *higher mental control functions* to distinguish them from the more basic mental control functions discussed in Chapter 5.

The concept of higher mental control is to be distinguished from cognition. Both involve the manipulation of knowledge and are related, but there are important differences.

The human prefrontal cortex is massive in comparison to that of most other living species and has often been regarded as the key to human distinctiveness. Intelligence was often equated with prefrontal function, but many observations proved this incorrect (Hebb and Penfield, 1940; Teuber, 1964). Studies of frontal brain injury and prefrontal leucotomy demonstrated that large amounts of prefrontal tissue could be damaged without altering intelligence, at least as measured by standard tests (Hebb and Penfield, 1940; Mettler, 1949; Stuss and Benson, 1986). Much earlier, H. Munk (1890) had demonstrated that damage to either occipital or parietal temporal brain areas produced far greater intellectual deficit than quantitatively similar frontal lobe damage. Others (Goltz, 1884; Loeb, 1886; Horsley and Schafer, 1888) also denied that the frontal lobes had important psychological or intellectual functions based on studies after prefrontal tissues had been destroyed.

Clinical reports, however, described serious consequences of frontal injury. Phineas Gage (Harlow, 1868) and the patients of L. Welt (1888), R. M. Brickner (1936), and S. S. Ackerly and A. Benton (1947) all suffered behavioral alterations following frontal lobe damage despite being basically intact physically and intellectually. Ample support came from the study of behavioral alterations following prefrontal leucotomy (Freeman, 1949; Moniz, 1937; Scoville, 1949), frontal brain tumors (Hécaen, 1964; Luria et al., 1964), and war-induced frontal brain injuries (Feuchtwanger, 1923; Kleist, 1934b; Lishman, 1968; Weinstein and Teuber, 1957). The reported behavioral disorders were variable, however. Premorbid intellectual, behavioral, and personality status was of obvious importance. Eventually some relatively consistent alterations, particularly personality disturbances, were documented, and a clinical impression of "frontal lobishness" gained acceptance.

More recent theories have provided a better conceptualization of frontal functions (Miller, Galanter, and Pribram, 1960; Pribram, 1973; Shallice and Evans, 1978; Teuber, 1964), at least partially supported by contemporary anatomical and clinical investigations. Krieg (1954), Nauta (1971, 1972), Pandya, Dye, and Butters (1971), Van Hoesen, Pandya, and Butters (1975), Goldman-Rakic (1984), and many others have demonstrated anatomical relationships between frontal lobe structures and other brain regions. Fuster (1980, 1989), Damasio (1979), Luria (1965, 1966, 1969), Stuss and Benson (1986), and others have written on the neural basis of frontal functions from a clinical viewpoint.

Stuss and Benson (1984, 1986) proposed that four higher control functions can be attributed to the prefrontal cortex. A fifth function was suggested by David Ingvar (1985).

Sequencing involves maintenance of the serial order of information (temporal grading), its organization into salient sets, and subsequent integration with previously learned data. It is the ability to maintain a serial relationship over time. Simple sequencing can be demonstrated in some higher primates, primarily through delayed response tasks (Fuster, 1980, 1989; Jacobsen and Nissen, 1937), but the ease of performing serial tasks that characterizes human thought processing is not present in other animals. The ability to handle sequential information, maintain it in accurate order for a finite period, and reorganize it for subsequent processing is of

Table 11.1 Manifestations of Prefrontal Damage (Frontal Lobishness)

Tactlessness	*Irritability
Poorly restrained behavior	Disinhibition
Decreased social concern	Coarseness
Jocularity	Hyperkinetic
Facetiousness	Hypokinetic
Witzelsucht	Flare with anger
Moria	Puerile (silly) attitude
Boastfulness	Disinhibition of social graces
Grandiosity	Inappropriate sexual advances
Decreased intiative	Sexual exhibitionism
Decreased attentiveness	Lewd conversation
Forgetfulness	Erotic behavior
Poor memory	*Euphoria
Indifference	Poor planning ability
*Apathy	Diminished concern for the future
Shallow effect	Capriciousness
Lack of spontaneity	Loss of abstract attitude
Abulia	Loss of esthetic sense
Asthenia	Impulsiveness
Akinesia	Distractability
Deterioration of work quality	Stimulus bound
Depression	Concreteness
Morose discontent	Perseveration
	Restlessness
Delusions: Grandiosity (strength, wealth, intelligence)	
Nihilism	
Paranoia	
Hypochondriasis	

*The unholy triad of frontal behavior disorder suggested by Geschwind (1977).

obvious importance. While closely associated with more basic mental attributes, and operating through them, the time-related function of sequencing appears to be an independent prefrontal activity (Goldman-Rakic, 1984).

Drive is closely related to the basic mental control functions discussed in Chapter 5. Clinical experience abundantly demonstrates that drive, motivation, and will tend to be altered by prefrontal damage. Drive can be considered a superordinate function that energizes and stimulates responses made through basal/posterior systems.

Executive (cognitive) control includes anticipation, planning of response, monitoring of the potential response, response selection, and then monitoring of the actual response (Freeman, Watts, and Hunt, 1942; Hunt, 1942; Lhermitte, 1986; Schrader and Robinson, 1945). It is primarily, if not exclusively, a human function that has developed with the enlarged prefrontal cortex. Clinical descriptions of patients with prefrontal damage routinely include evidence of disturbed executive control.

Future memory (Ingvar, 1985) is closely related to executive control but represents preplanning of potential future actions to a degree that the actual acts are eventually carried out as a memory of already formulated plans. This process is significantly compromised by prefrontal brain damage.

Self-awareness refers to the ability of the human mental system to monitor itself. It includes not only review of an immediate response and planned responses but the ability to consider both past and future potentials. Also referred to as *self-consciousness* or *self-analysis,* the reflective qualities of self-awareness stand atop the proposed hierarchy of mental control functions (Stuss and Benson, 1986).

Current data do not provide specific anatomical correlates for these proposed prefrontal functional systems, but clinical observations characterize higher mental control activities through descriptions of the dysfunctions caused by frontal lobe damage (Table 11.1).

CLINICAL EXAMPLES

One of the first, and still one of the finest, published reports of behavioral disorder following prefrontal damage is the classic case of Phineas Gage (Harlow, 1868).

Case 11.1

Phineas Gage, a young foreman on a railroad construction crew in New Hampshire, while unschooled, was said to have had a "well-balanced mind [and] was very energetic and persistent in executing all his plans and operations." On his job Gage used a pointed iron bar (3 feet 7 inches long, 1¼ inches at its widest point) to tamp blasting powder into a narrow hole. One day a spark ignited the powder, and the tamping iron was propelled directly upward, entering Gage's head in the left maxillary area and protruding through the top of his skull. Though unconscious for a short time at the accident site, he regained consciousness before arriving in the nearest community for medical attention. There the tamping iron was removed and, to everyone's surprise, Gage not only survived but was free of neurological disability such as paralysis, sensory loss, or visual field disturbance.

A striking alteration in Gage's personality was soon obvious, however. He had been a God-fearing, family-loving, teetotaling, and scrupulously honest working man, but his behavior changed so dramatically that his workmates said he was "no longer Gage." Harlow (1868) eloquently described this postaccident behavior:

> The equilibrium or balance, so to speak, between his intellectual faculties and animal propensities seems to have been destroyed. He is fitful, irreverent, indulging at times in the grossest profanity, manifesting but little deference for his fellows, impatient of restraint or advice when it conflicts with his desires, at times pertinaciously obstinate, yet capricious and vacillating, devising many plans of operation, which are no sooner arranged than they are abandoned in turn for others appearing more feasible. A child in his intellectual capacity and manifestations, he has the animal passions of a strong man. . . . (Harlow, 1868; Blumer and Benson, 1975)

Figure 11.1 illustrates the tamping iron and the skull defect as drawn from the display of Gage's skull and the iron at the Warren Museum of the Harvard Medical School. The author's conjecture as to the area of

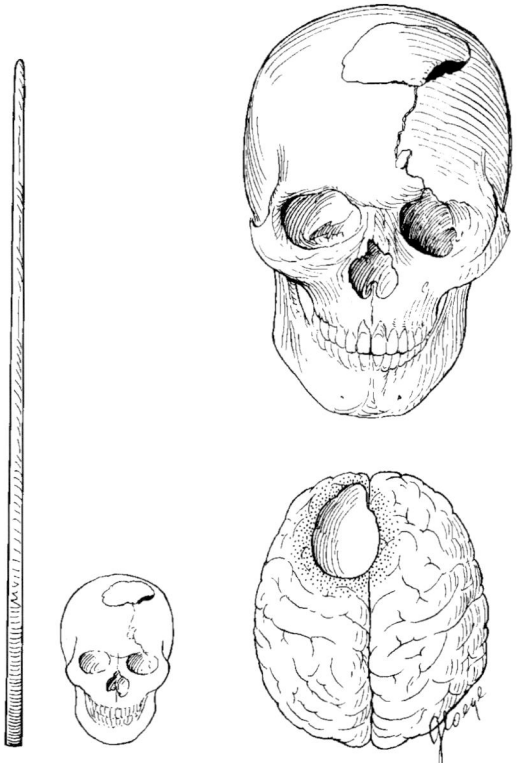

Fig. 11.1. Artistic representations of the case of Phineas Gage. On the *left*, both the skull and the tamping iron are drawn to scale. On the *right*, the upper image is an artist' rendition of the skull showing the left frontal defect. The lower image is an artistic rendition of the brain showing the area of suspected injury, including an area of tissue compression surrounding the absolute defect. Note that there is reversal of the skull/brain in the two right-sided illustrations. From Stuss and Benson, 1983.

brain destroyed (black) or significantly compressed (stippled) is on the right. This case demonstrates that considerable prefrontal tissue can be destroyed without altering basic neurological function but not without affecting higher control of behavior. Many similar cases were reported in the following century (Brickner, 1936; Faust, 1960; Goldstein, 1948b; Holmes, 1931; Kleist (1934b); Jastorwitz, 1888; Kretschmer, 1949; Lishman (1966, 1968) Oppenheim, 1889; Welt, 1888).

Case 11.2
A 53-year-old, garrulous, charismatic, and successful salesman sustained a compound fracture of the frontal skull in a traffic accident. Debridement of the left frontal pole was necessary. Recovery was slow, but there were only minimal neurological residuals—a slight limp and mild right hyperreflexia. The patient's Full Scale IQ was recorded at 118 in the postinjury state, and there was no evidence of

either aphasia or memory disturbance. Nonetheless, he remained under institutional care because of marked personality change. He was quiet, did not initiate conversation, and appeared remote and withdrawn. He readily responded to conversation, however, could discuss many topics intelligently, was expert at interpreting proverbs, gave detailed accounts of his life before the accident, could document the hospitals in which he had been treated and the names of the doctors and nurses in various treatment situations, and could accurately recite medical statements made about his current disability. Although frequently incontinent, he was unconcerned and almost never initiated an attempt to remedy the status. If asked directly, he denied any disability and insisted that he could return to work at any time, although he never requested discharge or even a weekend pass and was totally unconcerned about his wife and children or the fact that they no longer visited him. (Blumer and Benson, 1975)

In this case, prefrontal damage (almost certainly bilateral) produced a state of apathy that approached inertia. Basic physical and mental functions were intact, but the patient suffered severe loss of drive and executive control.

Case 11.3
A 32-year-old man was admitted to a VA for behavioral evaluation after having failed at an undemanding job. He had sustained a gunshot wound in Vietnam about five years before admission. The missile had entered the left temple and emerged through the right orbit. Infection necessitated surgical debridement of most of the orbital surface of the right frontal lobe. No basic neurological residua such as paralysis, sensory loss, language disturbance, memory loss, or cognitive disturbance could be detected. His IQ of 113 was considered a drop from an estimated premorbid IQ of 130. He was described as quiet, intelligent, and rigidly proper before the brain injury; he had graduated from West Point and attained the rank of captain in the U.S. Army, where he was regarded as a strict but even-handed officer.

When evaluated on admission, he was outspoken, facetious, brash, and disrespectful. Tendencies toward poorly controlled hedonic acts, including impulsive sexual advances, were noted. While showing no evidence of self-pity, he frequently described his current status with morbid jokes (e.g., "dummy's head") and made similarly disparaging remarks about others with whom he came in contact. His conversation was blatant, frank, often caustic, and embarrassingly unpleasant to those around him. His inability to monitor the content of his verbal output (verbal dysdecorum) had been severe enough to cause dismissal from the extremely elementary job provided by the VA. (Blumer and Benson, 1975)

In this case, frontal damage had produced a personality alteration featuring socially inappropriate behavior, both verbal and nonverbal. The patient's behavior was so impulsive and self-serving that it resembled that of antisocial personality disorder (American Psychiatric Association, 1987). Although he could recognize and discuss his behavioral and verbal output foibles, he could not control them. Verbal dysdecorum occurs most frequently following right frontal brain damage (Alexander, Benson, and Stuss, 1989).

Cases 11.2 and 11.3 illustrate the two types of personality abnormalities commonly described as sequelae of frontal injury (Table 11.1). Many frontally injured patients are apathetic and indifferent (e.g., Case 11.2) while others become impulsive (e.g., Case 11.3). Mixtures of the two behavioral disorders are the rule and are often associated with other mental control disturbances to result in the various behaviors listed in Table 11.1.

Case 11.4
A 30-year-old man was evaluated because of school failure. At age 23 years, while in his third year of college, depressed and under the influence of alcohol, he had attempted suicide with a 44-caliber revolver shot to his right frontotemporal area. He survived and made consistent neurological improvement until his behavior appeared grossly intact; neurological examination showed no residua, there was no significant depression, and both memory and language functions were intact. Psychological evaluation revealed a superior intelligence (Full Scale IQ of 123), and counselors persuaded him to reenter college. Despite limited classloads and considerable counseling, he consistently failed courses and on two occasions had to drop out of college. He insisted that he both understood and remembered the material presented in the courses but could not maintain sufficient interest to succeed. Figure 11.2 shows a CT scan demonstrating the areas of frontal lobe destruction in this case. (Stuss and Benson, 1986)

While this patient showed some evidence of the apathy and disinhibition of frontal damage, his greatest problem was an inability to maintain mental activity (concentration). Basic mental functions such as memory and language were fully intact, and his cognitive competency appeared

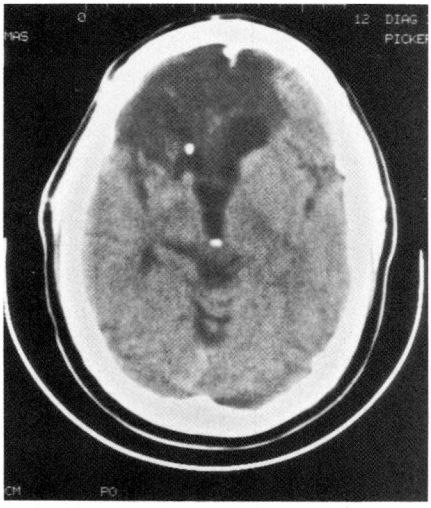

Fig. 11.2. X-ray CT scan demonstrating massive prefrontal damage, greater on the right than on the left, from Case 11.4. From Stuss and Benson, 1986.

adequate for college-level work. An inability to sustain interest in the course work and to inhibit distracting influences sabotaged his efforts. Both drive and executive control were disrupted.

Case 11.5

A middle-aged man was referred for behavioral evaluation after he had failed at a simple mail sorting job. He had suffered a severe closed head injury approximately 20 years earlier. On recovery he had worked in a clerical position but had never been promoted. He attributed his poor performance at mail sorting to a lack of interest. Neurological examination revealed no significant disturbances; there was neither aphasia nor amnesia. The patient achieved a Full Scale IQ of 138 and scored in the 99th percentile on the Raven Progressive Matrices, indicating that he possessed an exceptionally high IQ. When the Wisconsin Card Sort Test was administered, however, he performed poorly (achieving only four sorting criteria) and made innumerable perseverative errors (a control subject of similar age and educational background achieved ten sorting criteria). (Stuss and Benson, 1986)

In Case 11.5, a profound disturbance of the ability to maintain sequences of related material apparently resulted from prefrontal damage. Again, basic physical and mental functions were not disordered, but a mental disability marked by difficulty in maintaining sequences of material over time was present.

Case 11.6

A 51-year-old, right-handed man with a left frontal oligodendroglioma was treated by resection, chemotherapy, and radiotherapy with satisfactory regression. After six years of stability, the tumor recurred and was treated with chemotherapy, again producing tumor shrinkage. The patient's behavior following the second treatment course, however, suggested frontal symptomatology. There were no disturbances of basic language functions, calculating ability, memory, or ability to carry out motor activity (drive). A strong tendency to imitate the behavior of others was coupled with a strong urge to carry out activities suggested by the situation (environmental dependency syndrome). Thus, after a visit in his physician's living room, the patient was taken outside the door where the word museum was spoken; after returning to the room, he proceeded to gaze upon the wall hangings, statuary, and so forth, which he commented on as though viewing specimens in a museum. On another occasion, when taken into a bedroom where the covers had been pulled down, he immediately removed his clothing and got into bed. When a piece of his discarded clothing was picked up and shown to him, he arose, put his clothes back on, and left the room. When questioned several days later, he described these activities and intimated that he had acted appropriately. (Lhermitte, Pillon, and Serdaru, 1986)

Lhermitte and colleagues (Lhermitte, 1983, 1986; Lhermitte, Pillon, and Serdaru, 1986) reported a series of cases with significant frontal structural damage (unilateral right, unilateral left, and bilateral) and a strong tendency to imitate the behavior of others, to carry through an act even though inappropriate (utilization behavior), and to carry out an act appropriate for the environmental setting although not appropriate for the situation (environmental dependency). The authors suggested that such abnormal behavior following frontal damage with no memory, language, cognition, or sensorimotor disorder indicated release of parietal competency from frontal control. Moderate frontal damage led to imitative behavior, but, when the damage was severe, the behavior appeared to be "commanded" by the environmental situation.

Cases 11.2 through 11.6 illustrate that, while suffering little or no impairment of basic mental functions such as memory, language, cognition, or visual–spatial competency, individuals with prefrontal damage may have difficulty using these skills. They have lost executive control; in the words of Luria (1973), "knowledge is divorced from action." This problem is well illustrated by an anecdote concerning Case 11.2:

While being evaluated for the presence of diabetes insipidus, the patient was instructed: "Don't drink any water; don't go near the water fountain." Within a few minutes he was observed having a drink at the water fountain. When asked by the examiner what he had just been told, he immediately replied: "Don't drink any water; don't go near the water fountain." He had understood and remembered the instructions, but this knowledge could not be used to control his actions. (DFB)

Executive control disorder affects memory, as noted in Chapter 9. The memory disturbance that follows frontal damage is forgetfulness, a retrieval disturbance. In Case 11.2, the instructions were properly encoded but were not retrieved until a specific prompt was given. Knowledge was separated from action.

Case 11.7
A 57-year-old man had suffered a subarachnoid hemorrhage at age 49 years; an anterior communicating artery aneurysm was found and treated surgically. His postoperative course was unremarkable, but he failed to make adequate social improvement and was eventually placed in a custodial institution. About five years after the surgery he was referred to a neurobehavior unit for evaluation of his behavior.

He was oriented only to person, had almost no memory of recent events, and confabulated regularly. He was intermittently incontinent and neglected his hygiene. He was reclusive and tended to read a great deal. He masturbated openly and spent much time pacing the hallway singing old songs. When asked simple questions he responded with involved, almost always morbid, fictitious tales, usually involving his family. Thus, when asked about the (aneurysm surgery) scar on his frontal scalp he said that this dated from World War II when he had surprised a German girl who shot him in the head, killing him, but that surgery had brought him back to life. He often spoke of how his children had died in his arms or had been killed before his eyes. He would give lurid details of sexual experiences with his own daughters and vented many gruesome and rambling confabulations without any provoking question or other external stimulus.

IQ tests performed during this hospitalization showed a WAIS Full Scale IQ of 116, a Memory Quotient of 93, and a normal digit span. His performance on the Wisconsin Card Sort Test was severely impaired. Isotope cisternography demonstrated massive enlargement of the anterior ventricular horns and a lack of circulation of cerebrospinal fluid (normal pressure hydrocephalus). A right ventriculoperitoneal shunt was placed, but, after an initial improvement, he returned to his previous confabulatory state. Figure 11.3 is an early-generation CT scan showing the bilateral frontal cysts that remained after the ventricular enlargement had been reduced. (Stuss et al., 1978)

In addition to frontal behavioral disturbances (unconcern, lack of planning or foresight, lack of motivation), Case 11.7 presented a relatively unusual clinical disorder called *fantastic* or *spontaneous confabulation*. In this case the confabulation was associated with a significant memory disorder, but amnesia does not always accompany spontaneous confabulation; the one consistent finding in reports of this disorder is bifrontal structural damage (Stuss et al., 1978).

Case 11.8

While under the influence of alcohol, a 49-year-old man fell and sustained a head injury. He was seen in a local hospital, discharged home, readmitted, and, one week later, transferred to the Boston VA hospital. Carotid angiography demonstrated bilateral frontal avascular intracerebral hematomas. His condition consistently improved, and a nonsurgical approach was elected. Two weeks after admission he was transferred to the neurobehavior service for additional evaluation.

His mental condition had improved considerably so that he was oriented for time and could give details of the accident as related to him by others. A distinct, persistent abnormality of orientation for place was noted, however. He agreed that he was in the Boston VA hospital but insisted that he was in a branch of that hospital located in his home town. In fact, on close questioning he often stated

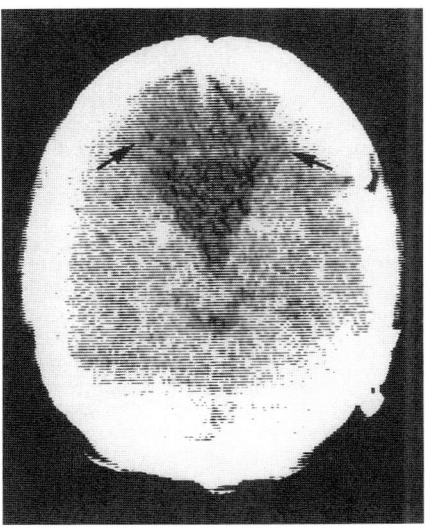

Fig. 11.3. X-ray CT scan of Case 11.7. This postoperative scan reveals the massive bifrontal tissue damage in this case of spontaneous confabulation. From Stuss et al., 1978.

that this unit of the hospital was actually located within his own home; to support this statement he recounted conversations he thought he had had with workmen in the upstairs hallway of his home at the time they were building the hospital branch.

Psychological testing revealed a WAIS Full Scale IQ of 114 and a Wechsler Memory Quotient of 137. His problem with orientation for place improved only slowly over a period of weeks. After he was taken to his own home by staff members and found no branch of the Boston VA located there, he admitted that he must have been mistaken. He insisted, however, that it still seemed that he was in a branch of the hospital located in his own home. On follow-up examination one month later this mental aberration had disappeared. (Benson, Gardner, and Meadows, 1976)

In Case 11.8, the hospital location was reduplicated, a phenomenon called *reduplicative paramnesia* (Benson, Gardner, and Meadows, 1976; Pick, 1903). While able to learn other current information, the patient was unable to accept the location of the hospital for several weeks but in other respects his mental state had returned to normal. Bifrontal intracerebral hematomas were present.

Case 11.9

A 44-year-old man suffered a head injury when he was struck by a car. Carotid arteriography disclosed large, right dorsal frontal and subfrontal subdural hematomas that were eventually removed. Recovery was only partial, and the patient was transferred to a VA hospital. His memory disturbance, incontinence, and ataxia slowly improved, and by ten months posttrauma he could go on weekend passes with his wife. At about this time a striking disturbance of orientation to person was noted. The patient insisted that he now lived with a second family that was almost identical to his "first" family and that this new family lived in a house exactly like the one he had lived in previously. He insisted that the second wife was an imposter who looked like his real wife and used the same name.

The patient's behavioral status, particularly his memory function, continued to improve, but because of the fixed delusion he remained hospitalized. He had no episodes of suspiciousness, paranoia, hallucinations, thought disorder, or ideas of reference and was never agitated or angry at anyone, including his wife. Approximately three years later he was transferred to the neurobehavior unit, where he was found to be oriented for time and place and could recount the details of his original injury and hospital admission. A mild right facial weakness was noted, but mild paresis and clumsiness were more prominent in the left limbs.

Disorientation for person was limited to his immediate family. He was fully oriented for time and place and easily learned and retained the names of the ward staff. He continued to insist that he had two families of identical composition; both wives had the same first name and the same maiden name, were similar in appearance and manner, came from the same town, and had brothers with identical names. Similarly, each family had five children with the same names and sex distribution, but the children of his original family were about one year younger than those in the second family. When directly questioned about the remarkable coincidence of two identical families he admitted that the situation sounded ridiculous. He even expressed amazement and disbelief at the coincidence but continued to insist that it was a true situation. When the examiners insisted that his perception of two separate families was incorrect, he would accept the logic of the argument, but when reinterviewed, even a few hours later, although able to repeat the earlier discussion, he would again insist that he had two families. He retained an unperturbed, jovial manner. His WAIS Full Scale IQ was 102, and his Wechsler Memory Quotient was 124. He performed poorly on some neuropsychological tests, most dramatically the Wisconsin Card Sort Test, and showed a mild, variable impairment on tests of visual–spatial function. The neuropsychological assessment suggested frontal pathology with indications of additional right hemisphere dysfunction. Figure 11.4 is a CT scan showing the bifrontal and right temporal parietal pathology. (Alexander, Stuss, and Benson, 1979)

Case 11.9 insisted that close relatives (his wife and his children) were imposters, substitutes provided by his real wife. This disorder, known as the *Capgras syndrome* (Capgras and Reboul-Lachaux, 1923), occurred in the face of relative preservation of mental functions.

While the manifestations of Cases 11.7, 11.8, and 11.9—spontaneous confabulation, reduplicative paramnesia, and Capgras syndrome—are substantively different, they share two salient features. Each is characterized by inability to monitor and/or correct a false mental impression, and in each case bilateral frontal damage was present.

Reduplicative paramnesia was originally described by Pick (1903) in an elderly demented patient who insisted that the hospital was located in her own home town. Similar cases have been reported, usually following head trauma (Paterson and Zangwill, 1944; Weinstein and Kahn, 1955; Weinstein, Kahn, and Sugarman, 1952), and more recently the presence of frontal brain dysfunction has been stressed (Benson, Gardner, and Meadows, 1976; Hakim, Verma, and Greiffenstein, 1988; Ruff and Volpe, 1981).

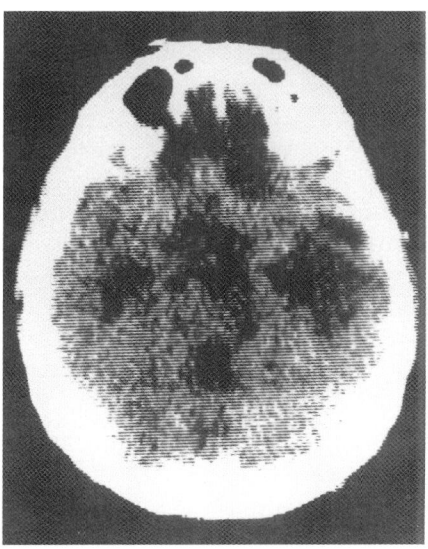

Fig. 11.4. X-ray CT scan of Case 11.9 demonstrating bifrontal and right temporal lucencies, the sites of significant brain damage. From Alexander, Stuss, and Benson, 1979.

Reduplication of family members or other familiar individuals (the Capgras syndrome), unlike reduplication of place, has usually been considered a psychiatric disorder (Enoch and Trethowan, 1979; Lehmann, 1975; Rudnick, 1982). Traditionally described as a delusional state (Capgras and Reboul-Lachaux, 1923), the syndrome tends to be regarded as a paranoid psychotic disorder (Ball and Kidson, 1968; Enoch, 1963; Merrin and Silberfarb, 1978). Some reviewers (Alexander, Stuss, and Benson, 1979; Christodoulou, 1977; Lewis, 1987; Merrin and Silberfarb, 1976; Quinn, 1981) have noted that in more than one-half of reported cases there is evidence of brain disorder, most often involving the frontal systems.

Spontaneous confabulation is a rarely reported phenomenon. The paper by Stuss et al. (1978) is one of the few providing a clinical–pathological correlation; in each of their five cases bilateral frontal damage was evident. In most clinical disorders involving confabulation there is little or no evidence of focal brain damage (see Chapter 9), and the confabulatory state is transient (Talland, 1965; Victor, Adams, and Collins, 1971). It has been suggested that all cases of confabulation are based on inadequate ability to self-correct (Mercer et al., 1977), and the possibility that this represents frontal malfunction has been raised (Stuss and Benson, 1986); but only in those cases with "fantastic" spontaneous confabulation persisting for prolonged periods is there clear structural damage to the frontal lobes (Berlyne, 1972).

In all three conditions—reduplicative paramnesia, Capgras syndrome, and spontaneous confabulation—decreased ability to monitor the obvious incorrectness of a belief and/or to act on corrected information represents the key dysfunction. Stuss and Benson (1986) suggested that the three syndromes have different phenomenology based on damage affecting specific basal/posterior functions but that all three show disturbed ability to monitor (self-criticize) one's own errors, a frontal executive control dysfunction.

If the frontal executive control system is accepted as crucial for self-awareness, several common psychiatric findings can be more readily explained. Illusions, delusions, and hallucinations all feature disordered critical awareness, an impaired ability to monitor the unreality of one's impressions or beliefs and to act accordingly. In some instances hallucinations are associated with recognized cerebral dysfunction (e.g., confusional state, aura of epilepsy), and evidence now relates the fixed delusional belief, at least in some elderly persons (late-life paraphrenia), with frontal pathology (Miller et al., 1986).

The clinical cases in this chapter show that a variety of complex problems featuring breakdown of mental control can follow frontal injury. Thus there is abundant evidence from the clinic that frontal control is a crucial component of human thought processing.

NEUROANATOMICAL SUBSTRATE

Anatomically, the frontal lobes can be subdivided in a variety of ways, none fully satisfactory. One traditional division is into motor, premotor, and prefrontal cortices (Luria, 1969), each of which receives input from a different area of the thalamus (Brodal, 1981; Nauta and Feirtag, 1986). A more satisfactory delineation relates to distant connections. Information comes to prefrontal structures via reciprocal connections with the unimodal association cortices of all sensory modalities and the posterior heteromodal association cortices through three major white matter bundles—the superior and inferior occipitofrontal fasciculi and the superior longitudinal fasciculus (Petrides and Pandya, 1984). These connections provide a flow of information pertaining to basic sensorimotor functions to the prefrontal cor-

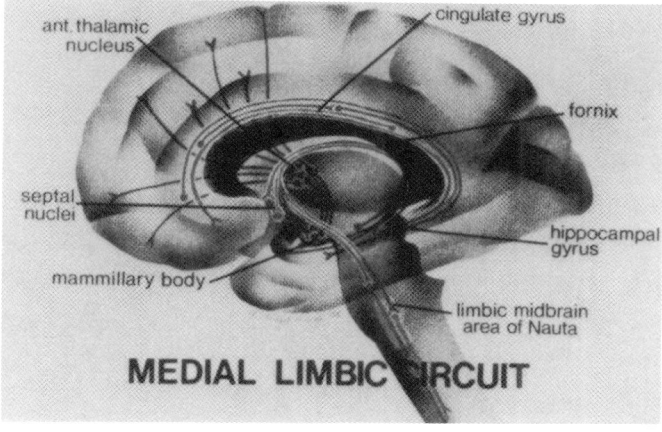

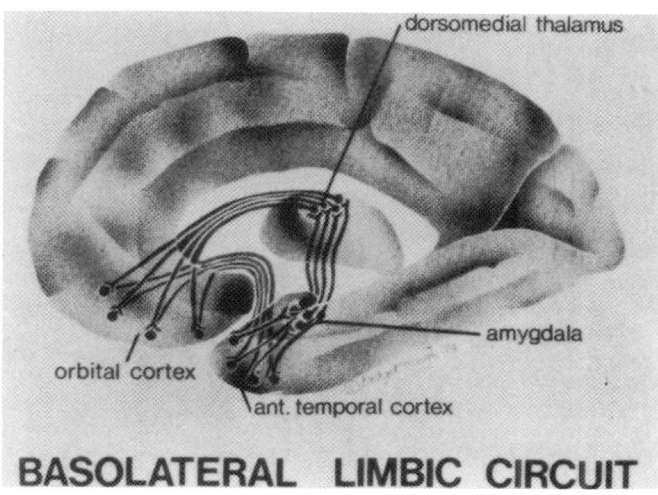

Fig. 11.5. Two proposed limbic circuits. The medial limbic circuit (*top*) demonstrates connections between the limbic circuit (see Fig. 9.2) and the diencephalic–hypothalamic–tegmental reticular structures. The basolateral limbic circuit (bottom) represents connections of the medial dorsal nucleus of the thalamus. From Livingston and Escobar, 1973.

tex. The posterior-lateral prefrontal cortex receives the heaviest projections from the inferior parietal area. More dorsal and ventral aspects of the prefrontal cortex interact with rostral, superior, and ventral temporal areas. Prefrontal association cortex also receives direct input from olfactory areas at the base of the brain, the only cortical area known to receive olfactory input (Nauta, 1971; Potter and Nauta, 1979).

The prefrontal lobes have connections with three limbic systems (Nauta, 1973): (1) the cortical–limbic regions (e.g., subiculum, entorhinal area, parahippocampal structures); (2) subcortical limbic structures (such as the thalamic and hypothalamic nuclei); and (3) the visceral–endocrine peripheral nervous system (via a series of ill-defined visceral–sensory pathways originating in the spinal cord and lower brain stem). Although the limbic structures are intimately interconnected, they are anatomically distinct and appear to influence prefrontal structures in an organized manner. Livingston and Escobar (1973) proposed two major limbic frontal circuits, a medial (primarily hypothalamic and mesencephalic) and a lateral (primarily thalamic) circuit (Fig. 11.5). In addition, Nauta (1971) stressed that the prefrontal cortex is the only area in the nervous system that receives and integrates information from both the somatosensory and the limbic–sensory systems, a factor of potential significance in cognitive control.

The prefrontal cortex also has rich efferent connections to subcortical

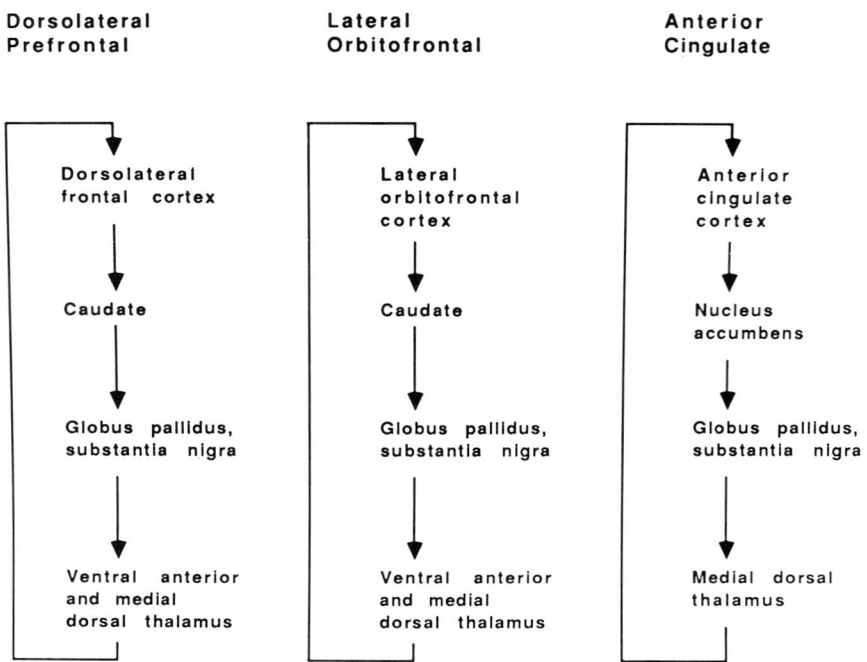

Fig. 11.6. Schematic diagrams of three prefrontal–subcortical circuits thought to influence thought processing. Adapted from Cummings, 1990.

motor centers (caudate, globus pallidus, putamen, substantia nigra, nucleus accumbens), most of which participate in a circuit by returning to prefrontal cortex via various thalamic nuclei. Figure 11.6 provides a flow-sheet illustration of three prefrontal–subcortical circuits that may be influential in thought processing.

More than any other region of the brain, the prefrontal area, composed entirely of association cortex, interconnects with both cortical and subcortical structures and with sensorimotor, limbic, and reticular structures. The vast flow of information to the prefrontal region provides the milieu necessary for a control mechanism.

THE NEURAL BASIS OF HIGHER MENTAL CONTROL

To correlate higher mental control with an anatomical base, the prefrontal functions described earlier will be utilized. It must be remembered, however, that the clear anatomical basis for function that is present in primary cortex and unimodal association areas is not available in the prefrontal cortex. Higher mental controls are supramodal in operation.

Drive

Considerable clinical evidence links medial sagittal frontal structures, particularly cingulate gyrus and supplementary motor area, with the initiation and maintenance of both motor and mental activity (Blumer and Benson, 1975; Botez and Barbeau, 1971; Damasio and Van Hoesen, 1983; Schiff et al., 1983). Damage to medial prefrontal structures tends to decrease both the speed and amount of human activity. The medial sagittal structures represent only part of a neural continuum that starts in the reticular activating system of the mesencephalon and includes selected nuclei of the thalamus, the hypothalamus, and the frontal subcallosal and septal areas. All involved areas are medial in location. Functionally, this midline frontal region represents a continuation of the tonic influences of basal brain structures discussed in Chapter 5. Damage or dysfunction at any site along this network tends to decrease motor activation, the state known as *psychomotor retardation* (Benson, 1990). Variations within this state—bradykinesia, hypokinesia, akinesia, apathy—are not site specific. The highest level of control over the initiation and maintenance of cerebral activation is located in the medial frontal lobe structures.

The opposite of psychomotor retardation, hyperactivity, represents a decreased ability to inhibit overt action and also occurs in frontally damaged patients. Clinical evidence suggests that the gross overactivity that can follow acquired brain damage (secondary mania) is associated with midline pathology, particularly involving the right hemisphere (Cummings, 1985a; Cummings and Mendez, 1984). Orbitofrontal damage is often associated with decreased ability to inhibit action (see Case 11.3).

While the two polar abnormalities of behavior—psychomotor retardation and hyperactivity—can occur independently, patients with frontal damage often have a mixture of these features. Poorly controlled reactions, often manifested as irritability, are coupled with apathy and euphoria, the unholy triad of frontal personality disorder described by Geschwind (1977).

Sequencing

Difficulty in organizing and maintaining serial information in meaningful sequences, the temporal organization of behavior (Fuster, 1989), is a common clinical observation following frontal lobe damage. Case 11.5 presented an individual who, while of superior intelligence, failed to perform any but simple, routine tasks because of his inability to handle sequences of information. Tests of sequential competence depend on basic sensorimotor functions and cannot produce clear results in the presence of more basic dysfunctions (e.g., aphasia, amnesia). Most human brain injuries that involve prefrontal and basal/posterior tissues result in defective sequencing.

Animal experiments and clinical observations indicate that the lateral aspects of the prefrontal cortex, primarily the dorsal convexity and possibly the lateral orbital cortex, are crucial for the acceptance and maintenance of mental data in a prescribed order. With improved testing and new imaging methods, a growing body of evidence supports the view that the lateral aspects of the prefrontal cortex control sequential processing (Fuster, 1985a,b; Goldman-Rakic, 1987, 1990; Petrides, 1991).

Executive (Cognitive) Control

Gathered under the umbrella term *executive control* are a number of mental functions almost universally attributed to prefrontal activity: anticipation, goal selection, response formulation, monitoring of the planned response, initiation of a response, and monitoring of the response and its consequences. These functions operate as supramodal controls over drive and sequencing as well as over the basic basal/posterior functions.

The ability to utilize information extracted from other neural systems, to anticipate needed responses, to select goals, to experiment, to modify and otherwise act on this information, and to monitor both potential and ongoing responses represents a high level of mental activity. Available clinical data, including the cases described in this chapter, indicate that executive control depends on intact prefrontal function. Prefrontal damage may disrupt executive control even when more basic mental functions are intact.

Future Memory

Ingvar (1985) noted that descriptions of cognitive control focus on responses to immediate stimulation but that many actions are planned for the future. For example, getting up to have a snack, reading a bit before going to bed, and stopping for groceries on the way home demand planning of future acts. The actions are thought out, even rehearsed mentally, so that when they are actually carried out the act is at least partially performed from memory (of the future). A prefrontal dominance for the ability to plan, rehearse, and then act on memories of future action is demonstrated by clinical case material. In particular, apparent surprise at a predictable occurrence and the failure to plan for the future characterizes many individuals with frontal brain damage.

Self-Awareness

The mental attribute called *self-awareness* (or *self-analysis*) has been recognized for centuries. Only recently, however, has a neural basis for awareness of self been suggested. Although related to cognitive control and future memory, self-awareness is a different mental process. Ruminating about long-term goals, conjecturing on changes that could have occurred if past experiences and responses had been different, fantasizing about imagined past or future experiences, and the ability to guide current activity to maximize future planned behaviors differ from basal/posterior processes and the executive control activities that manage them. The human is capable of forming and manipulating imagined constructs. Not only day-dreaming or fantasizing but virtually all planning for the future requires such constructs. These mental activities can be considered a higher level of executive control.

Clinical data firmly place executive control, future memory, and self-awareness among the prefrontal functions. Defects such as mental shallowness, inability to plan ahead, impaired self-concern, and unconcern about the effect of personal behavior on future relationships are routinely described as sequelae of frontal damage (Greenblatt and Solomon, 1966; Stuss and Benson, 1986).

Cases 11.7, 11.8, and 11.9 illustrate that prefrontal activity is instrumental in a related control function, reality testing. These cases and many others in the literature indicate that intact prefrontal functioning is necessary for successful monitoring of personal behavior and for the self-correcting inhibition needed for socially appropriate behavior. Disturbance of this prefrontal function can lead to the dramatic confabulatory and reduplicative phenomena illustrated in the cases, and it is probably a crucial factor in the occurrence of delusions and hallucinations, the disturbances of reality testing that characterize psychotic behavior.

While there is adequate clinical evidence to relate frontal lobe damage with the disturbances of function described in this chapter, neither the mechanisms nor the anatomical basis for frontal behavioral control are understood. Figure 11.7 presents the hierarchical scheme suggested by Stuss and Benson (1986) to depict the supramodal status of prefrontal control functions. At the bottom of the illustration are nine basic behavioral functions performed in basal/posterior brain areas (as outlined in Chapters 3–10). Above this are the prefrontal control functions. While

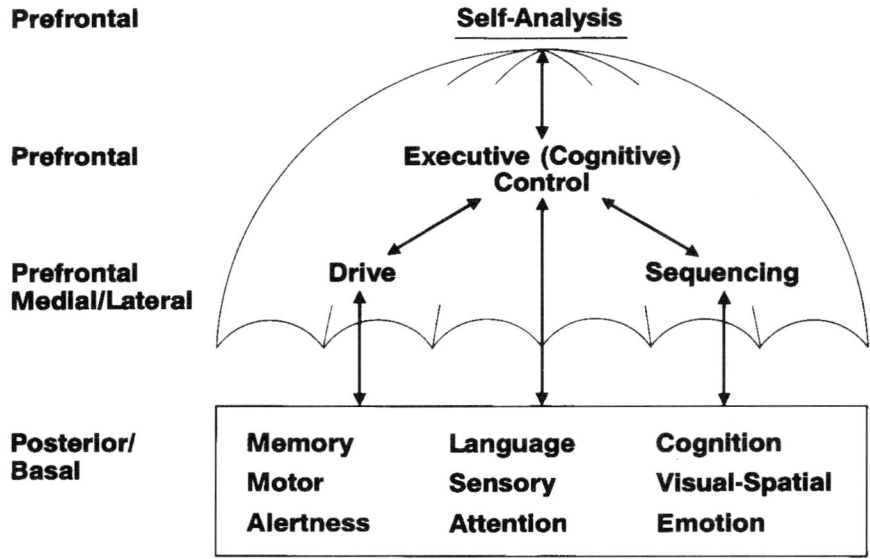

Fig. 11.7. Graphic representation of proposed control functions of prefrontal cortical processes on the more posterior–basally located primary brain functions. Adapted from Benson, 1989.

illustrating that prefrontal control operates only through more basic brain functions, the scheme leaves the neural mechanism obscure.

Anatomically, prefrontal cortex has widespread, direct connection with sensory, motor, and limbic structures. Through these connections the prefrontal cortical areas can monitor information from all levels of brain processing and accordingly activate, inhibit, or otherwise influence all these processes, including thinking.

The prefrontal cortex, while monitoring and capable of acting on basic sensory, motor, and limbic activity, is particularly involved in processing information from the neural circuits carrying cross-modal associations. With its widespread connections and vast information base, the prefrontal cortex occupies a prime position to monitor input, weigh potential response consequences, and initiate and monitor the selected response, the process called *executive control*.

12

The Neurology of Thought Disorders

> We must completely give up the idea of the psyche's being somehow connected with the brain. . . .
> —CARL JUNG, 1954

> . . . we may look forward to a day when paths of knowledge and, let us hope, of influence will be opened up, leading from organic biology and chemistry to the field of neurotic phenomena.
> —SIGMUND FREUD, 1938

AXIOMS/POSTULATES

Thought disorders are a diverse group of mental abnormalities that feature abnormal thought content, disturbed thought processing, or both.

Thought disorder occurs in a setting of inadequate monitoring and/or control of responses leading to psychosis or personality disorder.

While thought disorders may arise from structurally based neurological disorders, they often have no obvious neural basis.

Nevertheless, thought disorders arise from brain dysfunction, usually involving several different neural systems.

The term *thought disorder* has been widely but loosely applied to a variety of psychiatric disorders, particularly those featuring poor contact with reality. Of obscure etiology, they have been variously attributed to a loss of soul or to the devil himself (Fraser, 1911; Jaynes, 1976; Veith, 1965), to animal spirits (Nozaki, 1961), to social conditions (Lewin, 1935; Sartre, 1965), to family influences (Bowen, 1960; Laing, 1965), to maternal–childhood relationships (Sullivan, 1949), and to other environmental sources of emotional stress (Schachter and Singer, 1962). Until recently the brain has been largely excluded from consideration. Even psychopathologists who envisioned a neuropathological basis acknowledged that there was little evidence to support it (Bleuler, 1912/1950; Kraepelin, 1909). This is changing but there is still little firm footing for a neurology of the psychiatric thought disorders. This chapter will therefore focus on recognized neurological disorders that are associated with disturbances of thought.

VARIETIES OF THOUGHT DISORDER

The classic thought disorder, the only one worthy of the term for many psychiatrists, is schizophrenia. Eugen Bleuler (1912/1950) noted four major symptoms (the four As): ambivalence, autism, loose associations, and affective blunting. C. Schneider (1930) emphasized the loss of control of thought, as in thought broadcasting, mind reading, forced thinking, and delusional misinterpretation. These symptoms have been classed as "first rank" for the diagnosis of schizophrenia (Mellor, 1970; Taylor, 1972). Clinicians have been most impressed by perceptual and cognitive alterations such as hallucinations, illusions, and delusions (Fish, 1962), the so-called positive symptoms of schizophrenia (Andreason and Olsen, 1982). Negative symptom patterns featuring apathy and negativism are also recognized. There is a consensus that schizophrenia is not a single disorder (Bleuler, 1912/1950; Carpenter et al., 1976). Multiple varieties and etiologies exist, and many schizophreniform and/or schizophrenia-like disorders associated with organic factors have been described (Davison and Bagley, 1969; Hill, 1962; Slater, Beard, and Glithero, 1963). Even in these situations, however, the cause of the clinical phenomena remains nonspecific.

Disordered thought also occurs in affective illness—depression, mania, and cyclic combinations of the two. In severe depression, morbid thoughts become overwhelming; all physical and mental efforts tend to appear worthless and pleasureless (Mayer-Gross, Slater, and Roth, 1969). Depressive periods may alternate with periods of similarly extravagant elation and hyperactivity. In both the high and the low stages, abnormalities of thought processing and thought contents may be conspicuous (Beck, 1963; Hinchcliffe, Lancashire, and Roberts, 1971; Lishman, 1972). Exaggerated feelings of despair, hopelessness, and helplessness lead to delusions of worthlessness; these may alternate with an equally delusional, grandiose sense of power, wealth, or brilliance.

Obsessive-compulsive disorder, sociopathic personality, and other character disorders feature problems in thought management, particularly an impairment of monitoring one's own behavior. A neurological basis is recognized for a few personality disorders, including the frontal lobe personality and the interictal personality disorder of limbic epilepsy (Cases 6.2, 11.1, 11.2, 11.3) (Benson, 1987).

Thought disorder is a prominent manifestation of dementia. Aberrations of memory, language, cognition, and other mental functions result in disordered thought contents and thought processing. The prototypical dementia is Alzheimer's disease, in which plaques, neurofibrillary tangles, and granulovacuolar degeneration are found primarily in the neocortex (Alzheimer, 1907; Tomlinson, 1977). But it is now recognized that dementia may result from subcortical pathology (Cummings, 1990). In some types of dementia, e.g., multiinfarct dementia and posttraumatic dementia, the pathology is mixed and the clinical manifestations are particularly complex.

CLINICAL EXAMPLES

Case 12.1

A 29-year-old man was admitted to the Maudsley Hospital in London for treatment of intractable schizophrenia. He had been mute for almost a year but had remained clean, fed himself, and passively accepted verbal commands from hospital staff. Various treatment regimes including drugs and a course of electroshock therapy had not altered the mutism.

Several months after admission, the patient rather suddenly began to enter into conversation with staff and fellow patients. Questioning revealed that he had accurate memories of occurrences during the period of mutism. He explained that he had remained mute by direct order of God, adding that he had been selected by God to lead the Jewish people in Israel and, as a condition of this role, had been forbidden to communicate his thoughts to others. He had suddenly been released from the nontalking decree. He told of frequent direct communication with God, who gave him verbal commands that he immediately followed, and said that he and God often carried on conversations. During one interview, he suddenly stopped talking and remained silent for about four minutes; he then resumed talking, stating that he had received an order from God not to answer further questions but that a second order had cancelled that command. He remained passive and cooperative but did not improve sufficiently to allow hospital discharge. (DFB)

The delusional system within which this patient operated and the acknowledgement of command hallucinations with no evidence of focal brain damage, seizure disorder, or other neurological disease warranted a diagnosis of schizophrenia.

Case 12.2

A 17-year-old youth was admitted to the Maudsley Hospital for evaluation of drug abuse. At intake interview he admitted to consuming a variety of street drugs including heroin, cocaine, marijuana, LSD, and amphetamine plus other unknown preparations. During three weeks of drug-free observation his behavior was abnormal but without symptoms of withdrawal. Careful questioning established that, while he had sampled many drugs, none had been used in a quantity to suggest substance abuse. His behavioral abnormalities, however, remained striking. He frequently cleared his throat with a grunting noise, often stopped conversation for five to ten second pauses, and irregularly carried out a variety of complex, inappropriate movements. For example, while sitting during an interview he would suddenly stand, assume a stooped posture, circle in one direction, resume the stooped posture, sit down, and then resume the conversation. Facial grimacing occurred frequently, without apparent environmental cues. The patient denied delusions or hallucinations, admitted to no Schneiderian first-rank symptoms, and revealed little about his ongoing thoughts. He offered no explanation for the interruptions of verbal response or the movements and, indeed, often appeared perplexed by them. Laboratory studies including CT scan and EEG were within normal limits. Based on observation more than on interview, a diagnosis of catatonic schizophrenia was made. Psychotropic medication was started, and after several weeks the patient's behavior improved sufficiently for him to return to the care of his parents. (DFB)

In contrast to Case 12.1, this young man admitted neither delusions nor hallucinatory experiences, but his striking, often stereotyped movements and his perplexed attitude toward the mental compulsion to carry out these movements, again without evidence of overt neurological disorder, suggested a clinical diagnosis of catatonic schizophrenia. Both patients had abnormalities of movements and of thought processing. The presence of thought disorder was evident on a verbal plane in Case 12.1 but not in Case 12.2, where it was manifested primarily through disordered control of motor acts.

Only since the advent of psychotropic medications (the phenothiazines and their successors) has evidence of a biological basis for schizophrenia become available. As knowledge of the actions of the psychotropic medications advanced, biological theories of schizophrenia waxed and waned (Hartmann, 1976; McGeer and McGeer, 1976). An organic basis for schizophrenia is widely suspected, though the evidence is tentative. This includes demonstrations of ventricular enlargement (Weinberger et al., 1979), irregular hippocampal cell arrangement (Scheibel and Kovelman, 1981), abnormal cerebral blood flow (Ingvar and Franzen, 1974) and glucose metabolism (Buchsbaum et al., 1982, 1990), abnormal neuropeptide concentrations (Bissette, Nemeroff, and MacKay, 1986; Roberts et al., 1983), cholinergic disturbances (McGeer and McGeer, 1976), and irregular catecholamine activity (Bird, Spoke, and Iverson, 1979; Hartmann, 1976).

Case 12.3
A 20-year-old woman was seen at the Maudsley Hospital because of severe paranoia that interfered with her job performance. She was one of twins, right-handed, and without family history of either seizures or psychosis. Nocturnal seizures started at age 5 years, but were neither recognized nor treated until she was 15 years old. She was then started on anticonvulsant medication with partial seizure control. Several years later she became withdrawn, and her family thought she was hallucinating although she did not admit this. She did well in school but became emotionally rigid, did not date, and had neither sexual desire nor experience. She continued to have occasional seizures. EEG showed slowing over the left temporal cortex, and sphenoidal leads revealed spiking on the left. At age 20 years, following an episode of right focal motor status epilepticus, she was hospitalized for seizure control. The seizures were controlled but an attempt at office work failed because of growing paranoia, and she was readmitted to the Maudsley Hospital. She freely described her thought status, insisting that her thoughts could be read by others, that her own thinking was controlled by both radio and television announcers, and that their over-the-air conversation answered her unvoiced questions (although she acknowledged that many of the broadcasts were

prerecorded). Some thoughts were forced on her, and voices or noises were often incorporated into her own thought processes, often as obscene words. Objectively she was an intense, serious, humorless individual who was nonetheless warm, friendly, and fully cooperative.

During one interview, occasional movements involving her jaw and eyes were noted. The most prominent were episodes of rhythmic (approximately three per second) vertical jaw movements ranging from only one or two movements to thirty seconds of continuous movement. On rare occasions rapid lateral conjugate excursions of the eyes and, less often, of her head accompanied the jaw movements. The timing of movement onset was consistent. Movement would begin before she spoke a phrase or sentence, often while the examiner was still asking a question. Automatic or serial language tasks (e.g., counting, recitation of days of the week) did not elicit movements, nor did reading aloud. But if she was asked to comprehend written material, even silently, the lateral jaw movements appeared. Simple, memorized calculations (e.g., 4 + 5) were not accompanied by jaw movements, but complex calculations (e.g., 37 + 59) always were. Following the period of movement, she always presented the correct answer. She could write to dictation without jaw movements, but when she was asked to write her own ideas on paper the movements occurred. Familiar songs could be sung without the peculiar movements. Elementary idioms and simple proverbs were interpreted without movements, but more complex proverbs (those demanding subtle metaphorical interpretation) always provoked the jaw movements. Nonverbal tasks such as drawing to copy or command, rhythm tapping, alternate hand movements, or solving visual puzzles produced none of the movements. The jaw movements resembled those reported in some varieties of reflex epilepsy (seizure disorder triggered by a specific stimulus), particularly "reading epilepsy" (Daly and Forster, 1975; Forster, Paulsen, and Baughman, 1969), and appeared to be provoked by cognitive efforts.

A diagnosis of reflex epilepsy and schizophrenia-like disorder was made. The movements were controlled by increased anticonvulsant dosage, but the schizophrenia-like disorder did not respond to antipsychotic medications. After treatment with unilateral electroshock on a monthly basis, the patient improved enough to return to her family, although she remained disabled. (Courtesy of Dr. Brian Toone)

Case 12.3 is complicated but illustrates several important points. First, the clinical picture includes cardinal symptoms of schizophrenia: (1) foreign thoughts, particularly obscene thoughts, placed into her mind; (2) a tendency for extraneous noises (e.g., footsteps) to become words in her mind; and (3) a belief that the announcers on radio and television were responding to questions she was thinking. When compared with Cases 12.1 and 12.2, however, there are sharp differences. One is her warm, cooperative attitude, an affect unlike the distant and guarded responses characteristic of classic schizophrenia. Denis Hill (1953, 1962) and others (Pond, 1957; Trimble, 1977) have suggested that the warm affect present in schizophrenia-like disorders based on neurological disorder, particularly epilepsy, helps differentiate them from "nuclear" schizophrenia.

A second abnormality of thought is illustrated in Case 12.3. Seizures appeared to be triggered by specific cognitive operations. The patient developed jaw and eye movements only when challenged with a mental problem that demanded manipulation of knowledge. Her jaw movements resembled those described by D. Daly and F. Forster (1975) in cases of reading epilepsy and by I. Sherwin (1966) in language-induced epilepsy. Seizures triggered by decision making have been reported previously (Forster et al., 1975). The neural activity needed for cognitive manipulation appears to overflow into repetitive motor discharges—the jaw and eye movements. Case 12.3 suffered not only a thought disorder of schizophrenia-like proportions but also a thought-induced movement disorder, all in the context of a long-standing epileptic condition. In schizophrenic symptomatology, Case 12.3 is more closely related to Case 12.1, but in terms of movement abnormality she more closely resembled Case 12.2. The next two cases illustrate more direct organic causation of thought disorder.

Case 12.4

A 62-year-old man was admitted to the Boston VA hospital for rehabilitation of right hemiplegia and aphasia resulting from an acute cerebrovascular accident four weeks earlier. Considerable recovery had already occurred so that by the time of transfer he was ambulatory with aid, could feed and partially dress himself, and could move in and out of bed. His verbal output was nonfluent. Considerable effort was needed to produce a small quantity of poorly articulated speech, almost entirely limited to semantically specific words. Comprehension of spoken language was better but imperfect. Repetition, naming, and reading aloud were impaired. A diagnosis of Broca's aphasia secondary to a posterior inferior frontal lesion that extended into the caudate area on the left side was made.

With therapy the hemiplegia and language function improved. The patient originally appeared unconcerned about the extent of his problem and was passively cooperative. As he became more aware of both present and future limitations, he showed more frustration, became irritable, and had angry outbursts, usually directed at his wife or the nursing staff. About one month after admission, over a period of four or five days, his appetite and energy level decreased, he complained of insomnia, lost interest, and became uncooperative in both physical and language therapies. He admitted feeling depressed and expressed some suicidal ruminations. Suicide precautions were undertaken, treatment with antidepressants initiated, and the rehabilitation therapies altered. In a few days his appetite and energy level improved, he no longer admitted to suicidal thoughts, and his irritability decreased. He completed his therapy program without further serious affective problems. (DFB)

In Case 12.4, a reactive depression appeared relatively late in the course of recovery from anterior aphasia. Depression is a relatively common complication during aphasia rehabilitation (Benson, 1979b, 1992). More long-lasting depression can also occur, particularly when left frontal tissue is damaged (Robinson and Benson, 1981; Starkstein and Robinson, 1992).

Case 12.5

A 47-year-old man with known cardiac arrhythmia was hospitalized following the acute onset of garbled speech and mild right paresis. The paresis disappeared within a few days, and he was discharged home despite ongoing language difficulty. His behavior at home became intolerable; he had violent verbal tirades, primarily directed against his wife and child, and periodic outbursts of agitated activity, usually associated with search for a lost (presumed stolen) article or an incorrectly interpreted statement from his family or friends. In one violent outburst he did considerable damage to the home, purportedly in response to suspected infidelity on the part of his wife. He was readmitted to a hospital and then transferred to a VA aphasia therapy unit.

No basic neurological abnormality could be demonstrated. The patient was oriented to time and place and fully aware of the reason for hospital admission. He insisted that his suspicions about his wife were correct, despite her protests. His verbal output was fluent, somewhat pressured, and contained occasional semantic paraphasic substitutions. Comprehension of spoken language was severely limited, usually to a single word. He could read and understand sentence-length but not paragraph-length written material. A diagnosis of word deafness (almost pure word deafness) with severe paranoid response was made, and a deep left posterior temporal lobe locus of pathology was presumed. Psychotropic medications controlled the agitated behavior, and the patient became more tractable to language therapy. Nonetheless, he was released at his own insistence approximately four weeks after admission despite considerable residual language problems. (DFB)

In both Cases 12.4 and 12.5, disordered thought occurred in conjunction with acute focal brain damage that caused aphasia. Clinical experience has demonstrated that two major psychiatric conditions can be associated with aphasia (Benson, 1973, 1992). One is a depressive reaction, seen most commonly with anterior aphasia, featuring frustration, negativity, depressed mood, and, in extreme cases, catastrophic responses (e.g., uncontrolled weeping). The other occurs primarily in patients with posterior aphasia, particularly those with temporal lobe damage (e.g., Wernicke's aphasia and pure word deafness) and is characterized by unawareness and/or unconcern about the language disorder complicated by a tendency toward paranoia and impulsive behavior.

Two theories of the cause of these behavioral complications of aphasia have been advanced. The first is psychodynamic. Anterior aphasics, aware and concerned about their language disorder, become frustrated and depressed. Posterior aphasics, having less awareness of their own language problems, tend to blame others, and this leads to paranoia. The second theory is anatomical. Depression is more frequent after cerebrovascular accident than with other disorders producing similar physical disability (Folstein, Maiberger, and McHugh, 1977), and the depression associated with cerebrovascular accident is most frequent when damage involves the left frontal region (Robinson and Price, 1982; Robinson and Szetela, 1981). In contrast, paranoia and impulsivity are seen when temporal lobe damage produces aphasia (Benson, 1973, 1979b). Thus most pure word-deaf patients develop paranoid and impulsive responses, whereas the parietal damage underlying posterior aphasia (e.g., transcortical sensory aphasia) rarely produces these behavioral changes. Damage to temporal lobe structures would appear to involve control mechanisms that modulate impulsive responses.

Cases 12.4 and 12.5 show that depression sufficiently significant to be considered a thought disorder can follow focal brain damage. While the mechanism remains unsettled, the relationship is clear. That the thought disorder is not based entirely on language impairment is demonstrated by the findings of significant postcerebrovascular accident depression in many patients without serious language impairment (Robinson and Szetela, 1981; Starkstein et al., 1988).

Case 12.6

A 48-year-old woman (same as Case 3.6) was referred for consultation because of "atypical" facial pain. A dull, constant, aching sensation had insidiously developed in the right temporal region some eight years before. Neurologists, neurosurgeons, psychiatrists, otolaryngologists, ophthalmologists, dentists, osteopaths, chiropractors, Chinese herbalists, naturopaths and other practitioners were consulted, and innumerable studies were carried out, including carotid angiography. A broad variety of treatments such as drugs, spinal manipulations, exercise programs, and alcohol injection of the gasserian ganglion had been tried; none had provided relief. Over the years the woman's personality had changed; she became chronically unhappy, sarcastic and negative in conversation, and frankly described herself as cranky and bitchy. Her husband had deserted her, and each of her children had avoided her until they could eventually leave the home. By the time of the hospital consultation she was living as a recluse in a secluded mountain cabin. She insisted that before the onset of the facial pain she had been pleasant and affable, with a good sense of humor, and had enjoyed a caring marital relationship and a happy family life.

She was thin but healthy, and her conversation was difficult to tolerate. She was severely critical of medical practitioners but was almost equally nasty in comments about everyone. The neurological examination was entirely normal, as were EEGs and brain imaging studies. Her posterior molars seemed flattened. Dental consultation confirmed malocclusion and a diagnosis of Kosten's syndrome. She underwent the prolonged, unpleasant dental procedures needed to correct the malocclusion and, some months later, was reevaluated. At this time she was bright and cheerful and had pleasant things to say about the examiner, the dentist who had worked on her mouth, and the world in general. She had left her cabin, returned to the city, and was working at a job demanding considerable social interchange, something she could not have accomplished before the malocclusion was corrected. (DFB)

Case 12.6, to a somewhat exaggerated degree, suffered the personality disorder frequently associated with the chronic pain caused by arthritis, orthopedic problems, face pain, and low back pain and characterized by constant complaining and a generally negative, anhedonic temperament. Psychogenic explanations (Engel, 1959) seem less plausible since resolution of the chronic pain almost always reestablishes the former character traits. It is perhaps more probable that chronic volleys of pain impulses evoke recurrent neurotransmitter responses that change the cerebral chemical milieu and thus alter the individual's emotional status. As discussed in Chapter 3, pain is a subjective experience, a psychological state, even though a specific source of the pain can be determined in most instances. In a normal individual pain produces both a physical alteration—the recognition by the nervous system of the pain and its source—and a psychological response—the conscious realization of the discomfort. With chronic pain, alterations of emotional monitoring and control occur, often leading to a change in personality. It is possible that the psychological changes accompanying chronic pain reflect the altered biochemical milieu of the brain; thus the personality alteration accompanying chronic pain might be viewed as an organic thought disorder.

Case 12.7
A 22-year-old female college student was evaluated at a neurobehavior clinic for Tourette's syndrome. Occasional tic-like movements had been noted when she was young (probably by age 8 years) but had waxed and waned and had been accepted as "nervousness." The movements (primarily a sharp jerk of the head to the left) increased in her midteens, and various treatment regimes for anxiety control were tried. None succeeded. The woman's verbal output was distinctive. Soft grunting noises developed into expressions sounding like "slut," sometimes whispered, sometimes shouted, and often occurring in runs (coprolalia). A diagnosis of Tourette's syndrome was made.

Despite tic movements that involved head, neck, and both arms and the explosive verbalizations, this young woman was a successful music student and played the piano in public. She could willfully control the verbalizations and most of the motor tics, but an urge to move would build continuously until allowed to occur. In social circumstances demanding strict control, she would intermittently excuse herself to a private area (often the bathroom) to give vent to the pent-up movements and vocalizations. She also described compulsive behavior that included numerous rituals for dressing and undressing, strictly maintained positions for the articles on her desk and dresser, a rigidly disciplined piano practice schedule, and other fixed behavior patterns that ruled much of her life.

Treatment with low-dose haloperidol decreased the frequency and amplitude of the tics and stopped the coprolalia. The obsessive–compulsive traits were not altered, however. The patient disliked the feeling of mental clouding produced by the medication and used it only on selected occasions to provide temporary symptom control. (DFB)

Case 12.7 is considerably more difficult to evaluate. Obsessive–compulsive disorder (American Psychiatric Association, 1987) is accepted as a free-standing psychiatric disorder (Jenike, 1983), but the same mental and motor control problems are seen in Meige's syndrome, postencephalitic Parkinson's disease, and other "organic" disorders (Cummings, 1985b), as well as in Tourette's syndrome (Montgomery, Clayton, and Friedhoff, 1982). Evidence suggests that the obsessive–compulsive traits in Tourette's syndrome reflect changes in the biochemical milieu of the central nervous system (Cummings and Frankel, 1985; Nee et al., 1980). That the tics and the obsessive–compulsive personality are not based on a single neurochemical disturbance, however, is obvious from the presence of each without the other in many clinical conditions (Caine, 1985; Frankel et al., 1986) and from the response of one but not of the other to medication, as in Case 12.7. In a positron emission tomography scan study of depression with and without obsessive–compulsive features, Baxter and colleagues (1987) found decreased glucose metabolism in the left frontal brain of depressed individuals with obsessive–compulsive traits. From this viewpoint, obsessive–compulsive personality can be seen as a disorder of thought processing with a presumed relationship to neurochemical dysfunction that may be amenable to pharmacological therapy (Insel et al., 1983; Thoren et al., 1980). Successful treatment of Tourette's syndrome, however, often has little effect on the obsessive–compulsive traits, and successful treatment of obsessive–compulsive disorder usually has little effect on tics.

Case 12.8

At age 40 years, a working man was first evaluated because of spells of disorientation and absence. No motor manifestations had been observed, but the episodes were recognized by his workmates. Although EEGs were consistently normal, seizure disorder was suspected and he was treated with anticonvulsants. Eventually, despite increasing anticonvulsant treatment, the episodes interfered with work and he was forced to retire. Multiple EEGs were either completely normal or showed only mild, diffuse slowing. The man's behavior, however, became a major problem. He became intensely preoccupied and vociferous concerning patriotism. Statements such as "My country, right or wrong" and "The U.S.A., love it or leave it" epitomized his verbal output. He often cornered other patients, medical personnel, and even people on the street to harangue them about the impropriety of disagreeing with official U.S. government statements or actions. When these diatribes became too forceful, he would be admitted to the hospital. It was conjectured that he suffered an interictal personality disorder (Geschwind syndrome) even though no seizure focus could be defined.

His neurological examination remained fully normal, as did the basic mental status examination. During one EEG, under the observation of a neurologist, he sat up with his arms clasped across his chest and maintained this posture for approximately thirty seconds before again reclining. The EEG tracing before and immediately after the episode was entirely normal, showing no evidence of focal or diffuse slowing (muscle artifact obliterated the tracing during the episode). A carotid arteriogram revealed distortion of the middle cerebral branches, and a left temporal lobectomy was performed. The pathologist reported the specimen to be "normal temporal lobe." The patient expired ten days postoperatively. At autopsy, glioblastoma was found to fill the entire left hemisphere, starting 1 cm behind the frontal pole and continuing to 1.5 cm in front of the occipital pole. The necrotic center of the tumor was located beneath the left insula. In the left hemisphere, only the temporal lobe had escaped tumor invasion. (DFB)

Case 12.8 presented with a major personality alteration and a question as to seizure disorder. The personality disorder was characterized by circumstantiality and a viscous, adhesive, overinclusive verbosity (the patient was relatively unschooled, and hypergraphia was never observed). History revealed a long-standing lack of sexual drive plus increasing emotional and cognitive intensity. During some periods his behavior went beyond the realm of reality testing and verged on psychosis. This syndrome, particularly the circumstantiality, altered sexual activity, and intensification of emotional and intellectual expression, has been recorded in patients with epilepsy, almost always involving limbic structures (Bear and Fedio, 1977; Blumer, 1975; Geschwind, 1979). Bear (1979a) suggested that the personality disturbance was based on a temporal lobe hyperconnection due to the overdevelopment of pathways connecting anterior temporal lobe with frontal and diencephalic limbic regions. The clinical syndrome is the opposite of the Klüver-Bucy syndrome (see Case 6.1) based on structural damage to anterior temporal lobe (hypoconnection) (Blumer and Benson, 1982; Gastaut, Roger, and Roger, 1956). Most epileptics have no personality disorder, and the relation of the syndrome of circumstantiality/hyposexuality/intensified mental function to epilepsy remains controversial (Hermann and Riel, 1981; Trimble, 1983). While the issue is unsettled, the presence of a consistent cluster of findings (syndrome) in some individuals with long-standing seizure disorder involving limbic structures (Case 12.8) implies an organic etiology for a distinct personality disorder (Benson, 1987).

Case 12.9

A 56-year-old general surgeon (also presented as Case 10.4) was diagnosed with Alzheimer's disease. He had marked difficulty learning new material early in the disease course. Immediate recall was excellent, and his ability to retrieve overlearned information (e.g., his surgical skills) was adequate, but little current information was retained. He had considerable difficulty in the manipulation of knowledge and in performing visual–spatial skills, but his speech was clearly articulated and there was no defect in basic neurological functions. The clinical picture, the subsequent course, and the autopsy findings established the diagnosis of Alzheimer's disease, a disorder in which degeneration of cortical neurons predominates.

Case 12.10

A 51-year-old man was seen in the hospital for confirmation of a diagnosis of Huntington's disease. His father and one brother had previously been diagnosed with Huntington's disease, and his paternal grandfather had died in a mental institution. Problems were first noted seven or eight years before this examination but were not sufficiently severe to warrant medical attention for a number of years. A change in personality with a tendency to be withdrawn and negative was the first symptom noted by his family. Forgetfulness, restricted activities, and decreased competency in everyday activities and at his job were eventually noted. Finally, facial grimacing, mannerisms, and increasingly frequent jerking movements of the limbs appeared.

Examination revealed a significant chorea with irregular jerking movements of the head, neck, and trunk, sharp jerking movements of the limbs, sometimes partially disguised as purposeful movements such as rubbing the nose or patting a leg, plus almost constant facial grimacing. He often sat on his left hand, a learned posture to help control extraneous movements. His gait was wide based, cautious, and showed occasional dancing movements.

On mental status examination he was alert and oriented. His verbal output was marred by poor articulation, uneven inflection, and irregular rhythm so that understanding what he said demanded concentration. Despite this, he had full language competency, including a good vocabulary and adequate use of syntactic structures. His writing was almost illegible because of uncontrolled jerking movements of the pen. He could learn new information, although this was done somewhat slowly. When asked for the newly learned information after a passage of time, he almost always responded that he had forgotten, but if provided with vague structural hints (e.g., color) he would retrieve most of the information. Similar retrieval problems were demonstrated with questions concerning current political events, sporting events, and ward activities. He would deny knowledge, explaining that he had paid no attention. With a few broad hints, however, he could present considerable information, sometimes quite detailed, about these events. His interpretation of proverbs was concrete, and he had considerable difficulty explaining similarities and differences. The diagnosis of Huntington's disease was confirmed, and treatment with psychotropic medications (haloperidol) produced an appreciable decrease in the extraneous movements. (DFB)

Case 12.10 had marked problems with the mechanics of speech but relatively little difficulty in language function. Both cognition and visual–spatial functions were performed poorly but could be accomplished if some structure was offered. Similarly, he could learn and retain new material but had difficulty retrieving it unless given some cue. These mental changes, plus the chorea and the positive family history, confirmed the diagnosis of Huntington's disease.

Table 12.1. Differentiation of Cortical and Subcortical Dementia

	Cortical	Subcortical
Speech	Normal	Abnormal (hypophonic, dysarthric, mute)
Language	Abnormal (comprehension disturbance, paraphasia)	Normal, mild anomia
Memory	Abnormal (learning disorder)	Abnormal (retrieval disorder)
Cognition	Abnormal (failed)	Abnormal (slowed, needs prompting)
Visual–spatial skills	Abnormal (failed)	Abnormal (motorically disordered)
Personality	Abnormal (unconcerned, irritable)	Abnormal (depressed, apathetic, unmotivated)
Stance	Normal	Abnormal (stooped, twisted)
Gait	Normal	Abnormal (festinating, dancing)
Movements	Normal	Abnormal (choreic, tremulous, dystonic)
Activity	Normal	Abnormal (slow)

Adapted from Cummings and Benson, 1986.

In both Cases 12.9 and 12.10, the effects of dementia were a major problem. While both cases showed similar gross characteristics (disturbance of verbal output, memory, cognition, and visual–spatial skills plus altered personality), the features differed in ways that fit the patterns called *cortical* and *subcortical dementia*, respectively (Albert, Feldman, and Willis, 1974; Cummings and Benson, 1983, 1984; McHugh and Folstein, 1975). Case 12.9 was conspicuous for both unawareness of and unconcern about his difficulty; in contrast, Case 12.10 was apathetic, lacked personal direction, and suffered inability to motivate himself. Thought processing was clearly disordered in both cases, and thought contents were abnormal in Case 12.9. The different characteristics of the thought disorder reflect differences in the neuroanatomical bases of these two varieties of dementia. Table 12.1 lists ten clinical features that distinguish cortical from subcortical dementia (Cummings and Benson, 1986). Half of these features involve psychological functions, the other half motor; poor control of either produces a disturbance of mental processing.

NEUROANATOMICAL SUBSTRATE

The clinical examples, augmented by pertinent neurological and psychiatric literature, clearly show that no single anatomical site or sites underlie thought disorder. In fact, despite years of intense study, no focal central nervous system damage can be demonstrated in the overwhelming majority of psychotic disorders traditionally treated by psychiatrists. Careful clinical observations correlated with neuropathological studies consistently reaffirm this negative observation. The failure to demonstrate brain pathology fostered the belief that thought disorders are psychogenic, occurring independently of nervous system malfunction. The quotation from Jung at the start of this chapter presents a view shared by many psychiatrists through much of the twentieth century. Many clinical cases demonstrate, however, that phenomenologically similar disorders of thought processing can occur in patients with neurological diseases.

Two causes of thought disorder can be discerned in the cases of this chapter. In one, a neurochemical malfunction was suspected (Cases 12.1, 12.3, and 12.6). In the other, focal structural damage to the CNS apparently led to thought disorder (Cases 12.4 and 12.5). To hypothesize a neural relationship between these different sources of thought disorder, dysfunction in one or more of three anatomical networks can be proposed (Table 12.2), with at least two additional systems operating at a supraordinate level.

Limbic Systems

Dysfunction in the limbic system can produce striking disturbances in emotional responsivity, at times sufficiently unregulated to be considered psychotic (severely thought-disordered). Medial temporal structures (e.g., hippocampus, amygdala) are traditionally considered the source of basic

Table 12.2. Anatomical Networks Involved in Thought Disorders

Basic networks
Limbic (particularly medial temporal) systems
Hemispheric sensorimotor/cognition systems
Verbal regulation systems

Supraordinate networks
Neurotransmitter systems
Frontal control systems

limbic disturbance, but, as Case 12.8 illustrates, long-term involvement of other limbic structures in seizure discharges may be associated with striking behavioral abnormalities. After the work of Papez (1937), many attempts have been made to link limbic nuclei and/or circuits with normal and abnormal emotional behavior (MacLean, 1970). While some investigators have focused on individual nuclei or pathways (Poeck, 1969, 1982, 1985; Reeves and Plum, 1969), most envision multisynaptic neural circuits, as conceived by Papez, for many autonomic (MacLean, 1949) and emotional (Powell and Hines, 1974) functions. The proposed relationship of specific limbic circuits with behavior affords a biological basis for one factor in thought disorder (Livingston and Escobar, 1973).

Hemispheric Systems

A related but more far-ranging system involves sensory, motor, and cognitive processes. Acquired dysfunction of any of the posterior hemispheric structures can produce disordered processing of thought contents. Misperception of external stimuli as well as misinterpretation or misidentification of correctly perceived stimuli can foster false ideas and/or false beliefs, the hallmarks of traditional psychotic disorders. Misperception and/or misidentification are not uncommon; however, the unreality of the situation is usually recognized and the false impression refuted. Persistent misidentification, however, such as that seen with phantom limb problems (Weinstein, 1969) (Case 3.9), can lead to thought disorder unless tightly controlled.

A pair of cortical circuits has also been proposed as essential for proper mental function (Bear, 1983; Ungerleider and Mishkin, 1982). The dorsal, parietofrontal system carries out surveillance of both external and internal sensory input under limbic control, particularly through the regulation of arousal. The ventral, temporofrontal system has greater responsibility for decoding, interpreting, and responding to the signals, working under a frontal control system. Disturbance within either circuit can produce higher mental dysfunction, including thought disorder. Figure 12.1 is a graphic representation of the two proposed circuits.

Observed hemispheric variations in emotional behavior (Gainotti, 1972) have been explained by variations in the workload of the two proposed cortical circuits. In the left hemisphere much of the temporofrontal

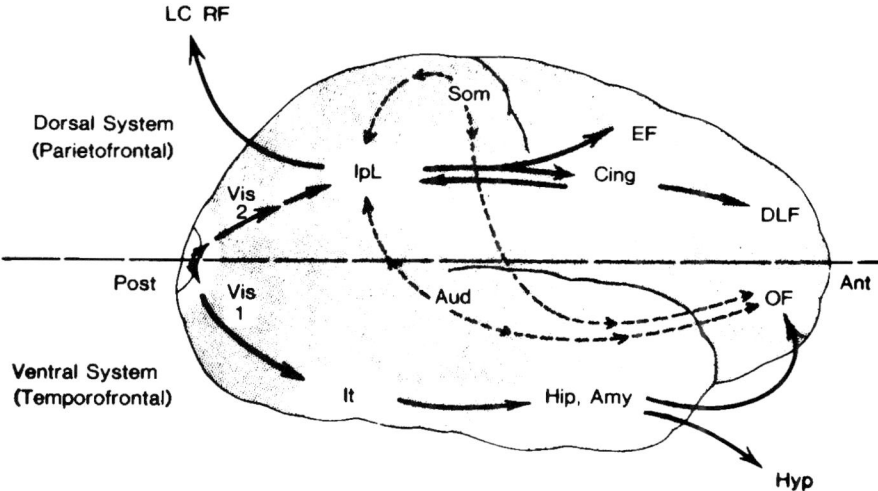

Fig. 12.1. A representation of two proposed mental processing systems: a superior (dorsal) system that monitors external stimuli and an inferior (ventral) system that monitors internal stimuli. From Bear, 1983. See original text for definition of abbreviations.

system is dedicated to language analysis and synthesis; damage within this circuit produces aphasia. The same circuit in the right hemisphere is thought to have more responsibility for the control of emotional behavior, and the observed differences in emotional responsivity following unilateral hemispheric damage are thus said to be based on decreased right hemisphere control. While the two sets of hypothesized neural circuits differ in structure and function, each presents a plausible mechanism for thought control; dysfunction in either of the circuits in either hemisphere may lead to thought disorder.

Verbal Regulation

Although rarely appreciated, a considerable regulation of thought can be traced to language (Luria, 1960; Luria and Homskaya, 1964; Stuss and Benson, 1986). Words, in both their semantic meaning and their syntactic relationship, can modulate human thought and action. For example, aphasia may lead to thought disorder of a psychotic nature (see Cases 12.4 and 12.5). In such cases mental activity appears to be influenced by the abnormal interpretation and/or use of verbal data.

Even more fundamental, normal discourse is strongly affected by choice of lexicon. Mark Twain (1961) noted that ". . . the difference between the right word and the almost-right word is the difference between lightning and the lightning bug." The connotative qualities of words are the stock-in-trade of politicians, ministers, salesmen, and others attempting to influence human behavior. Everyone uses words to influence others and is, in turn, influenced by words.

It is easy to see that abnormalities in the ability to handle verbal information might lead to thought disorder; it is far more difficult to establish an anatomical basis for the verbal regulation of thought. Two kinds of supraordinate systems must also be included in any attempt to propose a neural basis for thought disorder.

Neurotransmitter Systems

Anatomically, neurotransmitter systems have nuclei of origin in the brain stem, the basal forebrain, and the basal ganglia with receptors spread through the brain stem, basal ganglia, limbic areas, and cortex. While widespread, neither the nuclei nor the receptors are diffusely or evenly situated (Angevine and Cotman, 1981; McGeer, Eccles, and McGeer, 1978). Even small deviations in the fine balance of neurotransmitter activity might upset mental processing (Graybiel, 1990; Mandell, 1980). Most drugs currently used to treat psychiatric disorders act by influencing the chemical balance of one or more of the neurotransmitter systems. While precise correlations remain elusive, the effect of drugs on traditional thought disorders provides strong evidence of the importance of neurotransmitters in thought processing.

Different neurotransmitter abnormalities may be associated with different thought disorders. For instance, abnormal dopamine activity is present in such diverse disorders as parkinsonism, catatonia, and schizophrenia (Graybiel, 1990). Serotonin disturbance has been associated with anxiety states and sleep disorders (Jones, 1990). Decreased norepinephrine output has been noted in Alzheimer's disease, Parkinson's disease, and normal aging and disturbed acetylcholine function, affecting selected cortical neurons, has been reported in Alzheimer's disease (Cummings and Benson, 1992). While neurotransmitter disturbances are often associated with syndromes that feature thought disorder, the neurotransmitters are neither specific to a given process nor dedicated to an isolated neural system. Rather, it can be conjectured that neurotransmitters exert a control function in the regulation of thought processing.

Frontal Control Systems

As discussed in Chapter 11, the higher mental control systems of the frontal lobe play a crucial role in the regulation of thought. Masses of clinical data demonstrate that damage to these prefrontal neural systems disrupts mental review processes, in particular the ability to monitor reality. The individual who fails to recognize the unreality of misperceptions or misidentifications, faulty conceptions, or false interpretations and acts on them as though they are real is considered psychotic. Disturbed reality testing can result directly from frontal lobe structural damage (Cases 11.7, 11.8, and 11.9) but is more common following disturbance of frontal systems, the circuits connecting areas of the frontal cortex with a variety of other cortical and/or subcortical structures (Alexander, De Long, and

Strick, 1986). Damage to any of the frontal systems depicted in Figure 12.1 could permit the development of disorders of thought control.

THE NEURAL BASIS OF THOUGHT DISORDER

Thought disorder implies malfunction of some portion of the neural processing systems that underlie thought. This simple truism contains one crucial modifying phrase: "some portion." The specific symptomatology of a given clinical thought disorder indicates where the malfunction in the neural processes of thinking occurs but is often complicated by neighborhood signs reflecting the area or system involved and is colored, at least to some degree, by the individual's thought contents.

It can be proposed that clinical thought disorder stems from abnormalities in at least one of the three basic networks listed in Table 12.2, coupled with disturbance of at least one of the two supraordinate systems. The combination provides a crude neural basis for clinical thought disorder. For example, distorted reception of a simple sensory stimulus can cause misidentification of a neutral sound such as one's own name. If this occurs frequently (based on some disturbance in the auditory language perception/association system) and the reality or unreality of the stimulation is not monitored carefully (based on faulty prefrontal function), a reaction—turning and responding to the sound—can occur. If the reaction includes a socially unacceptable response (such as swearing at or threatening the misidentified sound source), psychotic behavior (thought disorder) is diagnosed.

As another example, Case 11.2 failed to carry out a verbal instruction ("Do not drink the water"), although he could remember and accurately recite the command; the verbal regulation of his behavior was disordered. This alone may not be adequate to explain his behavior, however. Although he correctly retained the information, he could not retrieve it out of context (forgetting, a disorder of cognitive association) and therefore acted without this knowledge (frontal control disorder). Simple thought disorder was based on frontal brain damage that affected two interacting neural systems (verbal regulation and frontal control).

Other examples of thought disorder suggest simultaneous involvement of interacting neural systems. The agitated paranoia of Case 12.5 occurred in the context of a temporal lobe lesion that produced word deafness (involvement of posterior hemispheric sensory function), but the behavioral disorder strongly suggested anterior temporal (limbic) dysfunction and/or decreased executive control (frontal system disinhibition). Similarly, while the aphasia in Case 12.4 was a sensorimotor dysfunction, evidence suggests that the depression that follows left frontal vascular infarction is based on a neurochemical alteration (Robinson and Chait, 1985). The simultaneous involvement of different interacting neural systems can be proposed as underlying the psychotic behavior sometimes associated with aphasia.

It is more difficult to pinpoint neural system dysfunction in traditional psychiatric disorders. That phenomenologically similar thought disorders occur in cases with and without demonstrable brain dysfunction implies a relationship between them (Geschwind, 1975b). It is reasonable to conjecture that the schizophrenic phenomena of Cases 12.1, 12.2, and 12.3 stemmed from pathology in several neural systems and that the differences in phenomenology among the three cases reflected variations in the degree to which different systems were involved. Among the problems each apparently had were abnormal perception (McGhie, Chapman, and Lawson, 1965), disordered neurotransmitter activity, and impaired cognitive control. The resulting disruption of self-critical faculties allowed disordered thought at the level of psychosis.

Theoretical Considerations

13

The Neural Basis of Thinking

> The mind is a cauldron and things bubble up and show for a moment, then slip back into the brew. You can't reach down and find anything by touch. You wait for some order, some relationship in the order in which they appear. Then yell Eureka! and believe that it was a process of cold, pure logic.
> —JOHN D. MCDONALD, 1968

> Has anyone measured the flight of thought? In a timeless flash it can embrace a hundred images, encompass a multitude of ideas.
> —NGAIO MARSH, 1941

> The stream of thought flows on; but most of its segments fall into the bottomless abyss of oblivion.
> —WILLIAM JAMES, 1890

AXIOMS/POSTULATES

Thinking (thought processing) is carried out by fixed, organized, integrated neural systems that simultaneously perform multiple mental activities.

A hierarchical organization of cortex, subject to subcortical influence, provides the neural matrix for thinking.

The vast majority of material processed for thinking does not reach conscious awareness; it is subject to degradation, low- and high-level gating procedures, and selective attention controls.

The stream of thought (unconscious, subconscious, and conscious) moves continuously and is always changing.

To envisage a neural model for the processing of thought, a number of controlling features must be considered. One concerns the limits imposed by the anatomical structures involved in higher cortical functions. A second, closely related factor is the increasingly complex operational characteristics of the cortical neural matrix. A third feature is the influence that

248   *Theoretical Considerations*

subcortical processes play on these cortical operations. Finally, a number of characteristics controlling these high-level functional systems deserve attention. This chapter will deal with each of these issues in turn.

NEUROANATOMICAL FOUNDATION OF HIGHER CORTICAL FUNCTION

Based on the clinical and anatomical correlations developed in this volume, four different types of neural function can be demonstrated for human cortex. They represent levels of neural processing of progressive complexity that are carried out in different cortical regions. By modifying Mesulam's terminology (1985), the four divisions can be called (1) primary cortex, (2) unimodal association cortex, (3) heteromodal association cortex, and (4) supramodal association cortex. Each occupies a relatively specific anatomical locus, and each appears to have distinct operational characteristics. A crude representation of the anatomical locus of the four types of cortex that carry out sensorimotor responses is given in Figure 13.1. The limbic cortex is also included but will not be discussed here.

Primary Cortex

Primary cortex refers to those brain areas that receive stimuli from external sources and transmit these impulses for cortical processing or, in the case of primary motor cortex, transmit the messages to lower neural levels. The primary cortical regions are relatively small, precisely defined regions dedicated to the processing of stimuli of one modality. The only cortical–cortical connections available to primary cortex are with adjacent unimodal association cortex and with homologous areas of primary cortex in the opposite hemisphere. The three areas devoted to sensory input are the primary visual (calcarine) cortex (Brodmann area 17), the primary

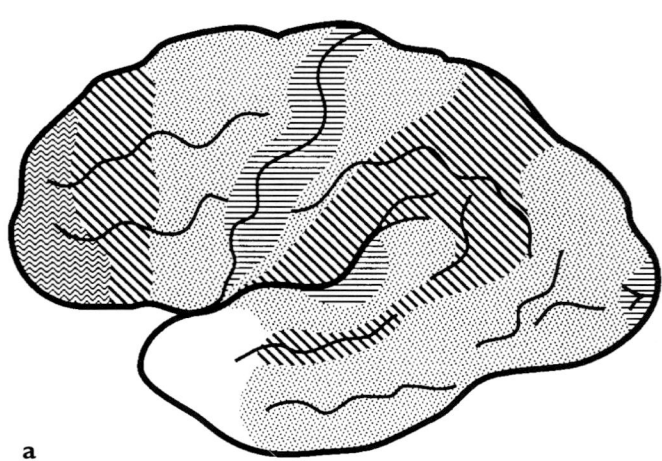

a

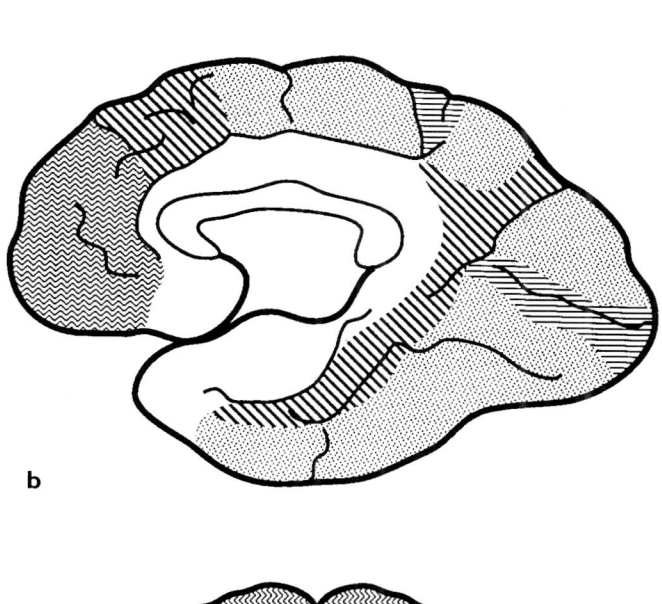
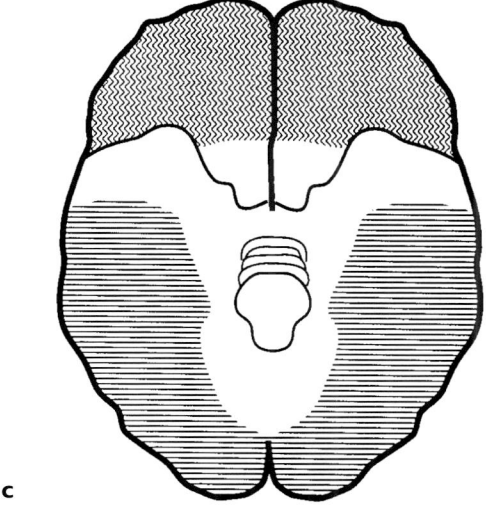

Fig. 13.1. Three views—*a*, lateral, *b*, midline sagittal, and *c*, inferior—of the human brain illustrating distribution of the four types of cortex: *horizontal lines*, primary cortex; *stippled area*, unimodal association cortex; *heavy diagonal lines*, heteromodal association cortex; and *wavy lines*, supramodal association cortex. Unshaded area is limbic or other cortex. See text for Brodmann designation contained in each cortical area. From Benson, 1993.

auditory area (Heschl's gyrus) (Brodmann areas 40 and 42), and the primary somesthetic area (Brodmann areas 3, 1 and 2). The primary motor area is designated as Brodmann area 4.

Unimodal Association Cortex

As the name implies, unimodal association cortex consists of association cortex dedicated to a single modality. The four major modalities—visual, auditory, somesthetic, and kinetic—each command a sizable area of cortex for unimodal operations. Smaller sensory systems (e.g., gustatory, olfactory) and the limbic systems occupy more limited cortical territory and do not appear to conform to the organization of the four major functions. The areas of unimodal association cortex devoted to these functions are (1) vision—Brodmann areas 18 and 19; (2) audition—Brodmann area 22; (3) somesthesis—Brodmann area 5 and 7; and (4) kinesis—Brodmann area 6 plus the posterior aspects of Brodmann area 8, Brodmann area 44, and the medial extension of Brodmann area 4, the supplementary motor area. Unimodal association cortex, unlike primary cortex, contains neurons with long axons connecting with neurons in heteromodal association cortex. The extensive cortical zone dedicated to unimodal associations allows progressively more complex processing of sensory stimuli in a single modality plus connections with multiple cross-modal association regions.

Heteromodal Association Cortex

The heteromodal association cortex has a rich matrix of connections that travel across modalities. Many names have been given to these cortical areas (*secondary, polymodal, cross-modal, multimodal, transmodal, heteromodal*), all indicating that in this region the interchange of information between modalities can be accomplished. Percepts formed from unimodal association cortex are intermixed in the heteromodal association cortex and then correlated with other percepts, primarily from memory stores. Extensive neuronal networks are necessary. The networks include multiple connections to both nearby and distant heteromodal and unimodal regions. Most information (memory) is stored within these cognitive networks and can be accessed at multiple points within the neural complexes. All but the most elementary cross-modal functions also require maintenance of serially presented material, a process defined as working memory (Goldman-Rakic, 1990), temporal gradient (Fuster, 1985a,b), or sequencing (Stuss and Benson, 1986).

The Brodmann areas regarded as heteromodal association cortex are areas 39 (angular gyrus), 40 (supramarginal gyrus), 36 (the superior portion of the second temporal gyrus), 7 (the anterior portion of the superior parietal lobe), and part of area 22 (Wernicke's area). Other cortical areas may perform cross-modal activities. Thus areas 37 (posterior temporal),

21 (inferior portion of the second temporal gyrus), and 20 (the inferior medial temporal lobe), while traditionally classed as unimodal association cortex, may have mixed modality functions. The region essential for the maintenance of serial order is the dorsal convexity of the prefrontal cortex, an area active in heteromodal processing. Prefrontal cross-modal regions include the anterior portion of Brodmann area 8 (frontal eye field), posterior area 9, and areas 45, 46, and possibly 47.

Supramodal Association Cortex

Supramodal association cortex represents a fourth level of cortical activity and includes the phylogenetically most recent portions of the prefrontal cortex. Clinical studies (see Chapter 11) indicate that supramodal association exerts executive control over other brain functions. The territory involved includes Brodmann areas 9, 10, 11, 12, 32, and possibly portions of area 47. All of these areas are located rostrally in the frontal lobes and occupy more orbital than dorsal–lateral or medial–frontal cortex (see Fig. 13.1).

HIERARCHY OF CORTICAL FUNCTIONS

While each of the four types of cortical activity is relatively distinct, the anatomical boundaries are far from absolute, and, as the cognitive functions increase in complexity, the boundaries between participating structures become ever more obscure. Nonetheless, based on clinical and anatomical correlations, the anatomical divisions described above (and illustrated in Fig. 13.1) appear relatively accurate. Overlap is considerable, but distinguishing operational features are consistent with a hierarchy of functions.

Primary cortex has been the subject of physiological studies since the early nineteenth century, and several functions have been clearly assigned to it. The relative preciseness of the motor (Fig. 4.10) and sensory homunculi (Fig. 3.6) have now been corroborated with equally precise divisions of visual and auditory primary cortices. Primary sensory cortex receives impulses from the thalamus and transfers this information to unimodal association cortex. It is probable that some steps in categorization of the neural impulses take place in the primary cortex, but these remain obscure. Reception and transfer can be considered the major operations.

Unimodal association cortex processes the vast array of impulses entering from primary cortex. Sensory impulses enter columns of neurons that are interconnected (Hubel and Wiesel, 1979; Mountcastle, 1986); within this unimodal matrix they are processed through functional stages such as discrimination, categorization, and comparison to produce a unimodal percept (see Chapter 3). Within unimodal association cortex, interconnected systems simultaneously process stimuli so that they may be categorized and compared with previously experienced single modality information. The final product, a unimodal percept, is available for additional, cross-modal processing. It is probable, however, that incompletely processed material from unimodal association cortex is also available for cross-modal association.

Heteromodal association cortex is far more difficult to define by its operational characteristics. While it can be considered an area in which information from the three sensory systems is intermixed, this is far too simplistic. Heteromodal association cortex interconnects neural processes from both adjacent and distant neural areas to form activated neural networks. The networks become the operational modules that accept, interchange and further process information; they can be considered cognitive networks. These networks appear to be defined, at least to a degree, by the type of information they process. Thus clinical observations demonstrate that certain areas of heteromodal association cortex perform language functions, others appear essential for visual–spatial and constructional tasks, and so on. The operational modules are not, however, sharply demarcated. A single anatomical region appears capable of participating in a variety of distinct, albeit related functions (i.e., a focal lesion may disrupt semantic interpretation of input from either auditory or visual systems).

In addition to the association of stimuli, heteromodal association cortex must maintain the serial order of successive stimuli. The ability of prefrontal heteromodal association cortex to accept, accurately maintain, and then select pertinent bits of information for future processing is firmly demonstrated by both animal and human studies (Goldman-Rakic, 1990).

Pathology involving heteromodal association cortex produces most of the well-known syndromes of higher cortical function. For instance, the syndromes of aphasia (Chapter 8) follow damage to heteromodal association cortex in a relatively circumscribed and consistent portion of the language-dominant hemisphere. Many disorders of higher cognitive function such as acalculia, right–left disorientation, and facial recognition disturbance result from focal pathology involving specific portions of heteromodal association cortex.

Memory must be considered here. Cross-modal associations utilize previously learned information, both unimodal percepts and mixed modality aggregates. While current investigations (Chapter 9) emphasize the role of the inner limbic core in new memory formation, the site of memory storage has remained enigmatic. Heteromodal cognitive networks, with their rich connections to unimodal association cortex, would seem crucial to this process and the probable participation of unimodal association cortex in memory storage may account for the extensive territory dedicated to this function.

The neural networks formed by heteromodal association cortex appear to perform most of the processing of thought content. It is probable that multiple cognitive networks are operating at all times in this region.

Table 13.1. Hierarchy of Higher Cortical Function

Anatomical Area	Function	Operational Characteristic
Primary cortex	Transfer of sensory or motor impulses	Reception and transmission of neural impulses
Unimodal association cortex	Discrimination, categorization, and comparison of single modality information to form unimodal percept	Interconnected, reverberating loops
Heteromodal association cortex	Formation and processing of complex multimodal percepts	Networks performing distributed processing
Supramodal association cortex	Control of cognitive networks	Selective inhibition

Supramodal association cortex appears essential for the control of high-level human cognition, but the operational mode remains obscure. It can be conjectured that supramodal cortex serves as a theater in which the many simultaneously active cognitive neural networks can be monitored, assessed, and controlled. The immediate (and future) significance of ongoing cognitive activities is weighed in the balance of input from limbic sources. Desired cognitive activity is selected, and less desired activity is inhibited; in this way supramodal cortex controls thought content and thought processing.

Additional activities of supramodal association cortex can be conjectured on the basis of clinical studies. Day-dreaming, fantasizing, anticipation, mental rehearsals, and the ability to be self-critical may be largely under the influence of supramodal cortex (see Chapter 11). While supramodal association cortex can be said to act at the highest level of thought processing, its function is one of control rather than processing. Table 13.1 presents a simplified view of the operating characteristics of each of the four types of higher cortical function.

SUBCORTICAL INFLUENCES

Extracortical brain structures can influence thought processing, sometimes in a broad way. Thus cortical tone (Chapter 5) can be considered a widely distributed subcortical influence. In many instances, however, subcortical influence is more focused. Two areas of cortex—primary and supramodal association—are the primary recipients of major subcortical connections. Unimodal association cortex and posterior heteromodal association cortex (that occupying the postcentral regions) receive little direct subcortical input. In contrast, the anterior heteromodal association cortex, particularly the dorsal–medial region, has robust connections with the basal ganglia and thalamus. Limbic input strongly influences supramodal association cortex and through this connection influences other higher cortical functions. Table 13.2 lists six subcortical areas

Table 13.2. Subcortical Systems with Prominent Frontal Influence

Thalamic projection
Basal ganglia/extrapyramidal motor
Reticular activating
Limbic-hypothalamic
Basal neurotransmitter
Adrenal–pituitary axis

known to influence prefrontal cortical operations. Pathology that affects any of these subcortical areas tends to produce frontal symptomatology.

GOVERNING CHARACTERISTICS OF FUNCTIONAL SYSTEMS

The many functional systems that combine to process thought have both neuroanatomical and psychological consistencies that can be accepted as operational characteristics.

Fixed

Each system operates over a relatively fixed neuroanatomical substrate and executes relatively consistent psychological functions (e.g., language, visual imagery, cognitive manipulation). Most thought processing demands activity by several of these systems. For example, language reception operates through a fixed neuroanatomical system, but to achieve the rich semantic and pragmatic aspects of linguistic communication multiple interactions with other systems must occur. Clinical case studies suggest that the anatomical base and the psychological characteristics of any single functional system do not vary significantly from individual to individual. Each functional system and each definable subactivity can be regarded as a stable and fixed operation.

Independent

Anatomically and psychologically, the functional systems are to a large extent independent of each other. This independence is particularly clear in the unimodal sensory and motor functions. In the more complex functional systems (e.g., memory, language, higher mental control), independence is less obvious, but for many basic mental functions (e.g., reading- see Chapter 8) a separate neuroanatomical network can be outlined and unique psychological characteristics distinguished.

Integrated

Integration of the anatomical structures and their psychological functions is a prerequisite for thought processing. Individual neural networks communicate at all levels of cortical activity and the ability to integrate information rapidly produces an enlarging matrix of activated neural structures.

Integration is based on associations. It is the association of elements within a unimodal sensory system (e.g., the combination of color, form, light intensity and direction of movement) that produces a unimodal percept available for higher level integration. As integration proceeds, however, individual elements become increasingly more difficult to identify. Complex functional systems such as language, cognition, and higher mental control receive inputs simultaneously from many independent functional systems, and the integration of these inputs with previously stored information is the essential activity for thought processing.

Interactive

Integration at both unimodal and heteromodal levels is followed by further intermixing of information. Percepts are not only integrated to produce heteromodal associations but also interact with each other and with stored information in higher level cognitive activities such as object recognition, categorization, problem solving, and decision making (Chapter 10). Individual visual percepts of color, form, and movement, coupled with an identifiable acoustic percept and eventually confirmed by a tactile percept, can define a baseball batted into the air and caught by the fielder. Motor adjustments by the fielder to place the body and mitt into the path of the ball depend on the processing of information from multiple unimodal sensory systems and its integration to produce an appropriate activation of the motor response system. Through multiple experiences (rehearsal) this complex feat becomes a relatively low-level interaction, performed as a nearly unconscious reflex. Identification (naming) of the baseball and determining what to do with the ball after it has been caught demand cross-reference with other stored information and then decision making by executive control. All of these interactions are based on cross-modal associations; many occur simultaneously.

The different functional systems involved in high-level interactions operate through neural structures with common junctions, forming a network capable of integrating multiple unimodal and heteromodal systems. While separate operations for the individual functional systems can be demonstrated, particularly in well-selected clinical or psychological studies, in real-life situations each system is influenced by the others. Interaction of multiple systems is essential to thought processing.

Successive

While it is useful to consider each operation performed within a functional system as a finite entity, the operations are actually reactivated with extreme frequency and slight variations in most processes. As an elementary example, visualization of a moving object (baseball) across a fixed background (playing field) is not a single image but rather a succession of images. Determination of trajectory and the consequent motor responses depend on the interpretation of a succession of images. Thus successive patterns of neural activity are needed to produce the complex image of the baseball's projected flight. In much of thought processing, successively occurring unimodal and heteromodal associations are combined to produce increasingly more complex interactions.

Multiple and Simultaneous

In the example of the ball player given above, the sound of the bat on the ball was registered, the moving baseball was visualized, the need for motor reaction was recognized, and the speed, direction, and degree of body movement needed to meet the ball's trajectory were calculated and carried out until a tactile impression of the ball in the mitt was processed. Simultaneously, however, the fielder was aware of the position of the base runners and was monitoring their posture and conjecturing their intended movements so that by the time he caught the ball the motor actions needed to throw it toward the appropriate infielder had been planned and mentally rehearsed and could be immediately initiated. Different cognitive channels had been simultaneously active and a variety of motor responses conceived. All of these cognitive activities occurred simultaneously or nearly so.

In ordinary life, barrages of percepts are constantly being processed by the brain. One may simultaneously experience music from a radio, conversation with another individual, proprioceptive stimuli relating to posture, plus feelings of hunger or thirst. At least some of these percepts (e.g., the music and the conversation) produce successions of intermodal associations. Emotional and/or intellectual associations based on previously experienced stimuli may occur simultaneously.

Each bit of information being processed represents a potential thought. Most percepts remain incomplete, however, needing successive, reinforcing stimulations to reach higher levels of association. As this occurs, the initial percepts interact to form a multimodal percept, a thought. Ongoing percept processing never fully ceases, except possibly in the deepest stages of sleep or anesthesia. The mass of information constantly being processed is overwhelming. For recognizable thought to take shape, stringent, directed control measures are essential.

CONTROL MECHANISMS

A number of mechanisms can be suggested as instruments for controlling the overabundance of available information. None is well understood, but there is at least some evidence to support each one.

Degradation

One powerful factor governing the quantity of information to reach conscious awareness stems directly from the basic physiology of nerve transmission. Individual neurons conduct impulses sequentially through successive stimulations (volleys). A neuron needs time for recovery between stimulations, and with successive firing the recovery time (refractory period) increases. For a stimulus to be perceived, a large pool of neurons must be activated simultaneously and successively. Unless the stimulus activates an enlarging network, the originally activated neurons will cease firing. Physiological degradation occurs naturally and is a basic mechanism for controlling the quantity of stimuli to be processed. Most information derived from the sensory systems disappears before advancing sufficiently to form a percept and long before entering thought formation.

Competition

Most newly received information cannot be maintained in the face of additional stimuli that compete for the same neural networks. In the psychology laboratory this phenomenon has been demonstrated by the presentation of excessive verbal information as a distractor to learning (Butters and Grady, 1977; Peterson and Peterson, 1959), and in the clinic it has been used to control pain. In each instance, competing stimuli decrease the degree of stimulation experienced.

Gating

A more directed mechanism for controlling the quantity of incoming stimuli has been proposed. Melzack and Wall (1965) coined the term *gating* to identify a mechanism that modulates the number of individual pain stimuli transmitted from the peripheral to the central nervous system. They proposed that inhibitory synapses where the peripheral nerve enters the central nervous system (spinal cord or brain stem) could decrease the stimulation load perceived by centrally located neurons following peripheral stimulation. Increasing volleys of stimuli, registering a peripheral source of pain, stimulate inhibitory neurons that modulate the quantity of impulses allowed to enter central nervous system channels. A great deal of evidence has been gathered to support the thesis of sensory gating (Wall, 1985).

At higher levels, similar gating mechanisms have been proposed in the hypothalamus (Damasio, 1979), the thalamus (Scheibel and Scheibel, 1967), basal ganglia (Schneider, 1984), and frontal lobes (Stuss and Benson, 1986; Fuster, 1980). Most are mere conjectures that reflect the obvious need to limit the quantity of stimuli bombarding brain structures and that have been extrapolated from a reasonably secure thesis based on peripheral nerve physiology. The best defined of the higher gating systems was proposed by M. Scheibel and A. B. Scheibel (1967), who noted that two sets of thalamic nuclei—interlaminar and reticularis—have synaptic connections with all of the thalamic nuclear aggregates and also with the brain stem and the prefrontal cortex (Fig. 13.2). The Scheibels conjectured that impulses from the mesencephalon (primarily limbic) and prefrontal

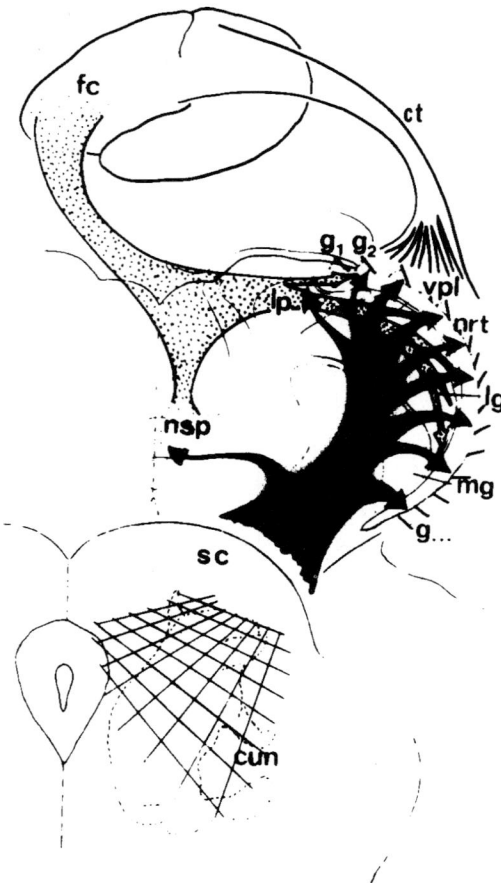

Fig. 13.2. Schematic illustration of some systems influencing the thalamic nucleus reticularis. The *heavy dark arrow* represents ascending pathways from mesencephalon (*sc; cun*), the *stippled area* represents projections from prefrontal cortex (*fc*) and medial thalamus (*nsp*), while the *clear projection* indicates descending cortical–thalamic (*ct*) connections. The combined interplay of these projections on the thalamic nucleus reticularis, which has connections with all other thalamic nuclei, is conjectured as a possible gating influence on sensorimotor networks. From Scheibel, 1980.

cortex (both sensorimotor and limbic), acting through the interlaminar and reticularis nuclei, could modulate the many sensory and motor activities conducted through the thalamus. The reticularis and interlaminar nuclei of the thalamus would thus provide a major potential mechanism (gate) for controlling the quantity of sensory data received by the cortex.

DIRECTED THOUGHT

In addition to the many intrinsic means to control the quantity of stimuli being processed, humans appear capable of providing personal direction to their thought processes. Attention may be directed by successive volleys of strong stimuli capable of overwhelming most other ideation. For instance, hunger or thirst can interfere with thought processing; if sufficiently strong, such feelings can dominate thought processes. Similar reactions occur with fear, depression, and elation, among other emotional states. These examples of strongly directed attention have potent emotional, probably limbic, components.

Much of directed attention, however, is not so obviously emotional. Individuals with musical interest can lose themselves completely in a concert, concentrating so intensely on the music that they are unaware of co-occurring visual or somesthetic stimuli. A good novel or a good drama can inhibit, at least temporarily, all thoughts except those associated with it. The mathematician solving a problem, the carpenter at his lathe, the salesman making a pitch, the batter at the plate, all demonstrate strongly directed attention. They exclude extraneous stimuli to concentrate on the object or action of interest. Selected attention can operate over several spheres simultaneously. Thus, it is possible to read a magazine or novel while listening to music, shifting attention from one to the other.

Conscious direction of attention is a powerful, valuable attribute but one that demands considerable effort. Unless accompanied by strong emotional force, directed attention tends to be short-lived. In most situations, attention wanders from item to item, maintaining interest in some, rapidly scanning others. Attention to the thoughts being processed runs an uneven, content-scattered course.

The content of thoughts being processed is strongly influenced by other elements being processed simultaneously. Thus, the image of the president's face or the sound of a well-known musical composition will excite totally different associations at different times, influenced by the robustness of contributing or competing images. Thought content is always open to considerable alteration, prejudiced by competing elements. An idea formed from relatively stable thought contents will change under differing influences and tends to recur in an altered state. This phenomenon, the constantly changing, always different contents of one's thought, and the many influences that play on thought processing, have proved difficult to conceptualize. One successful conceptualization is J.M. Barrie's metaphorical description of the complexity of thought when he attempted to portray a child's mental processing in the prose adaptation of his play "Peter Pan":

> I don't know whether you have ever seen a map of a person's mind. Doctors sometimes draw maps of other parts of you, and your own map can become intensely interesting, but catch them trying to draw a map of a child's mind, which is not only confused, but keeps going round all the time. There are zigzag lines on it, just like your temperature on a card, and these are probably roads in the island; for the Neverland is always more or less an island, with astonishing splashes of colour here and there, and coral reefs and rakish-looking craft in the offing, and savages and lonely lairs, and gnomes who are mostly tailors, and caves through which a river runs, and princes with six

elder brothers, and a hut fast going to decay, and one very small old lady with a hooked nose. It would be an easy map if that were all; but there is also first day at school, religion, fathers, the round pond, needlework, murders, hangings, verbs that take the dative, chocolate pudding day, getting into braces, say ninety-nine, threepence for pulling out your tooth yourself, and so on; and either these are part of the island or they are another map showing through, and it is all rather confusing, especially as nothing will stand still. (Barrie, 1911/1988)

SUMMATION

This volume has been an attempt to demonstrate the obvious: (1) thinking is a function of the brain and (2) many individual neural processes must be linked in order to process thought. Equally obvious, thinking is not a unitary process; no single brain operation, anatomical area, or psychological process carries out the activity. Thought processing proceeds on multiple levels that are simultaneously but asynchronously interactive. Dedicated sensory association loops interact to produce unimodal percepts, which in turn are combined with data from other sources via cross-modal associations. Basic cross-modal associations merge with information from other intermodal circuits in complex neural matrices. The results are monitored and manipulated by supramodal association mechanisms. While the latter activity, the control of complex neural circuits, requires high-level (executive) control, this function is not synonymous with thinking. *Thought processing* encompasses operations at all levels from elementary sensory transfer to the managed interplay of simultaneously active cortical and subcortical networks. *Thought content* is the information that is processed through this hierarchical chain and then retained, at least briefly. *Thinking* includes the contents and the processing of thought, both of which depend on multiple interacting brain structures.

References

Abrams, R., Taylor, M. A., Stoloruw, K. A. Catatonia and mania: patterns of cerebral dysfunction. *Biological Psychiatry* 14:111–117, 1979.

Ach, N. *Ueber die Willinstetigkeit und des Denken.* Gottingen, Vardenboeck, 1905.

Ackerly, S. S., Benton, A. L. Report of a case of bilateral frontal lobe defect. *Research Publications—Association for Research in Nervous and Mental Disease* 27:479–504, 1947.

Adams, H., Miller, D. Herpes simplex encephalitis: a clinical and pathological analysis of twenty-two cases. *Postgraduate Medical Journal* 49:393–397, 1973.

Adams, R. D., Victor, M. *Principles of Neurology.* New York, McGraw-Hill, 1989.

Adler, A. Disintegration and restoration of optic recognition in visual agnosia. *Archives of Neurology and Psychiatry* 51:243–259, 1944.

Ajax, E. T. Acquired dyslexia. *Archives of Neurology* 11:66–72, 1964.

de Ajuriaguerra, J., Tissot, R. The apraxias. In *Handbook of Clinical Neurology, Vol. 4: Disorders of Speech, Perception and Symbolic Behavior.* Vinken, P. J., Bruyn, G. W., eds. Amsterdam, North-Holland, 1969, pp. 48–66.

Akert, K., Gruesen, R. A., Woolsey, C. N. Klüver-Bucy syndrome in monkey with neocortical ablations of temporal lobe. *Brain* 84:480–497, 1961.

Albert, M. L. Subcortical dementia. In *Alzheimer's Disease: Senile Dementia and Related Disorders.* Katzman, R., Terry, R. D., and Bick, K. L., eds. New York, Raven Press, 1978, pp. 173–180.

Albert, M. L., Bear, D. Time to understand. A case study of word deafness with reference to the role of time in auditory comprehension. *Brain* 97:383–394, 1974.

Albert, M. L., Feldman, R. G., Willis, A. L. The sub-cortical dementia of progressive supranuclear palsy. *Journal of Neurology, Neurosurgery, and Psychiatry* 37:121–130, 1974.

Albert, M. L., Sparks, R., von Stockert, T., Sax, D. A case study of auditory agnosia: linguistic and non-linguistic processing. *Cortex* 8(4):427–445, 1972.

Alberts, M. S., Butters, N., Levin, J. Temporal gradients in the retrograde amnesia of patients with alcoholic Korsakoff's disease. *Archives of Neurology* 36:211–216, 1979.

Albin, R. L., Young, A. B., Penney, J. B. The functional anatomy of basal ganglia disorders. *Trends in Neuroscience* 12:366–375, 1989.

Alexander, G. E., De Long, M. R., Strick, P. L. Parallel organization of functionally segregated circuits linking basal ganglia and cortex. *Annual Review of Neuroscience* 9:357–381, 1986.

Alexander, M. P. Traumatic brain injury. *In Psychiatric Aspects of Neurologic*

Disease, vol. II. Benson, D. F., Blumer, D., eds. New York, Grune & Stratton, 1982, pp. 219–248.

Alexander, M. P., Benson, D. F. The aphasias and related disturbances. *In Clinical Neurology*, vol. 1. Joynt, R. J., ed. Philadelphia, J. B. Lippincott, 1991. Chap. 10, pp. 1–58.

Alexander, M. P., Benson, D. F., Stuss, D. T. Frontal lobes and language. *Brain and Language* 37:656–691, 1989.

Alexander, M. P., Freedman, M. Amnesia after anterior communicating artery aneurysm rupture. *Neurology* 34:752–757, 1984.

Alexander, M. P., Hiltbrunner, B., Fischer, R. S. Distributed anatomy of transcortical sensory aphasia. *Archives of Neurology* 46:885–892, 1989.

Alexander, M. P., Stuss, D. T., Benson, D. F. Capgras syndrome: a reduplicative phenomenon. *Neurology* 29:334–339, 1979.

Alzheimer, A. Uber eigenartige Erkrankung der Hirnrinde. *Allgemeine Zeitschrift für Psychiatrie* 64:146–148, 1907.

American Illustrated Medical Dictionary, 21st ed. Philadelphia, W. B. Saunders, 1947.

American Psychiatric Association. *Diagnostic and Statistical Manual of Mental Disorders*. Washington, DC, American Psychiatric Association, 1957.

American Psychiatric Association. *Diagnostic and Statistical Manual of Mental Disorders*, 2nd ed. Washington, DC, American Psychiatric Association, 1968.

American Psychiatric Association. *Diagnostic and Statistical Manual of Mental Disorders*, 3rd ed. Washington, DC, American Psychiatric Association, 1980a.

American Psychiatric Association. *A Psychiatric Glossary*, 5th ed. Washington, DC, American Psychiatric Association, 1980b.

American Psychiatric Association. *Diagnostic and Statistical Manual of Mental Disorders (Third Edition-Revised)*. Washington, DC, American Psychiatric Association, 1987.

Andreason, N. C., Olsen, S. Negative versus positive schizophrenia. *Archives of General Psychiatry* 39:789–794, 1982.

Angevine, J. B. Jr., Cotman, C. W. *Principles of Neuroanatomy*. New York, Oxford, 1981.

Anokhin, P. K. The multiple ascending influences of the subcortical centers on the cerebral cortex. In *Brain and Behavior*. Brazier, M.A.B., ed. Washington, DC, American Institute of Biological Sciences, 1961, pp. 139–170.

Anton, G. Blindheit nach Beiderseitiger Gehirnkrankung mit Verlust der Orientierrung in Raume. *Mittherlungen des Vereines der Artze in Stiermark* 33:41–46, 1896.

Arendt, H. *The Life of the Mind*. New York, Harcourt Brace Jovanovich, 1978.

Aristotle. De Anima. In *The Works of Aristotle*. Smith, J. A., translator. Oxford, Clarendon, 1931.

Arnheim, R. *Visual Thinking*. Berkeley, University of California Press, 1969.

Arrigoni, G., De Renzi, E. Constructional apraxia and hemispheric locus of lesion. *Cortex* 1:170–197, 1964.

Ashby, W. R. *Design for a Brain*. New York, John Wiley & Sons, 1952.

Auerbach, S. H., Alland, T., Naeser, M., Alexander, M. P., Albert, M. L. Pure word deafness: analysis of a case with bilateral lesions and a defect at the prephonemic level. *Brain* 105:271–300, 1982.

Aymes, E. W., Nielsen, J. M. Clinicopathologic study of vascular lesions of the anterior cingulate region. *Bulletin of the Los Angeles Neurological Societies* 20:112–130, 1955.

Babinski, J. Contribution a l'etude des Troubles mentaux dans l'Hemisphere Organique Cerebrale (Anosognosie). *Revue Neurologique* 22:845–847, 1914.

Babinski, J. Anosognosie. *Revue Neurologique* 25:365–366, 1918.

Bachman, D. L., Albert, M. L. The dopaminergic syndromes of dementia. In *Brain Pathology, vol. I: Cerebral Ageing and Degenerative Dementias*. Pilleri, G., Tagliavini, F., eds. Bern, Switzerland, University of Bern, 1984, pp. 91–119.

Baddeley, A. Working memory. *Science* 255:556–559, 1992.

Baddeley, A. D. Short term memory for word sequences as a function of acoustic, semantic and formal similarity. *Quarterly Journal of Experimental Psychology* 18:362–366, 1966.

Baddeley, A. D., Warrington, E. K. Memory coding and amnesia. *Neuropsychologia* 11:159–165, 1973.

Bahls, F. H., Chatrain, G. E., Mesher, R. A., Sumi, S. M., Ruff, R. L. A case of persistent cortical deafness: clinical, neurophysiologic, and neuropathologic observations. *Neurology* 38:1490–1493, 1988.

Bailey, C. H., Chen, M. Morphological basis of long-term habituation and sensitization in aplysia. *Science* 220:91–93, 1983.

Bain, A. *The Senses and the Intellect*. London: Longmans, Green, 1868.

Balint, R. Seelenlahmung des "Schauens," optische Ataxie, raumliche Storung der Auf merksamhiet. *Monatsschrift für Psychiatrie und Neurologie* 25:51–81, 1909.

Ball, J.R.B., Kidson, M. A. The Capgras syndrome: a rarity? *Australian and New Zealand Journal of Psychiatry* 2:44–45, 1968.

Ballantine, R. J., Cassidy, W. L., Flanagan, W. B., Marino, R. Stereotaxic anterior cingulotomy for neuropsychiatric illness and intractable pain. *Journal of Neurosurgery* 26:488–495, 1967.

Barbizet, J. Defect of memorizing of hippocampal-mamillary origin: a review. *Journal of Neurology, Neurosurgery, and Psychiatry* 26:127–135, 1963.

Barlow, H. B. Perception: What quantitative laws govern the acquisition of knowledge from the senses? In *Functions of the Brain*. Coen, C. W., ed. Oxford, Oxford University Press, 1985, pp. 11–43.

Barrett, A. M. A case of pure word-deafness with autopsy. *Journal of Nervous and Mental Disease* 37:73–92, 1910.

Barrie, J. M. *Peter Pan and Wendy*. New York, Clarkson N. Potter, Inc./Publishers (Crown), 1911/1988.

Bastian, H. C. On different kinds of aphasia. *British Medical Journal* 2:931–936, 985–990, 1887.

Bastian, H. C. *Aphasia and Other Speech Defects*. London, H. K. Lewis, 1898.

Battersby, W. S., Bender, M. B., Pollack, M., Kahn, R. L. Unilateral spatial agnosia (inattention). *Brain* 79:68–92, 1956.

Baxter, L. R., Phelps, M. E., Mazziotta, J. C., Guze, B. H., Schwartz, J. M., Selin, C. E. Local cerebral glucose metabolic rates in obsessive–compulsive disorder. *Archives of General Psychiatry* 44:211–218, 1987.

Baxter, L. R., Jr., Phelps, M. E., Mazziotta, J. C., Schwartz, J. M., Gerner, R. H., Selin, C. E., Sumida, R. M. Cerebral metabolic rates for glucose in mood disorders. *Archives of General Psychiatry* 42:441–447, 1985.

Baxter, L. R., Jr., Schwartz, J. M., Phelps, M. E., Mazziotta, J. C., Guze, B. H.,

Selin, C. E., Gerner, R. H., Sumida, R. M. Reduction of left prefrontal cortex glucose metabolism common to three types of depression. *Archives of General Psychiatry* 46:243–250, 1989.

Bay, E. Disturbances of visual perception and their examination. *Brain* 76:515–550, 1953.

Bear, D. Temporal lobe epilepsy: a syndrome of sensory-limbic hyperconnection. *Cortex* 15:357–384, 1979a.

Bear, D. The temporal lobes: an approach to the study of organic behavioral changes. In *Handbook of Behavioral Neurobiology, vol. 2: Neuropsychology*. Gazzaniga, M. S., ed. New York, Plenum Press, 1979b, pp. 75–95.

Bear, D. Hemispheric specialization and the neurology of emotion. *Archives of Neurology* 40:195–202, 1983.

Bear, D. M., Fedio, P. Quantitative analysis of interictal behavior in temporal lobe epilepsy. *Archives of Neurology* 34:454–467, 1977.

Beck, A. T. Thinking and depression: idiosyncratic content and cognitive disorders. *Archives of General Psychiatry* 9:324–333, 1963.

Bekhterev, V. M. *Objective Psychologie*. Leipzig, Tuebner, 1913.

Bekhterev, V. M. *General Principles of Reflexology*, 3rd ed. Leningrad, GIZ, 1917/1926.

Bender, M. B. Neuroophthalmology. In *Clinical Neurology*, 2nd ed. Baker, A. B., ed. New York, Hoeber-Harper, 1962, pp. 275–347.

Bender, M. B., Feldman, M., Sobin, A. J. Palinopsia. *Brain* 91:321–338, 1968.

Benedikt, M. Second life: Das Seelenbinnenleben des gesunden und kranken Menschen. *Wiener Klinik* 20:127–138, 1894.

Benson, D. F. Fluency in aphasia: correlation with radioactive scan localization. *Cortex* 3:373–394, 1967.

Benson, D. F. Psychiatric aspects of aphasia. *British Journal of Psychiatry* 123:555–566, 1973.

Benson, D. F. The third alexia. *Archives of Neurology* 34:326–331, 1977.

Benson, D. F. Neurologic correlates of anomia. In: *Studies in Neurolinguistics*, vol. 4. Whitaker, H., Whitaker, H. A., eds. New York, Academic Press, 1979a, pp. 298–328.

Benson, D. F. *Aphasia, Alexia, and Agraphia*. New York, Churchill Livingstone, 1979b.

Benson, D. F. Aphasia management: The neurologist's role. In *Seminars in Speech, Language and Hearing*. Wertz, R. T., ed. New York, Thieme-Stratton, Inc., 1981, pp. 237–247.

Benson, D. F. The neurology of human emotion. *Bulletin of Clinical Neurosciences* 49:23–42, 1984.

Benson, D. F. Alexia. In *Handbook of Clinical Neurology*, 2nd ed. Vol. 45, *Clinical Neurospychology*. Frederiks, J.A.M., ed. Amsterdam, Elsevier, 1985, pp. 433–455.

Benson, D. F. Aphasia and the lateralization of language. *Cortex* 22:71–86, 1986.

Benson, D. F. Epileptic personality disorder: the Geschwind syndrome. In Benson DF, ed. *Behavioral Disorders in Epilepsy—Course 219*. Minneapolis, American Academy of Neurology, 1987, pp. 77–98.

Benson, D. F. Disorders of visual gnosis. In *The Neuropsychology of Visual Perception*. Brown, J. W., ed. Hillsdale, N.J., Lawrence Erlbaum Associates, Inc., 1988a, pp. 59–78.

Benson, D. F. Classical syndromes of aphasia. In *Handbook of Neuropsychology*, vol. 1. Boller, F., Grafman, J., ed. Amsterdam, Elsevier, 1988b, pp. 267-280.

Benson, D. F. Approach to the patient with neurobehavioral disorders. In *Textbook of Internal Medicine*, vol 2, pt. X. Kelly, W. N., Paty, D. W., eds. Philadelphia, J. B. Lippincott, 1989, pp. 2507-2518.

Benson, D. F. Psychomotor retardation. *Neuropsychiatry, Neuropsychology, and Behavioral Neurology* 3:36-47, 1990.

Benson, D. F. The Geschwind syndrome. In *Neurobehavioral Problems in Epilepsy*. Smith, D. B., Treiman, D., Trimble, M., eds. New York, Raven Press, 1991, pp. 411-421.

Benson, D. F. Neuropsychiatric aspects of aphasia and related language impairments. In *Textbook of Neuropsychiatry*, 2nd ed. Yudofsky, S. C., Hales, R. E., eds. Washington, DC, American Psychiatric Press, 1992, pp. 311-327.

Benson, D. F. Progressive frontal dysfunction. In *Dementia*. Brun, A., ed. Basel, Karger, 1993.

Benson, D. F., Barton, M. I. Disturbances in constructional apraxia. *Cortex* 6:19-46, 1970.

Benson, D. F., Blumer, D. Amnesia: a clinical approach to memory. In *Psychiatric Aspects of Neurologic Disease*, vol. 2. Benson, D. F., Blumer, D., eds. New York, Grune & Stratton, 1982, pp. 251-277.

Benson, D. F., Cummings, J. L. Agraphia. In *Handbook of Clinical Neurology*, 2nd ed. Vol. 45, *Clinical Neuropsychology*. Frederiks, J.A.M., ed. Amsterdam, Elsevier Press, 1985, pp. 457-472.

Benson, D. F., Davis, R. J., Snyder, B. D. Posterior cortical atrophy. *Archives of Neurology* 45:789-793, 1988.

Benson, D. F., Denckla, M. B. Verbal paraphasia as a source of calculation disturbance. *Archives of Neurology* 21:96-102, 1969.

Benson, D. F., Gardner, H., Meadows, J. C. Reduplicative paramnesia. *Neurology* 26:147-151, 1976.

Benson, D. F., Geschwind, N. Shrinking retrograde amnesia. *Journal of Neurology, Neurosurgery, and Psychiatry* 30:457-461, 1967.

Benson, D. F., Geschwind, N. The alexias. In *Handbook of Clinical Neurology*, vol. 4. Vinken, P. J., Bruyn, G. W., eds. Amsterdam, North-Holland, 1969, pp. 112-140.

Benson, D. F., Geschwind, N. Developmental Gerstmann syndrome. *Neurology* 20:293-300, 1970.

Benson, D. F., Geschwind, N. Psychiatric conditions associated with focal lesions of the central nervous system. In *American Handbook of Psychiatry*, vol. 4. Arieti, S., Reiser, M. F., eds. New York, Basic Books, 1975, pp. 208-243.

Benson, D. F., Geschwind, N. The aphasias and related disturbances. In *Clinical Neurology*. Baker, A. B., Joynt, R. J., eds. Philadelphia, Harper & Row, 1985. Chap. 10 pp. 1-85.

Benson, D. F., Greenberg, J. P. Visual form agnosia. *Archives of Neurology* 20:82-89, 1969.

Benson, D. F., Marsden, C. D., Meadows, J. C. The amnesic syndrome of posterior cerebral artery occlusion. *Acta Neurologica Scandinavica* 50:133-145, 1974.

Benson, D. F., McDaniel, K. D. Memory disorders. In *Neurology in Clinical Practice*, Vol. II. Bradley, W. G., Daroff, R. B., Fenichel, G. M., Marsden, C. D., eds. Boston, Butterworth-Heinemann, 1991.

Benson, D. F., Patten, D. H. The use of radioactive isotopes in the localization of aphasia-producing lesions. *Cortex* 3:258–271, 1967.

Benson, D. F., Segarra, J. M., Albert, M. L. Visual agnosia—prosopagnosia. *Archives of Neurology* 30:307–310, 1974.

Benson, D. F., Sheremata, W. A., Buchard, R., Segarra, J., Price, D., Geschwind, N. Conduction aphasia. *Archives of Neurology* 28:339–346, 1973.

Benson, D. F., Stuss, D. T. Frontal lobe influences on delusions: a clinical perspective. *Schizophrenia Bulletin* 16:403–411, 1990.

Benson, D. F., Tomlinson, E. B. Hemiplegic syndrome of the posterior cerebral artery. *Stroke* 2:559–564, 1971.

Benson, D. F., Weir, W. Acalculia: acquired anarithmetria. *Cortex* 8:465–474, 1972.

Benton, A. L. *Right–Left Discrimination and Finger Localization: Development and Pathology.* New York, Hoeber, 1959.

Benton, A. L. The fiction of the "Gerstmann syndrome." *Journal of Neurology, Neurosurgery and Psychiatry* 24:176–181, 1961.

Benton, A. L. Constructional apraxia and the minor hemisphere. *Confinia Neurologica* 29:1–16, 1967.

Benton, A. L. Reflections on the Gerstmann syndrome. *Brain and Language* 4:45–62, 1977.

Benton, A.L. Gerstmann's syndrome. *Archives of Neurology* 49:445–447, 1992.

Benton, A. L., Van Allen, M. W. Impairment in facial recognition in patients with cerebral disease. *Cortex* 4:344–358, 1969.

Bergson, H. *Matter and Memory.* New York, MacMillan, 1911.

Berkeley, G. *The Principles of Human Knowledge.* London, Nelson, 1710/1942.

Berlyne, N. Confabulation. *British Journal of Psychiatry* 120:31–39, 1972.

Bianchi, L. The functions of the frontal lobes. *Brain* 18:497–522, 1895.

Bianchi, L. *The Mechanism of the Brain and the Functions of the Frontal Lobes.* New York, William Wood & Co., 1922.

Biemond, A. The conduction of pain above the level of the thalamus opticus. *AMA Archives of Neurology and Psychiatry* 75:231, 1956.

Binet, A. *Psychologie des Grands Calculateurs et Joueurs d'Eches.* Paris, Hachette, 1894.

Binet, A. *L'Etude Experimentale de L'Intelligence.* Paris, Schleicher Freres, 1903.

Bird, E. D., Spoke, E.G.S., Iverson, L. L. Increased dopamine concentration in limbic areas of the brain from patients dying with schizophrenia. *Brain* 102:347–360, 1979.

Birren, J. E. Translation in gerontology—from lab to life: psychophysiology and speed of response. *American Psychologist* 29:808–815, 1974.

Bisiach, E., Berti, A. Unilateral misrepresentation of distributed information: paradoxes and puzzles. In *Neuropsychology of Visual Perception.* Brown, J. W., ed. Hillsdale, N.J., Lawrence Erlbaum Associates, 1989, pp. 145–161.

Bisiach, E., Luzzatti, C. Unilateral neglect of representational space. *Cortex* 14:29–33, 1978.

Bisiach, E., Luzzatti, C., Perani, D. Unilateral neglect, representational schema and consciousness. *Brain* 102:609–618, 1979.

Bissette, G., Nemeroff, C. B., MacKay, A.V.P. Neuropeptides and schizophrenia. In *Progress in Brain Research, vol. 66, Peptides and Neurological Disease.* Emson, P. C., Rossor, M., Tohyama, M., eds. Amsterdam, Elsevier, 1986, pp. 161–174.

Black, F. W. Cognitive deficits in patients with unilateral war-related frontal lobe lesions. *Journal of Clinical Psychology* 32:366–372, 1976.
Bleuler, E. *Dementia Praecox*. Zinkin, J., translator. New York, International Universities Press, 1912/1950.
Bleuler, E. *Textbook of Psychiatry*. New York, Dover, 1951.
Bleuler, M. Acute mental concomitants of physical diseases. In *Psychiatric Aspects of Neurologic Disease*. Benson, D. F., Blumer, D., eds. New York, Grune & Stratton, 1975, pp. 37–61.
Blumer, D. Temporal lobe epilepsy and its psychiatric significance. In *Psychiatric Aspects of Neurologic Disease*. Benson, D. F., Blumer, D., eds. New York, Grune & Stratton, 1975, pp. 171–197.
Blumer, D., Benson, D. F. Personality changes with frontal and temporal lobe lesions. In *Psychiatric Aspects of Neurologic Disease*. Benson, D. F., Blumer, D., eds. New York, Grune & Stratton, 1975, pp. 151–170.
Blumer, D., Benson, D. F. Psychiatric manifestations of epilepsy. In *Psychiatric Aspects of Neurologic Disease*, vol. 2. Benson, D. F., Blumer, D., eds. New York, Grune & Stratton, 1982, pp. 25–47.
Bodamer, J. Die Prosop-Agnosie. *Archiv für Psychiatrie und Nerven Krankheiten* 179:6–53, 1947.
Bogen, J. E. The other side of the brain. II. An appositional mind. *Bulletin of the Los Angeles Neurological Societies* 34:135–162, 1969.
Bogen, J. E. Further discussion on split brains and hemispheric capabilities. *British Journal of the Philosophy of Science* 28:281–286, 1977.
Bogen, J. E. The callosal syndrome. In *Clinical Neuropsychology*. Heilman, K. M., Valenstein, E., eds. New York, Oxford University Press, 1979, pp. 308–359.
Bogen, J. E. Mental duality in the intact brain. *Bulletin of Clinical Neurosciences* 51:3–29, 1986.
Bogen, J. E. Physiological consequences of complete or partial commissural section. In *Surgery of the Third Ventricle*. Apuzzo, M.L.J., ed. Baltimore, Williams & Wilkins, 1987, pp. 175–191.
Bogen, J. E., Gazzaniga, M. S. Cerebral commissurotomy in man: minor hemisphere dominance for certain visuospatial functions. *Journal of Neurosurgery* 23:394–399, 1965.
Bogen, J. E., Vogel, P. J. Cerebral commissurotomy: a case report. *Bulletin of the Los Angeles Neurological Societies* 27:169, 1962.
Bolton, N. *The Psychology of Thinking*. London, Methuen, 1972.
Bonhoeffer, K. Die Korsakowshe symptomenkomplex in Seinen beseikungen zu den verscheidenen Krankheitsformen. *Allgemeine Zeitschrift für Psychiatrie* 61:744–752, 1904.
Bonhoeffer, K. Die Psychosen im Gefolge von akuten Infektionen, Allgemeinerkrankungen und inneren Erkrankungen. In *Handbuch der Psychiatrie*. Aschaffenburg, G., ed. Leipzig und Wein, Franz Deuticke, 1912, pp. 3–118.
Bornstein, B. Prosopagnosia. In *Problems of Dynamic Neurology*. Halpern, L., ed. Jerusalem, Jerusalem Post Press, 1963, pp. 283–318.
Botez, M. I., Barbeau, A. Role of subcortical structures, and particularly of the thalamus, in the mechanism of speech and language. *International Journal of Neurology* 8:300–320, 1971.
Botez, M. I., Gravel, J., Attig, E., Vezina, J. L. Reversible chronic cerebellar ataxia after phenytoin intoxication: possible role of cerebellum in cognitive thought. *Neurology* 35:1152–1157, 1985.

Bouillaud, J. Recherches cliniques propres a de montrer que la perte de la parole correspond a 'la lesion des lobules anterieurs du cerveau et a confirmer l'opinion de M. Gall sur la siege de l'organe du langage articule. *Archives Generale de Medicine* 8:25–45, 1825.

Bourne, L. E., Jr. *Human Conceptual Behavior.* Boston, Allyn-Bacon, 1966.

Bourne, L. E., Ekstrand, B. R., Dominowski, R. L. *The Psychology of Thinking.* Englewood Clifts, N.J., Prentice-Hall, 1971.

Bowen, M. A family concept of schizophrenia. In *The Etiology of Schizophrenia.* Jackson, D. D., ed. New York, Basic Books, 1960, pp. 346–372.

Bowsher, D. The reticular formation and ascending reticular system: Anatomical considerations. *British Journal of Anesthesiology* 33:174–182, 1961.

Brain, R. Visual disorientation with special reference to lesions of the right cerebral hemisphere. *Brain* 64:244–272, 1941.

Bremer, F. Cerveau "isole" et physiologie du sommeil. *Comptes Rendes Societe de Biologie* 118:1235–1241, 1935.

Brickner, R. M. *The Intellectual Functions of the Frontal Lobes.* New York, MacMillan, 1936.

Bridger, W. H. Cognitive factors in perceptual dysfunction. In *Proceedings of the Association for Research in Nervous and Mental Disease, vol. 48, Perception and Its Disorders.* Hamburg, D. A., Pribram, K. H., Stunkard, A. J., eds. Baltimore, Williams & Wilkins, 1970, pp. 255–265.

Brierley, J. B. The neuropathology of amnesic states. In *Amnesia.* Whitty, C.W.M., Zangwill, O. L., eds. New York, Appleton-Century-Crofts, 1966, pp. 150–180.

Brinkman, C. Lesions in supplementary motor area interfere with a monkey's performance of a bimanual coordination task. *Neuroscience Letters* 27:267–270, 1981.

Brion, S., Pragier, C., Guerin, R., Teitgen, M.M.C. Korsakoff syndrome due to bilateral softening of fornix. *Revue Neurologique* 120:255–262, 1969.

Broadbent, D. E. The role of auditory localization in attention and memory span. *Journal of Experimental Psychology* 47:191–196, 1954.

Broadbent, D. E. *Perception and Communication.* Elmsford, NY, Pergamon Press, 1958.

Broadbent, D. E. *Decision and Stress.* New York, Academic Press, 1971.

Broca, P. Remarques sur le siège de la faculté du langage articulé, suivies d'une observation d'aphemie. *Bulletin Societé Anatomique de Paris* 2:330–357, 1861.

Broca, P. Sur la faculté du langage articulé. Bulletin Societé Anthropologie (Paris) 6:337–393, 1865.

Brodal, A. *Neurological Anatomy.* New York, Oxford University Press, 1981.

Brodmann, K. Beitrage zur histologischen Lokalisation der grosshirnrinde. VI. Die Cortexgliederung der Menschen. *Journal of Psychology and Neurology* 10:231–246, 1908.

Brooks, V. B., Thach, W. T. Cerebellar control of posture and movements. In *Handbook of Physiology,* vol. II, pt. 2. Bethesda, American Physiological Association, 1981, pp. 877–946.

Brown, J. R. Short-term memory. *British Medical Bulletin* 20:8–11, 1964.

Brown, J. W. *Aphasia, Agnosia, and Apraxia.* Springfield, IL, Thomas, 1972.

Brown, J. W., ed. *The Neuropsychology of Visual Perception.* Hillsdale, NJ, Lawrence Erlbaum Associates, 1988.

Bruner, J. S., Goodnow, J. J., Austin, G. A. *A Study of Thinking.* New York, John Wiley, 1956.
Buchsbaum, M. S. The frontal lobes, basal ganglia and temporal lobes as sites for schizophrenia. *Schizophrenia Bulletin* 16:379–390, 1990.
Buchsbaum, M. S., Ingvar, D. H., Kessler, R., Waters, R. N., Cappelletti, J., van Kammen, D. P., King, C., Johnson, J. L., Manning, R. G., Flynn, R. W., Mann, L. S., Bunney, W. E., Jr., Sokoloff, L. Cerebral glucography with positron tomography—use in normal subjects and patients with schizophrenia. *Archives of General Psychiatry* 39:251–259, 1982.
Bumke, O. *Die Diagnose der Geisteskrankheiten.* Weisbaden, Bergmann, 1919.
Buschke, H., Grober, E. Genuine memory deficits in age-associated memory impairment. *Developmental Neuropsychology* 2:287–307, 1986.
Butler, S. Thought and language. In *The Importance of Language.* Black, M., ed. Ithaca, NY, Cornell University Press, 1890/1962, pp. 13–35.
Butters, N., Barton, M., Brody, B. A. Role of the right parietal lobe in the mediation of cross-modal associations and reversible operations in space. *Cortex* 6:174–190, 1970.
Butters, N., Brody, B. The role of the left parietal lobe in the mediation of intra- and cross-modal associations. *Cortex* 4:328–343, 1968.
Butters, N., Grady, M. The role of temporal processing factors in the short-term memory performance of patients with Korsakoff's and Huntington's diseases. *Neuropsychologia* 15:701–706, 1977.
Caine, E. D. Gilles de la Tourette's syndrome. *Archives of Neurology* 42:393–397, 1985.
Caine, E. D., Ebert, M. H., Weingartner, H. An outline for the analysis of dementia: the memory disorder of Huntington's disease. *Neurology* 27:1087–1092, 1977.
Cairns, H., Oldfield, R. C., Pennybacker, J. B., Whitteridge, D. Akinetic mutism with epidermoid cyst of the III ventricle. *Brain* 64:273–290, 1941.
Campbell, R., Landis, T., Regard, M. Facial recognition and lip reading: a neurological dissociation. *Brain* 109:509–521, 1986.
Cannon, W. B. The James-Lange theory of emotion: a critical examination and an alternative theory. *American Journal of Psychiatry* 34:106–124, 1927.
Cantu, R. C., Drew, J. H. Pathological laughing and crying associated with a tumor ventral to the pons. *Journal of Neurosurgery* 24:1024–1026, 1966.
Capgras, J., Reboul-Lachaux, J. L'illusion des sosies dans un délire systematisé clinique. *Bulletin de la Societé Clinique de Medicine Mentale* 11:6–16, 1923.
Caplan, L. R., Schoene, W. C. Clinical features of subcortical arteriosclerotic encephalopathy (Binswanger disease). *Neurology* 28:1206–1215, 1978.
Carpenter, W. T., Jr., Bartko, J. J., Carpenter, C. L., Strauss, J. S. Another view of schizophrenic subtypes. *Archives of General Psychiatry* 33:509–516, 1976.
Cellerier, G. Cognitive strategies in problem solving. In *Language and Learning: The Debate Between Jean Piaget and Noam Chomsky.* Piatelli-Palmarini, M., ed. Cambridge, Mass., Harvard Press, 1980, pp. 67–72.
Cermak, L. S., O'Connor, M. C. The anterograde and retrograde retrieval ability of a patient with amnesia due to encephalitis. *Neuropsychologia* 21:213–234, 1983.
Chan, J. H., Ross, E. D. Left handed mirror writing following right anterior cerebral artery infarction. *Neurology* 38:59–63, 1988.

Charcot, J. M. *Clinical Lectures on Diseases of the Nervous System*, vol. 3. London, New Sydenham Society, 1889.
Chase, M. H., ed. *The Sleeping Brain*. Association for the Psychophysiologic Study of Sleep. Los Angeles, Brain Information Service, 1972.
Chedru, F., Geschwind, N. Disorders of higher cortical functions in acute confusional states. *Cortex* 8:395–411, 1972.
Cherry, E. C. Some experiments on the recognition of speech with one and two ears. *Journal of the Acoustical Society of America* 25:975–979, 1953.
Chomsky, N. *Syntactic Structures*. The Hague, Mouton, 1957.
Chomsky, N. *Aspects of the Theory of Syntax*. Cambridge, MA, MIT Press, 1965.
Chomsky, N. *Language and Mind*. New York, Harcourt Brace Jovanovich, 1972.
Chomsky, N. *Reflections on Language*. New York, Pantheon, 1975.
Chomsky, N. *Rules and Representations*. New York, Columbia University Press, 1980.
Christodoulou, G. N. The syndrome of Capgras. *British Journal of Psychiatry* 130:555–564, 1977.
Chu, N., Bloom, F. E. Norepinephrine-containing neurons: changes in spontaneous discharge patterns during sleeping and waking. *Science* 179:907–910, 1973.
Clark, T. The Masters Movement: age conquers some but it doesn't conquer all. *Runner's World* 14:80–95, 1979.
Cloninger, C. R. A systematic method for clinical description and classification of personality variants. *Archives of General Psychiatry* 44:573–588, 1987.
Cogan, D. G. Lesions involving conjugate lateral movements. In *Neurology of the Ocular Muscles*. Cogan, D. G., ed. Springfield, IL, Charles C. Thomas, 1966, pp. 69–75.
Cohn, R. Dyscalculia. *Archives of Neurology* 4:301–307, 1961.
Coltheart, M. Deep dyslexia: a review of the syndrome. In *Deep Dyslexia*. Coltheart, M., Patterson, K., and Marshall, J. C., eds. London, Routledge & Kegan Paul, 1980, pp. 22–47.
Condillac, E. *Traite' des sensations*, vols. I and II. Paris, Londres, 1754.
Corbetta, M., Miezin, F. M., Dobmeyer, S., Shulman, G. L., Petersen, S. E. Attentional modulation of neural processing of shape, color, and velocity in humans. *Science* 248:1556–1559, 1990.
Corkin, S. Acquisition of motor skill after bilateral medial temporal-lobe excision. *Neuropsychologia* 6:255–265, 1968.
Craik, F. I. M. Age differences in human memory. In *Handbook of the Psychology of Aging*. Birren, J. E., Schaie, K. W., eds. New York, Van Nostrand Reinhold, 1977, pp. 384–420.
Critchley, M. *The Parietal Lobes*. London, Edward Arnold & Co., 1953.
Critchley, M. The problem of visual agnosia. *Journal of the Neurological Sciences* 1:274–290, 1964.
Critchley, M. The enigma of the Gerstmann's syndrome. *Brain* 89:183–198, 1966.
Critchley, M. Aphasiological nomenclature and definitions. *Cortex* 3:3–25, 1967.
Critchley, M. Thinking and speaking: verbal symbols in thought. In *Aphasiology*. Critchley, M., ed. London, Edward Arnold, Ltd., 1970a, pp. 159–173.
Critchley, M. Non-articulate modalities of speech and their disorders. In *Aphasiology*. Critchley, M., ed. London, Edward Arnold, Ltd., 1970b, pp. 325–347.

Crook, T., Bartus, R. T., Ferris, S. H., Whitehouse, P., Cohen, G. D., Gershon, S. Age associated memory impairment: Proposed diagnostic criteria and measures of clinical change. *Developmental Neuropsychology* 2:261–276, 1986.

Crosby, E. C., Humphrey, E., Lauer, E. W. *Correlative Anatomy of the Nervous System.* New York, MacMillan, 1962.

Cummings, J. L. Organic delusions: phenomenology, anatomic correlations, and review. *British Journal of Psychiatry* 46:184–197, 1985a.

Cummings, J. L. *Clinical Neuropsychiatry.* Orlando, FL, Grune & Stratton, 1985b.

Cummings, J. L., ed. *Subcortical Dementia.* New York, Oxford University Press, 1990.

Cummings, J. L., Benson, D. F. *Dementia: A Clinical Approach.* Boston, Butterworths, 1983.

Cummings, J. L., Benson, D. F. Subcortical dementia. *Archives of Neurology* 41:874–879, 1984.

Cummings, J. L., Benson, D. F., Dementia of the Alzheimer's type: an inventory of diagnostic clinical features. *Journal of the American Geriatrics Society* 34:12–19, 1986.

Cummings, J. L., Benson, D. F. *Dementia: A Clinical Approach.* 2nd ed. Boston, Butterworth-Heinemann, 1992.

Cummings, J. L., Benson, D. F., Hill, M. A., Read, S. Aphasia in dementia of the Alzheimer type. *Neurology* 35:394–397, 1985.

Cummings, J. L., Frankel, M. Gilles de la Tourette's syndrome and the neurological basis of obsessions and compulsions. *Biological Psychiatry* 20:1117–1126, 1985.

Cummings, J. L., Mendez, M. F. Secondary mania with focal cerebrovascular lesions. *American Journal of Psychiatry* 141:1084–1087, 1984.

Cummings, J. L., Syndulko, K., Goldberg, Z., Treiman, D. Palinopsia reconsidered. *Neurology* 32:444–447, 1982.

Cummings, J. L., Tomiyasu, U., Read, S., Benson, D. F. Amnesia with hippocampal lesion after cardiopulmonary arrest. *Neurology* 34:679–681, 1984.

Cutting, J. A study of anosognosia. *Journal of Neurology, Neurosurgery, and Psychiatry* 41:548–555, 1978.

Daly, D. Ictal affect. *American Journal of Psychiatry* 115:97–108, 1958.

Daly, R. F., Forster, F. M. Inheritance of reading epilepsy. *Neurology* 25:1051–1054, 1975.

Damasio, A. R. The frontal lobes. In *Clinical Neuropsychology.* Heilman, K. M., Valenstein, E., eds. New York, Oxford University Press, 1979, pp. 360–412.

Damasio, A. R. The frontal lobes. In *Clinical Neuropsychology.* 2nd ed. Heilman, K. M., Valenstein, E., eds. New York, Oxford University Press, 1985, pp. 339–376.

Damasio, A. R. Disorders of complex visual processing: agnosias, achromatopsia, Balint's syndrome, and related difficulties of orientation and construction. In *Principles of Behavioral Neurology.* Mesulam, M. M., ed. Philadelphia, F. A. Davis, 1985, pp. 259–288.

Damasio, A. R., Damasio, H. The anatomic basis of pure alexia. *Neurology* 33:1573–1583, 1983.

Damasio, A. R., Damasio, H., Chui, H. Neglect following damage to frontal lobe or basal ganglia. *Neuropsychologia* 18:123–131, 1980.

Damasio, A. R., Damasio, H., Van Hoesen, G. W. Prosopagnosia: anatomic basis and behavioral mechanisms. *Neurology* 32:331–341, 1982.

Damasio, A. R., Graf-Radford, N. R., Eslinger, P. J., Damasio, H., Kassell, N. Amnesia following basal forebrain lesions. *Archives of Neurology* 42:263–271, 1985.

Damasio, A. R., Van Hoesen, G. W. Structure and function of the supplementary motor area, abstracted. *Neurology* 30:359, 1980.

Damasio, A. R., Van Hoesen, G. W. Emotional disturbances associated with focal lesions of the limbic frontal lobe. In *Neuropsychology of Human Emotion*. Heilman, K. M., Satz, P., eds. New York, Guilford Press, 1983, pp. 85–110.

Damasio, A. R., Van Hoesen, G. W. Neuroanatomical correlates of amnesia in Alzheimer's disease. In *Biological Substrates of Alzheimer's Disease*. Scheibel, A. B., Wechsler, A. F., eds. Orlando, FL, Academic Press, 1986, pp. 65–71.

Damasio, H., Damasio, A. R. The anatomical basis of conduction aphasia. *Brain* 103:337–350, 1980.

Damasio, H., Damasio, A. R. *Lesion Analysis in Neuropsychology*. New York, Oxford University Press, 1989.

Darkins, A. W., Benson, D. F., Fromkin, V. A. A characterization of the prosodic loss in Parkinson's disease. *Brain and Language* 34:315–327, 1988.

Darley, F. L., Aronson, A. E., Brown, J. R. *Motor Speech Disorders*. Philadelphia, Saunders, 1975.

Davison, C., Kelman, H. Pathologic laughing and crying. *Archives of Neurology and Psychiatry* 42:595–643, 1939.

Davison, K., Bagley, R. Schizophrenia-like psychoses associated with organic disorders of the central nervous system: a review of the literature. In *Current Problems in Neuropsychiatry*. Harrington, R. N., ed. Ashford, Kent, Headley Brothers, 1969, pp. 113–183.

Dee, H. L. Visuoconstructive and visuoperceptive deficit in patients with unilateral cerebral lesions. *Neuropsychologia* 8:305–314, 1970.

Dejerine, J. Sur un cas de cécité verbale avec agraphie, suivi d'autopsie. *Memoires Societé Biologigue* 3:197–201, 1891.

Dejerine, J. Contribution a l'etude anatomoclinique et clinique des differentes varieties de cécité verbale. *Memoires Societé Biologique* 4:61–90, 1892.

Dejerine, J. *Semiologie des affections du systeme nerveux*. Paris, Masson, 1914/1977, pp. 42–43.

DeKosky, S., Heilman, K. M., Bowers, D. Recognition and discrimination of emotional faces and pictures. *Brain and Language* 9:206–214, 1980.

DeLay, J., Brion, S., Elissalde, B. Corps mamillaire et syndrome de Korsakoff. Etude anatomique de huit cas de syndrome de Korsakoff d'origine alcoolique sans alteration significative du cortex cerebral. I. Etude anatomoclinique. *La Presse Medicale* 66:1849–1852, 1958a.

DeLay, J., Brion, S., Elissalde, B. Corps mamillaire et syndrome de Korsakoff. Etude anatomique de huit cas. de syndrome de Korsakoff d'origine alcoolique sans alteration significative du cortex cerebral. II. Tubercules mamillaire et mecanisme de la memoire. *La Presse Medicale* 66:1965–1968, 1958b.

Dement, W. C. Daytime sleepiness and sleep "attacks." In *Advances in Sleep Research*. Guilleminault, C., Dement, W. C., Passouant, P., eds. New York, Spectrum, 1976, pp. 17–42.

Dempsey, E. M., Morrison, R. S. The electrical activity of a thalamo-cortical relay system. *American Journal of Psychiatry* 138:283–296, 1943.

Dennis, M. Capacity and strategy for syntactic comprehension after right or left hemidecortication. *Brain and Language* 10:287–317, 1980.

Denny-Brown, D. The nature of apraxia. *Journal of Nervous and Mental Disease* 126:9–32, 1958.

Denny-Brown, D. *The Basal Ganglia.* London, Oxford University Press, 1962.

Denny-Brown, D. The physiological basis of perception and speech. In *Problems of Dynamic Neurology.* Halpern, L., ed. Jerusalem, Hebrew Hadassah Medical School, 1963, pp. 30–62.

Denny-Brown, D., Banker, B. Q. Amorphosynthesis from left parietal lesion. *Archives of Neurology and Psychiatry* 71:302–313, 1954.

Denny-Brown, D., Meyer, J. S., Horenstein, S. The significance of perceptual rivalry resulting from parietal lesion. *Brain* 75:433–471, 1952.

Denny-Brown, D., Yanagisawa, N. The role of the basal ganglia in the initiation of movements. In *The Basal Ganglia.* Yahr, M. D., ed. New York, Raven Press, 1976, pp. 115–148.

De Renzi, E. Prosopagnosia in two patients with CT scan evidence of damage confined to the right hemisphere. *Neuropsychologia* 24:385–389, 1986.

De Renzi, E., Pieczuro, A., Vignolo, L. Ideational apraxia: a quantitative study. *Neuropsychologia* 6:41–52, 1968.

De Renzi, E., Spinnler, H. Facial recognition in brain damaged patients. *Neurology* 16:145–152, 1966.

De Renzi, E., Vignolo, L. A. The token test: a sensitive test to detect receptive disturbances in aphasics. *Brain* 85:665–678, 1962.

Descartes, R. (Torrey H.A.P., transl.). The Philosophy of Descartes in Extracts From His Writings. New York, Holt, 1892.

Desimone, R., Ungerleider, L. G. Neural mechanism in visual processing in monkeys. In *Handbook of Neuropsychology,* vol. 2. Boller, F., and Grafman, J., eds. Amsterdam, Elsevier, 1989, pp. 267–299.

Desmedt, J. E., Noel, P. Average cerebral evoked potentials in the evaluation of lesions of sensory nerves and of the somatosensory pathway. In *New Developments in Electromyography and Clinical Neurophysiology,* vol. 2. Desmedt, J. E., ed. Basel, Karger, 1973, pp. 352–371.

Dewey, J. *Leibnitz's New Essays Concerning Human Understanding—A Critical Exposition.* Chicago, C. C. Griggs and Co., 1888.

Dixon, W. F. *Subliminal Perception: The Nature of a Controversy.* London, McGraw-Hill, 1971.

Dorland's Illustrated Medical Dictionary. Philadelphia, W. B. Saunders, 1974.

Ebbinghaus, H. *Memory—A Contribution to Experimental Psychology.* New York, Dover Publications, 1885/1964.

Eccles, J. C. Conscious experience and memory. In *Brain and Conscious Experience.* Eccles, J. C., ed. Berlin, Springer-Verlag, 1966, pp. 314–344.

Eccles, J. C., Itoh, M., Szentagothai, J. *The Cerebellum as a Neural Machine.* New York, Springer-Verlag, 1967.

Efron, R. What is perception? *Boston Studies in the Philosophy of Science* 4:137–173, 1968.

Efron, R. *The Decline and Fall of Hemispheric Specialization.* Hillsdale, N.J., Lawrence Erlbaum Associates, 1990.

Elliott, F. A. Neurological aspects of antisocial behavior. In *The Psychopath: A*

Comprehensive Study of Anti-Social Disorders and Behavior. Reid, W., ed. New York, Brunner/Mazel, 1978a, pp. 146–189.
Elliott, F. A. Neurological factors in violent behavior (the dyscontrol syndrome). In *Violence and Responsibility.* Sadoff, R. L., ed. New York, Spectrum, 1978b.
Elliott, F. A. Violence: the neurological contribution: an overview. *Archives of Neurology* 49:595–603, 1992.
Ellis, A. W., Young, A. W. *Human Cognitive Neuropsychology.* Hillsdale, NJ, Lawrence Erlbaum Associates, 1988.
Engel, G. L. "Psychogenic" pain and the pain-prone patient. *American Journal of Medicine* 26:899–918, 1959.
Engel, G. L., Romano, J. Delirium: a syndrome of cerebral insufficiency. *Journal of Chronic Disease* 9:260–277, 1959.
Engel, J., Jr. *Seizures and Epilepsy.* Philadelphia, F. A. Davis Company, 1989.
Enoch, M. D. The Capgras syndrome. *Acta Psychiatrica Scandinavica* 39:437–462, 1963.
Enoch, M. D., Trethowan, W. H. *Uncommon Psychiatric Syndromes.* Bristol, Wright, 1979.
Erasmus, D. *The Praise of Folly.* New York, Walter Black, 1514/1942.
Ettlinger, G. Analysis of cross-modal effects and their relationship to language. In *Brain Mechanisms Underlying Speech and Language.* Millikan, C., Darley, F., eds. New York, Grune & Stratton, 1967, pp. 53–60.
Ettlinger, G. Apraxia considered as a disorder of movements that are language-dependent: evidence from cases of brain bisection. *Cortex* 5:285–289, 1969.
Farah, M. J. *Visual Agnosia.* Cambridge, MA, MIT Press, 1990.
Faust, C. Die psychischen und psychische Spatfolgen nach Hirnverletzungen. In *Psychiatrie der Gegenwart,* Band II. Gruhle, H. W., Jung, B. R., Mayer-Gross, W., Müller, M., eds. Berlin, Springer, 1960, pp. 552–645.
Feldman, M. J., Drasgow, J. *The Visual–Verbal Test Manual.* Beverly Hills, CA, Western Psychological Services, 1960.
Ferrier, D. *The Functions of the Brain.* London, Smith & Elder, 1886.
Feuchtwanger, E. *Die funktionen des Stirnhirns ihre pathologie und psychologie. Monographien aus dem Gesamtgebiete der Neurologie und Psychiatrie* 38:1–193, 1923.
Fish, F. *Schizophrenia.* Bristol, John Wright & Sons, 1962.
Flechsig, P. Developmental (myelogenetic) localization of the cerebral cortex in the human subject. *Lancet* 2:1027–1029, 1901.
Flor-Henry, P. Schizophrenic-like reactions and affective psychoses associated with temporal lobe epilepsy: etiological factors. *American Journal of Psychiatry* 126:400–403, 1969.
Flor-Henry, P., Koles, Z. J. EEG studies in depression, mania and normals: evidence for partial shifts of laterality in the affective psychoses. *Advances in Biological Psychiatry* 4:21–43, 1980.
Fodor, J. A. *The Language of Thought.* Cambridge, Harvard University Press, 1975.
Fodor, J. *The Modularity of Mind.* Cambridge, MA, MIT Press, 1983.
Foerster, O. The motor cortex in man in the light of Hughlings Jackson's doctrines. *Brain* 59:135–159, 1936a.
Foerster, O. Motorische felder und bahnen. In *Handbuch der Neurologie,* vol. 6. Bumke, O., Foerster, O., eds. Berlin, Julius Springer, 1936b, pp. 1–357.

Folstein, M. F., Maiberger, R., McHugh, P. Mood disorder as a specific complication of stroke. *Journal of Neurology, Neurosurgery, and Psychiatry* 40:1018–1020, 1977.
Forster, F. M., Paulsen, W. A., Baughman, F. A., Jr. Clinical therapeutic conditioning in reading epilepsy. *Neurology* 19:717–723, 1969.
Forster, F. M., Richards, J. F., Panitch, H. S., Huisman, R. E., Paulsen, R. E. Reflex epilepsy evoked by decision making. *Archives of Neurology* 32:54–56, 1975.
Fowler, O. S., Fowler, L. N. *The Illustrated Self-Instructor in Phrenology and Physiology.* New York, Fowlers and Wells, Publishers, 1849.
Frankel, M., Cummings, J. L., Robertson, M. M., Trimble, M. R., Hill, M. A., Benson, D. F. Obsessions and compulsions in Gilles de la Tourette's syndrome. Neurology 36:378–382, 1986.
Fraser, J. G. *The Golden Bough,* volume II, *Taboo and the Perils of the Soul,* 3rd ed. London, MacMillan, 1911.
Freedman, M., Alexander, M. P., Naeser, M. A. The anatomical basis of transcortical motor aphasia. *Neurology* 34:409–417, 1984.
Freedman, A. M., Kaplan, H. I., Sadock, B. J. *Comprehensive Textbook of Psychiatry/II,* 2nd ed. Baltimore, Williams & Wilkins, 1975.
Freeman, R. L., Galaburda, A. M., Cabal, R. D., Geschwind, N. The neurology of depression: cognitive and behavioral deficits with focal findings in depression and resolution after electroconvulsive therapy. *Archives of Neurology* 42:289–291, 1985.
Freeman, W. Transorbital leucotomy: the deep frontal cut. *Proceedings of the Royal Society of Medicine* 42:8–12, 1949.
Freeman, W., Watts, J. W., Hunt, T. *Psychosurgery.* Baltimore, Thomas, 1942.
French, J. D. Brain lesions associated with prolonged unconsciousness. *Archives of Neurology and Psychiatry* 68:727–740, 1952.
French, J. D. The reticular formation. *Journal of Neurosurgery* 15:97–115, 1958.
Freud, S. *Psychopathology of Everyday Life.* In *The Basic Writings of Sigmund Freud.* Brill, A. A., translator. New York, Modern Library, 1938, pp. 35–178.
Freud, S. *On Aphasia.* Stengl, E., translator. New York, International Universities Press, Inc., 1891/1953.
Freud, S. *Project for a Scientific Psychology.* In: *Complete Psychological Works of Sigmund Freud.* Strachey, J., translator. London, Hogarth, 1966.
Fuster, J. M. *The Prefrontal Cortex: Anatomy, Physiology, and Neuropsychology of the Frontal Lobe.* New York, Raven Press, 1980.
Fuster, J. M. Temporal organization of behavior. *Human Neurobiology* 4:57–60, 1985a.
Fuster, J. M. The prefrontal cortex, mediator of cross-temporal contingencies. *Human Neurobiology* 4:169–179, 1985b.
Fuster, J. M. *The Prefrontal Cortex, Second Edition.* New York, Raven Press, 1989.
Gado, M., Hughes, C. P., Danziger, W., Chi, D., Jost, G., Berg, L. Volumetric measurements of the cerebrospinal fluid spaces in demented subjects and controls. *Radiology* 144:535–538, 1982.
Gainotti, G. Emotional behavior and hemispheric side of lesion. *Cortex* 8:41–45, 1972.
Gall, F. *Sur les fonctions du cerveau et sur celles se chacune de ses parties.* Paris, Bailliere, 1825.

Gall, F. J., Spurzheim, G. *Recherches sur le systeme nerveux et general et sur celui cerveau en particulier.* Paris, Schoell, 1809.
Gall, F. J., Vimant, Broussais. *On the Function of the Cerebellum.* Edinburgh, Machlachlan and Stewart, 1838.
Galton, F. Psychometric experiments. *Brain* 2:149–162, 1879a.
Galton, F. Psychometric facts. *The Nineteenth Century* 5:425–433, 1879b.
Gamper, E. Schlaff—Delirium tremens—Korsakawsches. *Zentralblatt für Neurologie* 51:236–239, 1928.
Gardner, H. *Frames of Mind.* New York, Basic Books, 1983.
Gardner, H. *The Mind's New Science.* New York, Basic Books, 1985.
Gardner, R. A., Gardner, B. Teaching sign-language to a chimpanzee. *Science* 165:664–672, 1969.
Gastaut, H., Broughton, R. *Epileptic Seizures.* Springfield, IL, Charles C. Thomas, 1972.
Gastaut, H., Roger, J., Roger, A. Sur la signification de certaines epileptiques. A propos d'une observation electroclinique d'etal de mal temporal. *Revue Neurologique* 94:298–301, 1956.
Gazzaniga, M. S. *The Bisected Brain.* New York, Appleton-Century-Crofts, 1970.
Gazzaniga, M. S. *The Social Brain.* New York, Basic Books, 1985.
Gazzaniga, M. S., Sperry, R. W. Language after section of the cerebral commissures. *Brain* 90:131–148, 1967.
Gelenberg, A. J. The catatonic syndrome. *Lancet* 1:1339–1341, 1976.
Gerstmann, J. Fingeragnosia: Eine um schniebene Storung der Orienterung am eigenen Korper. *Wiener Klinische Wochenschrift* 31:1010–1012, 1924.
Gerstmann, J. Fingeragnosia and isolierte Agraphie, ein neues Syndrom. *Zeitschrift für die gesamte Neurologie und Psychiatrie* 108:152–177, 1927.
Gerstmann, J. Zur symptomatologie der Hirnlasionen im Uebergangsgebiet de interen Parietal und mittleren Occipital-windung. *Nervenarzt* 3:691–695, 1931.
Geschwind, N. The anatomy of acquired disorders of reading. In *Reading Disability: Progress and Research Needs in Dyslexia.* Money, J., ed. Baltimore, Johns Hopkins Press, 1962, pp. 115–129.
Geschwind, N. Disconnexion syndromes in animals and man. *Brain* 88:237–294, 585–644, 1965.
Geschwind, N. The varieties of naming errors. *Cortex* 3:97–112, 1967a.
Geschwind, N. The apraxias. In *Phenomenology of Will and Action.* Strauss, E. W., Griffith, R. M., eds. Pittsburgh, Duquesne University Press, 1967b, pp. 91–102.
Geschwind, N. The apraxias: neural mechanisms of disorders of learned movement. *American Scientist* 63:188–195, 1975a.
Geschwind, N. The borderland of neurology and psychiatry: some common misconceptions. In *Psychiatric Aspects of Neurologic Disease.* Benson, D. F., Blumer, D. eds. New York, Grune & Stratton, 1975b, pp. 1–8.
Geschwind, N. *Lectures in Neurobehavior.* Boston, Harvard Medical School, 1977.
Geschwind, N. Behavioral changes in temporal lobe epilepsy. *Psychological Medicine* 9:217–219, 1979.
Geschwind, N. Disorders of attention: a frontier on neuropsychology. In *The Neuropsychology of Cognitive Function.* Broadbent, D. S., Weiskrantz, L., eds. London, The Royal Society, 1982, pp. 173–185.

Geschwind, N., Fusillo, M. Color naming defects in association with alexia. *Archives of Neurology* 15:137–146, 1966.
Geschwind, N., Kaplan, E. A human deconnection syndrome. *Neurology* 12:675–685, 1962.
Gibbs, M., Ng, K. T. Psychobiology of memory: towards a model of memory formation. *Biobehavioral Review* 1:113–136, 1977.
Gibson, J. J. *The Ecological Approach to Visual Perception.* Boston, Houghton-Mifflin, 1979.
Gilhooly, K. J. *Thinking: Directed, Undirected, and Creative.* New York, Academic Press, 1982.
Gilman, S. The cerebellum: its role in posture and movement. In *Scientific Basis of Clinical Neurology.* Swash, M., Kennard, C., eds. Edinburgh, Churchill Livingstone, 1985, pp. 36–55.
Glassman, J. N., Dryer, D., McCartney, J. R. Complex-partial status epilepticus presenting as gelastic seizures: a report. *General Hospital Psychiatry* 8:61–64, 1985.
Gloning, I., Gloning, K., Hoff, H. *Neuropsychological Symptoms and Syndromes in Lesions of the Occipital Lobe and the Adjacent Areas.* Paris, Gauthier-Villars, 1968.
Gloning, I., Gloning, K., Seittelberger, F., Tschabitscher, H. Ein Fall von reiner Wortblindheit mit Obduktionsbefund. *Weiner Zeitschrift für Nervenheilkunde* 12:194–215, 1955.
Goldberg, G., Mayer, N. H., Toglia, J. V. Medial frontal cortex infarction and the alien hand sign. *Archives of Neurology* 38:683–686, 1981.
Goldman-Rakic, P. The frontal lobes: uncharted provinces of the brain. *Trends in Neuroscience* 7:425–429, 1984.
Goldman-Rakic, P. S. Circuitry of the frontal association cortex and its relevance to dementia. *Archives of Gerontology and Geriatrics* 6:299–309, 1987.
Goldman-Rakic, P. S. Cellular and circuit basis of working memory in prefrontal cortex of nonhuman primates. *Progress in Brain Research* 85:325–336, 1990.
Goldstein, K. Das Wesen der Amnestischen Aphasie. *Schweizer Archiv für Neurologie und Psychiatrie* 15:163–175, 1924.
Goldstein, K. *Human Nature in the Light of Psychopathology.* New York, Schocken, 1940.
Goldstein, K. *Language and Language Disturbances.* New York, Grune & Stratton, 1948a.
Goldstein, K. *Aftereffects of Brain Injury in War.* New York, Grune & Stratton, 1948b.
Goldstein, M. Auditory agnosia for speech (pure word deafness): a historical review with current implications. *Brain and Language* 1:195–204, 1974.
Goldstein, M. N., Brown, M., Hollander, J. Auditory agnosia and cortical deafness: analysis of a case with three year follow-up. *Brain and Language* 2:324–332, 1975.
Goltz, F. L. Zur Physiologie der Grosshirns. *Archiv für Psychiatrie,* 1884 (cited in Bianchi, L. *The Mechanism of the Brain and the Functions of the Frontal Lobes.* New York, William Wood, 1922).
Goodglass, H. Studies on the grammar of aphasics. In *Developments in Applied Psycholinguistics Research.* Rosenberg, S., Kaplan, J. H., eds. New York, MacMillan Co., 1968, pp. 177–208.

Goodglass, H. *Selected Papers in Neurolinguistics.* Munchen, Wilhelm Fink, 1978.
Goodglass, H., Kaplan, E. *The Assessment of Aphasia and Related Disorder.* Philadelphia, Lea and Febiger, 1972.
Goodglass, H., Klein, B., Carey, P., Jones, K. Specific semantic word categories in aphasia. *Cortex* 2:74–89, 1966.
Gordon, H. W., Bogen, J. E. Hemispheric lateralization of singing after intracarotid sodium amylobarbitone. *Journal of Neurology, Neurosurgery, and Psychiatry* 37:727–738, 1974.
Gorham, D. R. A proverbs test for clinical and experimental use. *Psychological Reports* 1:1–12, 1956.
Graf, P., Schacter, D. L. Implicit and explicit memory for new associations in normal and amnesic subjects. *Journal of Experimental Psychology of Learning, Memory, and Cognition* 11:386–396, 1985.
Grafman, J., Salazar, A. M., Weingartner, H., Vance, S. C., Ludlow, C. Isolated impairment of memory following a penetrating lesion of the fornix cerebri. *Archives of Neurology* 42:1162–1168, 1985.
Grant, D. A., Berg, E. A. A behavioral analysis of reinforcement and ease of shifting to new responses in a Weigl-type card-sorting problem. *Journal of Experimental Psychology* 38:404–411, 1948.
Graybiel, A. M. Neurotransmitters and neuromodulators in the basal ganglia. *Trends in Neuroscience* 13:244–254, 1990.
Greenblatt, M., Solomon, H. C. Studies of lobotomy. In *Research Publications—Association for Research in Nervous and Mental Disease,* vol. 36, *The Brain and Human Behavior.* Solomon, H. C., Cobb, S., and Penfield, W., eds. New York, Hafner, 1966, pp. 19–34.
Greenblatt, S. H. Alexia without agraphia or hemianopsia. *Brain* 96:307–316, 1973.
Greenblatt, S. H. Neurosurgery and the anatomy of reading: a practical review. *Neurosurgery* 1:6–15, 1977.
Greenblatt, S. H. Localization of lesions in alexia. In *Localization in Neuropsychology.* Kertesz, A., ed. New York, Academic Press, 1983, pp. 324–356.
Greenfield, J. G., Blackwood, W., Meyer, A., McMenemey, W. H., Norman, R. M. *Neuropathology.* London, Edward Arnold, Ltd., 1958.
Grewel, F. Acalculia. *Brain* 75:397–407, 1952.
Grimm, R. J., Nashner, L. M. Long loop dyscontrol. In *Progress in Clinical Neurophysiology,* vol. 4, *Cerebral Motor Control in Man: Long Loop Mechanisms.* Desmedt, J. E., ed. Basel, Karger, 1978, pp. 70–84.
Gross, C. G. Visual functions of inferotemporal cortex. In *Handbook of Sensory Physiology,* vol. II, pt. 3b: *Visual Centers in the Brain.* Jung, R., ed. New York, Springer, 1973, pp. 451–482.
Grüsser, O. J., Landis, T. *Visual Agnosias and Other Disturbances of Visual Perception and Cognition.* London, Macmillan Press, 1991.
Guberman, A., Stuss, D. The syndrome of bilateral paramedian thalamic infarction. *Neurology* 33:540–546, 1983.
Guilleminault, C., Dement, W. C., Passouant, P. Narcolepsy. In *Advances in Sleep Research.* Guilleminault, C., Dement, W. C., Passouant, P., eds. New York, Spectrum, 1976, p. 689.
Hachinski, V. C., Lassen, N. A., Marshall, J. Multi-infarct dementia: a cause of mental deterioration in the elderly. *Lancet* 3:207–210, 1974.
Hakim, H., Verma, N. P., Greiffenstein, M. F. Pathogenesis of reduplicative

paramnesia. *Journal of Neurology, Neurosurgery, and Psychiatry* 51:839–841, 1988.

Halstead, W. C. Function of the frontal lobe in man: the dynamic visual field, abstracted. *Archives of Neurology and Psychiatry* 49:633, 1943.

Hamburger, D., Pribram, K. H., Stunkard, A. J., eds. *Research Publications— Association for Research in Nervous and Mental Disease*, vol. 53, *Perception and Its Disorders*. Baltimore, Williams & Wilkins, 1970.

Hanada, Y., Kawamura, H. Sleep-waking electrocorticographic rhythms in chronic cerveau isolé rats. *Physiological Behavior* 26:725–728, 1981.

Harlow, J. Recovery from the passage of an iron bar through the head. *Publications of the Massachusetts Medical Society* 2:329–346, 1868.

Harner, R. N. EEG evaluation in the patient with dementia. In *Psychiatric Aspects of Neurologic Disease*. Benson, D. F., Blumer, D., eds. New York, Grune & Stratton, 1975, pp. 63–82.

Harris, R. *The Language Myth*. London, Duckworth, 1981.

Hartmann, E. Schizophrenia: a theory. *Psychopharmacology* 49:1–5, 1976.

Hathaway, S. R., McKinley, J. G. *Minnesota Multiphasic Personality Inventory*, 2nd ed. New York, New York Psychological Corporation, 1951.

Hauri, P. *The Sleep Disorders*, 2nd ed. Kalamazoo, The Upjohn Company, 1982.

Hausser, C. O., Robert, F., Giard, N. Balint's syndrome. *Canadian Journal of Neurological Sciences* 7:157–161, 1980.

Head, H. *Aphasia and Kindred Disorders*. London, Cambridge University Press, 1926.

Hebb, D. O., Penfield, W. Human behavior after extensive bilateral removal from the frontal lobes. *Archives of Neurology and Psychiatry* 44:421–438, 1940.

Hécaen, H. Clinical symptomatology in right and left hemisphere lesions. In *Interhemispheric Relations and Cerebral Dominance*. Mountcastle, V. B., ed. Baltimore, Johns Hopkins Press, 1962, pp. 215–243.

Hécaen, H. Mental symptoms with tumors of the frontal lobe. In *The Frontal Granular Cortex and Behavior*. Warren, J. M., Akert, K., eds. New York, McGraw-Hill, 1964, pp. 335–352.

Hécaen, H. Apraxias. In *Handbook of Clinical Neuropsychology*. Filskov, S. B., Boll, T. J., eds. New York, John Wiley and Sons, 1981, pp. 257–286.

Hécaen, H., Albert, M. L. *Human Neuropsychology*. New York, John Wiley and Sons, 1978.

Hécaen, H., Angelergues, R. Localization of symptoms in aphasia. In *Disorders of Language*. DeReuck, A.V.S., O'Connor, M., eds. London, Churchill Livingstone, 1964, pp. 223–246.

Hécaen, H., Angelergues, R., Houillier, S. Les varieties cliniques des acalculies au cours des lesion retrorolandiques: Approche statistique du probleme. *Revue Neurologique* 105:85–103, 1961.

Hécaen, H., Assal, G. A comparison of constructive deficits following right and left hemispheric lesions. *Neuropsychologia* 8:289–303, 1970.

Hécaen, H., de Ajuriaguerra, J. Balint's syndrome. *Brain* 77:373–400, 1954.

Hécaen, H., Penfield, W., Bertrand, C., Malmo, R. The syndrome of apractagnosia due to lesions of the minor cerebral hemisphere. *Archives of Neurology and Psychiatry* 75:400–434, 1956.

Hécaen, H., Tzavaras, A. Etude neuropsychologique des troubles de la reconaissance des visages humains. *Bulletin de Psychologie* 276:754–762, 1969.

Hedderly, F. *Phrenology: A Study of Mind*. London, Fowler & Co., 1970.

Heilman, K. Ideational apraxia—a redefinition. *Brain* 96:861–864, 1973.
Heilman, K. Apraxia. In Clinical Neuropsychology. Heilman, K., Valenstein, E., eds. New York, Oxford University Press, 1979, pp. 159–185.
Heilman, K. M., Scholes, R., Watson, R. T. Auditory affective agnosia: disturbed comprehension of affective speech. *Journal of Neurology, Neurosurgery, and Psychiatry* 38:69–72, 1975.
Heilman, K. M., Sypert, G. W. Korsakoff's syndrome resulting from bilateral fornix lesions. *Neurology* 27:490–493, 1977.
Heilman, K. M., Valenstein, E. Frontal lobe neglect in man. *Neurology* 22:660–664, 1972.
Heilman, K. M., Valenstein, E., Watson, R. T., Damasio, A. R. Localization of neglect. In *Localization in Neuropsychology*. Kertesz, A., ed. New York, Academic Press, 1983, pp. 371–392.
Heilman, K. M., Valenstein, E., Watson, R. T. The neglect syndrome. In *Handbook of Clinical Neurology*, 2nd ed., vol. 45, *Clinical Neuropsychology*. Vinken, P. J., Bruyn, G. W., Klawans, H. L., eds. Amsterdam, Elsevier, 1985a, pp. 151–183.
Heilman, K. M., Valenstein, E., Watson, R. T. Behavioral aspects of neurology: attentional, intentional, and emotional disorders. In *Clinical Neurology*. Baker, A. B., Joynt, R. J., eds. Philadelphia, Harper & Row, 1985b. (Chap. 22) pp. 1–38.
Heilman, K. M., Van den Abell, T. Right hemispheric dominance for mediating cerebral activation. *Neuropsychologia* 17:315–321, 1979.
Heilman, K. M., Watson, R. T., Valenstein, E. Neglect and related disorders. In *Clinical Neuropsychology*, 2nd ed. Heilman, K. M., Valenstein, E., eds. New York, Oxford University Press, 1985c, pp. 243–293.
Heimburger, R. F., Demyer, W., Reitan, R. M. Implications of Gerstmann's syndrome. *Journal of Neurology, Neurosurgery, and Psychiatry* 27:52–57, 1961.
von Helmholtz, H.L.F. *Handbuch der Physiologischen Optik*. Leipzig, Voss, 1856–66.
Henschen, S. E. *Klinishe und Anatomische Beitrage zur Pathologie der Gehirns*. Stockholm, Almquist and Wiksell, 1922.
Herbart, J. F. *Lehrbuch für Psychologie*. Konigsberg, Unzer, 1816.
Hermann, B. P., Riel, P. Interictal personality and behavior traits in temporal lobe and generalized epilepsy. *Cortex* 17:125–128, 1981.
Hermann, B. P., Stevens, J. Interictal behavioral correlates of the epilepsies. In *A Multidisciplinary Handbook of Epilepsy*. Springfield, IL, Charles C. Thomas, 1980, pp. 272–307.
Hier, D. B., Davis, K. R., Richardson, E. P., Mohr, J. P. Hypertensive putaminal hemorrhage. *Annals of Neurology* 1:152–159, 1977.
Hier, D. B., Mogil, S. I., Rubin, N. P., Kameros, G. R. Semantic aphasia: a neglected entity. *Brain and Language* 10:120–131, 1980.
Hilgard, E. *Divided Consciousness: Multiple Controls in Human Thought and Action*. New York, John Wiley and Sons, 1977.
Hilgard, E. R., Bower, G. H. *Theories of Learning*, 3rd. ed. New York, Meredith Corporation, 1966.
Hill, D. Psychiatric disorders of epilepsy. *Medical Press* 229:473–475, 1953.
Hill, D. The schizophrenia-like psychoses of epilepsy. *Proceedings of the Royal Society* 55:315–316, 1962.

Hinchcliffe, M. K., Lancasshire, M., Roberts, F. J. Depression: defense mechanism in speech. *British Journal of Psychiatry* 118:471–472, 1971.
Hinshelwood, J. *Letter-, Word-, and Mind-Blindness*. London, H. K. Lewis, 1900.
Hinsie, L. E., Campbell, R. J. *Psychiatric Dictionary*, 4th ed. Toronto, Oxford University Press, 1970.
Hinton, G. E., Anerson, J. A. *Parallel Models of Associative Memory*. Hillsdale, NJ, Lawrence Erlbaum Associates, 1981.
Hirst, W., Volpe, B. T. Temporal order judgments with amnesia. *Brain and Cognition* 1:294–306, 1982.
Hobbes, T. *Human Nature*. London: Bowman, 1650/1840.
Hobson, J. A. The cellular basis of sleep cycle control. *Advances in Sleep Research* 1:217–250, 1974.
Hobson, J. A., Lydic, R., Baghdoyan, H. A. Evolving concept of sleep cycle generation: from brain centers to neuronal populations. *Behavior and Brain Science* 9:371–448, 1986.
Hofstadter, D. R. Artificial intelligence: subcognition as computation. In *The Study of Information: Interdisciplinary Message*. Mechlup, F., Mansfeld, U., eds. New York, John Wiley and Sons, 1983, pp. 263–285.
Hollander, B. *The Mental Functions of the Brain, an Investigation Into Their Localization and Their Manifestations in Health and Disease: The Revival of Phrenology*. London: Richards, 1901.
Holmes, G. Disturbances of vision by cerebral lesions. *British Journal of Ophthalmology* 2:353–384, 1918.
Holmes, G. Palsies of the conjugate ocular movements. *British Journal of Ophthalmology* 5:241–250, 1921.
Holmes, G. Discussion on the mental symptoms associated with cerebral tumours. *Proceedings of the Royal Society of Medicine* 24:997–1008, 1931.
Horel, J. A., Keating, E. G., Misantine, L. J. Partial Klüver-Bucy syndrome produced by destroying temporal neocortex or amygdala. *Brain Research* 94:347–359, 1975.
Horsley, V., Schafer, E. A. Functions of the cerebral cortex. *Philosophical Transactions of the Royal Society of London* 179:1–45, 1888.
Howes, D. Application of the word frequency concept of aphasia. In *Disorders of Language: A Ciba Foundation Symposium*. DeReuck, A.V.S., O'Connor, M., eds. London, Churchill Livingstone, 1964, pp. 47–78.
Hubel, D. H., Wiesel, T. N. Receptive fields and functional architecture of monkey striate cortex. *Journal of Physiology* 195:215–343, 1968.
Hubel, D. H., Wiesel, T. N. Brain mechanisms of vision. *Scientific American* 241:150–162, 1979.
Humphrey, G. *Thinking: An Introduction to Experimental Psychology*. New York, John Wiley and Sons, 1963.
Hunt, T. Intelligence. In *Psychosurgery*. Freeman, W., Watts, J. W., eds. Springfield, IL, Charles C. Thomas, 1942, pp. 153–164.
Hyman, B. T., Van Hoesen, G. W., Damasio, A. R., Barnes, C. L. Alzheimer's disease: cell specific pathology isolates the hippocampal formation. *Science* 225:1168–1170, 1984.
Ingvar, D. H. "Memory of the future": an essay on the temporal organization of conscious awareness. *Human Neurobiology* 4:127–136, 1985.
Ingvar, D. H., Franzen, G. Distribution of cerebral activity in chronic schizophrenia. *Lancet* 2:1484–1486, 1974.

Innocenti, G. M. What is so special about callosal connections? In *Two Hemispheres—One Brain? Functions of the Corpus Callosum.* Lépore, F., Ptito, M., Jasper, H. H., eds. New York, Alan R. Liss, 1986, pp. 75–81.

Insel, T. R., Murphy, D. L., Cohen, R. M., Alterman, I., Kilts, C., Linniola, M. Obsessive–compulsive disorder: a double-blind trial of clomipramine and clorgyline. *Archives of General Psychiatry* 40:605–612, 1983.

Ironside, R. Disorders of laughter due to brain lesions. *Brain* 79:589–609, 1956.

Isserlin, M. Die Pathologische Physiologie der Sprache. *Ergebnisse der Physiologie* 29:129–249, 1929; 33:1–102, 1931; 34:1065–1144, 1932.

Iwata, M. Neural mechanisms of reading and writing in the Japanese language. *Functional Neurology* 1:43–52, 1986.

Jackson, J. H. Clinical remarks on cases of defects of expression (by words, writing, signs, etc.) in diseases of the nervous system. *Lancet* 1:604–605, 1864.

Jackson, J. H. On the physiology of language. *Medical Times and Gazette* II:275, 1868. Reprinted in *Brain* 38:59–64, 1915.

Jackson, J. H. Remarks on non-protrusion of the tongue in some cases of aphasia. *Lancet* 1:716, 1878. Reprinted in *Brain* 38:104–106, 1915.

Jackson, J. H. Selected Writings of J. Hughlings Jackson. Taylor, J., ed. London, Hodder and Stoughton, 1932.

Jacobs, B. L. Overview of the activity of brain monoaminergic neurons across the sleep–wake cycle. In *Sleep: Neurotransmitters and Neuromodulators.* Wauquier, A., Gaillard, J. M., Mount, J. M., Radulovachi, M., eds. New York, Raven Press, 1985, pp. 1–14.

Jacobs, L. Visual allesthesia. *Neurology* 30:1059–1063, 1980.

Jacobs, L., Feldman, M., Dimond, S. P. Palinacousis: persistent or recurring auditory sensations. *Cortex* 9:275–287, 1973.

Jacobsen, C. F., Nissen, H. W. Studies of cerebral function in primates. IV. The effects of frontal lobe lesions on the delayed alternation habit in monkeys. *Journal of Comparative Psychology* 23:101–112, 1937.

Jacobson, E. *The Human Mind: A Physiological Clarification.* Springfield, IL, Charles C. Thomas, 1982.

Jacoby, L. L. On interpreting the effects of repetition: solving a problem versus remembering a solution. *Journal of Verbal Learning and Verbal Behavior* 19:649–667, 1978.

James, W. *The Principles of Psychology.* London, Macmillan, 1890.

Janet, P. *The Major Symptoms of Hysteria.* New York, Hafner, 1920/1965.

Jastorwitz, M. Beitrage zur Lokalisation im Grosshirn und uber deren praktishe Verwerthung. *Deutsche Medizinische Wochenschrift* 14:81, 1888.

Jaynes, J. *The Origin of Consciousness in the Breakdown of the Bicameral Mind.* Boston, Houghton Mifflin Co., 1976.

Jeannerod, M. *The Brain Machine.* Cambridge, MA, Harvard Press, 1985.

Jenike, M. A. Obsessive–compulsive disorder. *Comprehensive Psychiatry* 24:99–115, 1983.

Jenkins, J. J. Language and thought. In: *Approaches to Thought.* Voss, J. F., ed. Columbus, Ohio, Merill, 1969, pp. 211–237.

Jennett, W. B. *Head Injuries and the Temporal Lobe. Current Problems in Neuropsychiatry,* Spec. Publ. No. 4. Herrington, R. N., ed. Ashford, Kent, England, Headley Brothers, Ltd., 1969.

Johnson-Laird, P. N., Wason, P. C. *Thinking: Readings in Cognitive Science.* Cambridge, Cambridge University Press, 1977.

Jones, B. E. Influences of the brainstem reticular formation, including intrinsic monoaminergic and cholinergic neurons, on forebrain mechanisms of sleep and waking. In *The Diencephalon and Sleep.* Mancia, M., Marini, G., eds. New York, Raven Press, 1990, pp. 31–48.

Jones, H. S., Oswald, I. Two cases of healthy insomnia. *Electroencephalography and Clinical Neurophysiology* 24:378–380, 1968.

Jouvet, M. Recherches sur les structures nerveuses et mechanismes responsibles des differentes phases du sommeil physiologique. *Archives of Italian Biology* 100:125–206, 1962.

Jouvet, M. The role of monoamines and acetylcholine containing neurones in the regulation of the sleep wake cycle. *Review of Physiology* 64:166–307, 1972.

Jung, C. G. *Diagnostische Associationsstudien.* Leipzig, J. A. Barth, 1906.

Jung, C. G. *Collected Works.* New York, Pantheon Books, 1954.

Kahn, R. L., Zarit, S. H., Hilbert, N. M., Niederehe, G. Memory complaint and impairment in the aged. *Archives of General Psychiatry* 32:1569–1573, 1975.

Kant, I. *Kritik der reinen Vernunft.* Riger, Hartknock, 1781.

Kapur, N., Coughlan, A. K. Confabulation and frontal lobe dysfunction. *Journal of Neurology, Neurosurgery, and Psychiatry* 43:461–463, 1980.

Katz, J. J., Fodor, J. A. The structure of semantic theory. *Language* 39:170–210, 1963.

Katzman, R. Normal pressure hydrocephalus. In *Dementia,* 2nd ed. Wells, C. E., ed. Philadelphia, F. A. Davis, 1977, pp. 69–92.

Kaul, S. N., Di Boulay, G. H., Kendell, B. E., Russell, R.W.R. Relationship between visual field defect and arterial occlusion in the posterior cerebral circulation. *Journal of Neurology, Neurosurgery, and Psychiatry* 37:1022–1030, 1974.

Kawamura, M., Hirayama, K., Shinohara, Y., Watanabe, Y., Sugishita, M. Alloaesthesia. *Brain* 110:225–236, 1987.

Keating, E. G., Horel, J. A. Effects of prestriate and striate lesions on performance of simple visual tasks. *Experimental Neurology* 35:322–336, 1972.

Kennard, M. Alterations in response to visual stimuli following lesions of the frontal lobe in monkeys. *Archives of Neurology and Psychology* 41:1153–1165, 1939.

Kertesz, A. *Aphasia and Associated Disorders.* New York, Grune & Stratton, 1979.

Kertesz, A. ed. *Localization in Neuropsychology.* New York, Academic Press, 1983.

Kertesz, A., Benson, D. F. Neologistic jargon—a clinico-pathological study. *Cortex* 6:362–386, 1970.

Kertesz, A., McCabe, P. Recovery patterns and prognosis in aphasia. *Brain* 100:1–18, 1977.

Kertesz, A., Sheppard, A., MacKenzie, R. Localization in transcortical sensory aphasia. *Archives of Neurology* 39:475–478, 1982.

Kety, S. S. Brain catecholamines, affective states and memory. In *The Chemistry of Mood, Motivation, and Memory.* McGaugh, J. L., ed. New York, Plenum Press, 1972, pp. 65–80.

King, E. The nature of visual field defects. *Brain* 90:647–668, 1967.

Kirshner, H. S. *Behavioral Neurology: A Practical Approach.* New York, Churchill Livingstone, 1986.

Kirshner, H. S., Webb, W. G. Word and letter reading and the mechanism of the third alexia. *Archives of Neurology* 39:84–87, 1982.
Klee, A. Akinetic mutism. *Journal of Nervous and Mental Disease* 133:536–553, 1961.
Kleist, K. *Gehirnpathologie.* Leipzig, Barth, 1934a.
Kleist, K. *Kriegverletzungen des Gehirns in ihrer Bedeutung fur Hirnlokalisation und Hirnpathologie.* Leipzig, Barth, 1934b.
Klüver, H., Bucy, P. C. Psychic blindness and other symptoms following temporal lobectomy in rhesus monkeys. *American Journal of Physiology* 119:352–353, 1937.
Klüver, H., Bucy, P. C. Preliminary analysis of function of the temporal lobes in monkeys. *Archives of Neurology and Psychiatry* 43:979–1000, 1939.
Koestler, A. *The Act of Creation.* New York: Macmillan Company, 1967.
Köhler, W. *The Mentality of Apes.* Winter, E., translator. London, Kegan Paul, 1924.
Kraepelin, E. *Psychiatrie.* Leipzig, Barth, 1909.
Kraepelin, E. *Manic Depressive Insanity and Paranoia.* Edinburgh, E. & S. Livingstone, 1921.
Kremer, M., Russell, W. R., Smyth, G. E. A mid-brain syndrome following head injury. *Journal of Neurology, Neurosurgery, and Psychiatry* 10:49–60, 1947.
Kretschmer, E. Die orbitalhirn und Zwischenhirnsyndrome nach Schadelbasisfrakturen. *Allgemeine Zeitschrift für Psychiatrie und ihre Grenzengebiete* 124:358–360, 1949.
Krieg, W.J.S. *Connections of the Frontal Cortex of the Monkey.* Springfield, IL, Charles C. Thomas, 1954.
Kruper, D. C., Palton, R. A., Koskoff, Y. D. Visual discrimination in hemicerebrectomized monkeys. *Physiological Behavior* 7:173–179, 1971.
Külpe, O. *Grundiss der Psychologie.* Leipzig, Englemann, 1893.
Kuypers, H.G.J.M. Anatomy of the descending pathways. In *Handbook of Physiology, Section 1, The Nervous System,* vol. II, pt. 1, *Motor Control.* Brooks, V. B., ed. Bethesda, American Physiological Society, 1981, pp. 612–626.
Kuypers, H.G.J.M. The anatomical and functional organization of the motor system. In *Scientific Basis of Clinical Neurology.* Swash, M., Kennard, C., eds. Edinburgh, Churchill Livingstone, 1985, pp. 3–18.
Laing, R. D. *The Disordered Self.* New York, Penguin, 1965.
Landis, T., Assal, G., Perret, E. Opposite cerebral hemispheric superiorities for visual associative processing of emotional facial expressions and objects. *Nature* 278:739–740, 1979.
Landis, T., Cummings, J. L., Benson, D. F., Palmer, E. P. Loss of topographic familiarity: an environmental agnosia. *Archives of Neurology* 43:132–136, 1986a.
Landis, T., Cummings, J. L., Christen, L., Bogen, J. E., Imhof, H.-G. Are unilateral right posterior cerebral lesions sufficient to cause prosopagnosia? Clinical and radiological findings in six additional patients. *Cortex* 22:243–252, 1986b.
Larson, G. *The Prehistory of the Far Side: 10th Anniversary Exhibit.* Kansas City, Universal Press Syndicate, 1986.
Lashley, K. S. *Brain Mechanism and Intelligence.* Chicago, University of Chicago Press, 1929.

Lashley, K. S. In search of the engram. *Symposia of the Society of Experimental Biology* 4:454–482, 1950.

Leary, T., Coffey, H. S. Interpersonal diagnosis: some problems of methodology and validation. *Journal of Abnormal and Social Psychology* 50:110–124, 1955.

LeDoux, J. E., Wilson, D. H., Gazzaniga, M. S. A divided mind: observations on the conscious properties of the separated hemispheres. *Annals of Neurology* 2:417–421, 1977.

Lehmann, H. E. Unusual psychiatric disorders and atypical psychoses. In *Comprehensive Textbook of Psychiatry II*. Freedman, A. M., Kaplan, H. I., Sadock, B. J., eds. Baltimore, Williams & Wilkins, 1975, pp. 1724–1736.

Leiner, H. C., Leiner, A. L., Dow, R. S. Reappraising the cerebellum: what does the hindbrain contribute to the forebrain? *Behavioral Neuroscience* 103:998–1008, 1989.

Leischner, A. Die Storungen der Schriftsprache (Agraphie und Alexia). Stuttgart, Georg Thieme Verlag, 1957.

Lenneberg, E. H. *Biological Foundations of Language*. New York, John Wiley & Sons, 1967.

Lessell, S. Higher disorders of visual function: positive phenomena. In *Neuroophthalmology*, vol. 8. Glaser, J. S., Smith, J. L., eds. St. Louis, Mosby, 1975, pp. 27–44.

Levine, D. N. Prosopagnosia and visual object agnosia: a behavioral study. *Brain and Language* 5:341–365, 1978.

Levine, D. N., Calvanio, R. Visual discrimination after lesion of the posterior corpus callosum. *Neurology* 30:21–30, 1980.

Lewin, K. *A Dynamic Theory of Personality: Selected Papers by Kurt Lewin*. New York, McGraw-Hill, 1935.

Lewis, S. Brain imaging in a case of Capgras syndrome. *British Journal of Psychiatry* 150:117–121, 1987.

Lezak, M. D. *Neuropsychological Assessment*. New York, Oxford University Press, 1976.

Lhermitte, F. "Utilization" behavior and its relation to lesions of the frontal lobes. *Brain* 106:237–255, 1983.

Lhermitte, F. Human autonomy and the frontal lobes. Part II. Patient behavior in complex and social situations: the "environmental dependency syndrome." *Annals of Neurology* 19:335–343, 1986.

Lhermitte, F., Chain, F., Escourolle, R., Ducarne, B., Pillon, B. Etude anatomo-clinique d'un case de prosopagnosie. *Revue Neurologique* 126:329–346, 1972.

Lhermitte, F., Gautier, J. C. Aphasia. In *Handbook of Clinical Neurology*, vol. 4. Vinken, P. J., Bruyn, G. W., eds. Amsterdam, North-Holland, 1969, pp. 84–104.

Lhermitte, F., Pillon, B., Serdaru, M. Human autonomy and the frontal lobes. Part I. Imitation and utilization behavior: a neuropsychological study of 75 patients. *Annals of Neurology* 19:326–334, 1986.

Lichtheim, L. On aphasia. *Brain* 7:434–484, 1885.

Lidsky, T. I., Manetto, C., Schneider, J. S. A consideration of sensory factors involved in motor functions of the basal ganglia. *Brain Research Reviews* 9:133–146, 1985.

Lieberman, A., Benson, D. F. Control of emotional expression in pseudobulbar palsy. *Archives of Neurology* 34:717–719, 1977.

Liepmann, H. *Das Krankheitsbild der Apraxie* ('motorischen Asymbolie'). Berlin, Karger, 1900.
Liepmann, H. Der weitere Krankheitsverlauf bei dem einseitag Apraktischen und der Gehirnbefund auf Grund von Serienschnitten. *Monatsschrift für Psychiatrie und Neurologie* 17:289–311, 1905.
Liepmann, H. *Drei Aufsatze aus dem Apraxiegebiet*. Berlin, Karger, 1908.
Lilly, R., Cummings, J. L., Benson, D. F., Frankel, M. The human Klüver-Bucy syndrome. *Neurology* 33:1141–1145, 1983.
Lindquist, G., Norlen, G. Korsakoff's syndrome after operation on ruptured aneurysm of the anterior communicating artery. *Acta Psychiatrica Scandinavica* 42:24–34, 1966.
Lindsley, D. B. The reticular system and perceptual discrimination. In *Reticular Formation of the Brain*. Jasper, H. H., ed. Boston, Little-Brown, 1958, pp. 513–534.
Lipowski, Z. J. *Delirium: Acute Brain Failure in Man*. Springfield, IL, Charles C. Thomas, 1980.
Lipowski, Z. J. *Delirium: Acute Confusional States*. New York, Oxford University Press, 1990.
Lishman, W. A. Psychiatric disability after head injury: the significance of brain damage. *Proceedings of the Royal Society of Medicine* 59:261–266, 1966.
Lishman, W. A. Brain damage in relation to psychiatric disability after head injury. *British Journal of Psychiatry* 114:373–410, 1968.
Lishman, W. A. Split minds: a review of the results of brain bisection in man. *British Journal of Hospital Medicine* 3:477–484, 1969.
Lishman, W. A. Amnesic syndromes and their neuropathology. In *Recent Developments in Psychogeriatrics*. Kay, B.W.K., Walk, A., eds. Ashford, Kent, England, Headley Bros., 1971a.
Lishman, W. A. Emotion, consciousness and will after brain bisection in man. *Cortex* 7:181–192, 1971b.
Lishman, W. A. Selective factors in memory. Part 2: affective disorder. *Psychological Medicine* 2:248–253, 1972.
Lishman, W. A. *Organic Psychiatry*, 2nd ed. Oxford, Blackwell, 1987.
Lissauer, H. Ein Fall von Seelenblindheit nebst einem Beitrage zur Theorie derselben. *Archiv für Psychiatrie* 21:2–50, 1889.
Livingston, K. E., Escobar, A. Tentative limbic system models for certain patterns of psychiatric disorders. In *Surgical Approaches in Psychiatry*. Laitinen, L. V., Livingston, K. E., eds. Baltimore: University Park Press, 1973, pp. 245–252.
Ljungberg, T., Ungerstedt, U. Sensory inattention produced by 6-hydroxydopamine-induced degeneration of ascending dopamine neurons in the brain. *Experimental Neurology* 53:585–600, 1976.
Locke, J. *An Essay Concerning Human Understanding*. Oxford, Clarendon Press, 1687/1934.
Loeb, J. Beitrage Physiologies der Grosshirns. *Pflugers Archive Physiologie* 39, 1886 (cited in Bianchi, L. *The Mechanism of the Brain and the Functions of the Frontal Lobes*. New York, William Wood, 1922).
Lugaresi, E., Medori, R., Mantagna, P., Baruzzi, A., Cortelli, P., Lugaresi, A., Tinuper, P., Zucconi, M., Gambetti, P. Fatal familial insomnia and dysautonomia with selective degeneration of thalamic nuclei. *New England Journal of Medicine* 315:997–1003, 1986.
Luria, A. R. *Traumatic Aphasia*. The Hague, Mouton, 1947/1970.

Luria, A. R. Disorders of "simultaneous perception" in a case of bilateral occipital-parietal brain injury. *Brain* 82:437–449, 1959.
Luria, A. R. Verbal regulation of behaviour. In *The Central Nervous System and Behavior: The Third Macy Conference*. Brazier, M.A.B., ed. Madison, NJ, Madison Printing Co., 1960, pp 359–423.
Luria, A. R. Two kinds of motor perseveration in massive injuries of the frontal lobes. *Brain* 88:1–10, 1965.
Luria, A. R. *Higher Cortical Functions in Man*. New York, Basic Books, 1966.
Luria, A. R. Frontal lobe syndromes. In *Handbook of Clinical Neurology*, vol. 2. Vinken, P. J., Bruyn, G. W., eds. Amsterdam, North-Holland, 1969, pp. 725–757.
Luria, A. R. *The Working Brain*. Haigh, B., translator. New York, Basic Books, 1973.
Luria, A. R., Homskaya, E. D. Disturbance in the regulative role of speech with frontal lobe lesions. In *The Frontal Granular Cortex and Behavior*. Warren, J. M., Akert, K., eds. New York, McGraw-Hill, 1964, pp. 353–371.
Luria, A. R., Pribram, K. H., Homskaya, E. D. An experimental analysis of the behavioral disturbance produced by a left frontal arachnoidal endothelioma. *Neuropsychologia* 2:257–280, 1964.
Luria, A. R., Tsvetkova, L. S. The programming of constructive activity in local brain injuries. *Neuropsychologia* 2:95–108, 1964.
Luria, A. R., Tsvetkova, L. S. Towards the mechanisms of "dynamic aphasia." *Acta Neurologica et Psychiatrica Belgica* 67:1045–1057, 1967.
Lyman, R. S., Kwan, S. T., Chao, W. H. Left occipital brain tumor with observations on alexia and agraphia in Chinese and English. *Chinese Medical Journal* 54:491–516, 1938.
MacLean, P. D. Psychosomatic disease and the "visceral" brain: recent developments bearing on the Papez theory of emotion. *Psychosomatic Medicine* 11:338–353, 1949.
MacLean, P. D. The limbic system and its hippocampal formation. *Journal of Neurosurgery* 11:29–44, 1954.
MacLean, P. D. Contrasting functions of limbic and neocortical systems of the brain and their relevance to psychophysiological aspects of medicine. *American Journal of Medicine* 25:611–626, 1958.
MacLean, P. D. The triune brain, emotion, and scientific bias. *The Neurosciences, Second Study Program*. New York, Rockefeller University Press, 1970, pp. 336–349.
Macrae, D., Trolle, E. The defect of function in visual agnosia. *Brain* 79:94–110, 1956.
Magoun, H. W. Caudal and eephalic influences of the brain stem reticular formation. *Physiological Review* 30:459–474, 1950.
Magoun, H. W. *The Waking Brain*. Springfield, IL, Charles C. Thomas, 1963.
Malamud, N. *Atlas of Neuropathology*. Berkeley, University of California Press, 1957.
Malamud, N., Skillicorn, S. A. Relationship between the Wernicke and the Korsakoff syndrome. *Archives of Neurology and Psychiatry* 76:586–596, 1956.
Malcolm, N. *Problems of Mind*. New York, Harper, 1971.
Maletzky, B. M. The episodic dyscontrol syndrome. *Diseases of the Nervous System* 36:178–185, 1973.

Malmo, R. B. Psychological aspects of frontal gyrectomy and frontal lobotomy in mental patients. *Research Publications—Association for Research in Nervous and Mental Diseases.* 27:537–564, 1948.

Mandell, A. J. Toward a psychobiology of transcendence: God in the brain. In *The Psychobiology of Consciousness.* Davidson, R. J., Davidson, J. M., eds. New York, Plenum, 1980, pp. 379–464.

Mandler, J. M., Mandler, G. *Thinking: From Association to Gestalt.* New York: John Wiley & Sons, 1964.

Marcie, P., Hécaen, H. Agraphia: writing disorders associated with unilateral cerebral disorders. In *Clinical Neuropsychology.* Heilman, K. M., Valenstein, E., eds. New York, Oxford University Press, 1979, pp. 92–127.

Marie, P. Revision de la question de l'aphasie. *Semaine Medicale* 26:241–247, 493–500, 565–571, 1906.

Marin, O.S.M. CAT scans of five deep dyslexic patients. In *Deep Dyslexia.* Coltheart, M., Patterson, K., Marshall, J. C., eds. London, Routledge & Kegan Paul, 1980, pp. 407–411.

Mark, V. H., Sweet, W., Ervin, F. Deep temporal lobe stimulation and destructive lesions in episodically violent temporal lobe epileptics. In *Neural Basis of Violence and Aggression.* Field, W. S., Sweet, W. H., eds. St. Louis, Warren Green, 1975, pp. 379–391.

Marlowe, W. B., Mancall, E. L., Thomas, T. J. Complete Klüver-Bucy syndrome in man. *Cortex* 11:53–59, 1975.

Marr, D., Nishihara, K. Representation and recognition of the spatial organization of three-dimensional shapes. *Proceedings of the Royal Society of London* 200:269–294, 1978.

Marsden, C. D. The mysterious motor function of the basal ganglia. *Neurology* 32:512–539, 1982.

Marsden, C. D. The basal ganglia. In *The Scientific Basis of Clinical Neurology.* Swash, M., Kennard, C., eds. Edinburgh, Churchill Livingstone, 1985, pp. 56–73.

Marsh, N. *Death and the Dancing Footman.* Boston, Little, Brown & Co., 1941.

Marshall, J. C., Newcombe, F. Syntactic and semantic errors in paralexia. *Neuropsychologia* 4:169–176, 1966.

Marshall, J. C., Newcombe, F. The conceptual status of deep dyslexia: an historical perspective. In *Deep Dyslexia.* Coltheart, M., Patterson, K., Marshall, J. C., eds. London, Routledge & Kegan Paul, 1980, pp. 1–21.

Martin, J. J., Yap, M. Nei, I. P., Tan, T. E. Selective thalamic degeneration—report of a case with memory and mental disturbances. *Clinical Neuropathology* 2:156–162, 1983.

Martin, J. P. Fits of laughter (sham mirth) in organic cerebral disease. *Brain* 73:453–464, 1950.

Martin, J. P. *The Basal Ganglia and Posture.* London, Pitman Medical, 1967, pp. 1–152.

Martin, P. R., Weingartner, H., Gordon, E. K., Burns, R. S., Linnoila, M., Kopin, I. J., Ebert, M. H. Central nervous system catecholamine metabolism in Korsakoff's psychosis. *Annals of Neurology* 15:184–187, 1984.

Mayer, A., Orth, J. A qualitative investigation of associations. *Zeitschrift fur Psychologie und Physiologie der Sinnesorgane* 26:1–3, 1901.

Mayer-Gross, W. Some observations on apraxia. *Proceedings of the Royal Society of Medicine* 28:1203–1212, 1935.

Mayer-Gross, W., Slater, E., Roth, M. *Clinical Psychiatry*, 3rd ed. London, Bailliere, Tindall and Cassell, 1969.

Mayeux, R., Benson, D. F. Phantom limb and multiple sclerosis. *Neurology* 29:724–726, 1979.

Mazziotta, J. C., Phelps, M. E., Wapenski, J. A. Human cerebral motor system metabolic responses in health and disease. *Cerebral Blood Flow and Metabolism* 5(Suppl. 1):S213–S214, 1985.

McCullough, W. S., Pitts, W. H. A logical calculus of the ideas imminent in nervous activity. *Bulletin of Mathematical Physics* 5:115–133, 1943.

McDaniel, K. Thalamic degeneration. In *Subcortical Dementia*. Cummings, J L., ed. New York, Oxford University Press, 1990, pp. 132–144.

McDonald, J. D. *The Girl in the Brown Paper Wrapper*. New York, Lippincott, 1968.

McEntee, W. J., Biber, M. P., Perl, D. P., Benson, D. F. Diencephalic amnesia: a reappraisal. *Journal of Neurology, Neurosurgery, and Psychiatry* 39:436–441, 1976.

McFarland, H. R., Fortin, D. Amusia due to right temporoparietal infarct. *Archives of Neurology* 39:725–727, 1982.

McFie, J., Piercy, M. F., Zangwill, O. L. Visual–spatial agnosia. *Brain* 73:167–190, 1950.

McFie, J., Zangwill, O. L. Visual constructive disabilities associated with lesions of the left cerebral hemisphere. *Brain* 83:243–260, 1960.

McGaugh, J. L., Gold, P. E. Modulation of memory by electrical stimulation of the brain. In *Neural Mechanisms in Learning and Memory*. Rosenzweig, M. R., Bennett, E. L., eds. Cambridge, MIT Press, 1976, pp. 549–560.

McGeer, P., Eccles, J. C., McGeer, E. *Molecular Neurobiology of the Mammalian Brain*. New York, Plenum Press, 1978.

McGeer, P. L., McGeer, E. G. Possible changes in striatal and limbic cholinergic systems in schizophrenia. *Archives of General Psychiatry* 34:1319–1323, 1976.

McGeogh, J. A. Forgetting and the law of disuse. *Psychological Review* 39:352–370, 1932.

McGhie, A., Chapman, J., Lawson, J. S. The effect of distraction on schizophrenic performance. I. Perception and immediate memory. *British Journal of Psychiatry* 111:383–390, 1965.

McGinn, C. *The Character of Mind*. London, Oxford University Press, 1982.

McHugh, P. R., Folstein, M. F. Psychiatric syndromes of Huntington's chorea: a clinical and phenomenologic study. In *Psychiatric Aspects of Neurologic Disease*. Benson, D. F., Blumer, D., eds. New York, Grune & Stratton, 1975, pp. 267–285.

McIntyre, M., Pritchard, P. B., Lambrusco, C. T. Left and right temporal lobe epileptics: a controlled investigation of some psychological differences. *Epilepsia* 17:377–386, 1976.

McKhann, G., Drachman, D., Folstein, M., Katzman, R., Price, D., Stadlan, E. M. Clinical diagnosis of Alzheimer's disease: Report of the NINCDS-ADRDA Work Group, Department of Health and Human Services Task Force on Alzheimer's Disease. *Neurology* 34:939–944, 1984.

McKenna, P., Warrington, E. K. Category-specific naming preservation: a single case study. *Journal of Neurology, Neursurgery, and Psychiatry* 41:571–574, 1978.

McNeill, D. L., Tidmarsh, D., Rastall, M. L. A case of dysmnesic syndrome following cardiac arrest. *British Journal of Psychiatry* 111:697–699, 1965.

Meadows, J. C. The anatomical basis of prosopagnosia. *Journal of Neurology, Neurosurgery and Psychiatry* 37:489–501, 1974.
Mellor, C. S. First rank symptoms of schizophrenia. *British Journal of Psychiatry* 117:15–23, 1970.
Melzack, R., Wall, P. D. Pain mechanisms: a new theory. *Science* 150:971–979, 1965.
Mendez, M. F. Visuoperceptual function in visual agnosia. *Neurology* 38:1754–1759, 1988.
Mendez, M. F., Benson, D. F. Atypical conduction aphasia—a disconnection syndrome. *Archives of Neurology* 42:886–891, 1985.
Mercer, B., Wapner, W., Gardner, H., Benson, D. F. A study of confabulation. *Archives of Neurology* 34:429–433, 1977.
Merrin, E. L., Silberfarb, P. M. The Capgras phenomenon. *Archives of General Psychiatry* 33:965–968, 1976.
Mesulam, M.-M. A cortical network for directed attention and unilateral neglect. *Annals of Neurology* 10:309–325, 1981.
Mesulam, M.-M. Attention, confusional states and neglect. In *Principles of Behavioral Neurology*. Mesulam, M.-M., ed. Philadelphia, F. A. Davis, 1985a, pp. 125–168.
Mesulam, M.-M. Patterns in behavioral neuroanatomy: association areas, the limbic system and hemispheric specialization. In *Principles of Behavioral Neurology*. Mesulam, M.-M., ed. Philadelphia, F. A. Davis, 1985b, pp. 1–70.
Mesulam, M.-M. Large-scale neurocognitive networks and distributed processing for attention, language and memory. *Annals of Neurology* 28:597–613, 1990.
Metter, E. J. *Speech Disorders*. New York, Spectrum, 1985.
Mettler, F. A., ed. *Columbia-Greystone Associates—Selective Partial Ablation of the Frontal Cortex: A Correlative Study of Its Effects on Human Psychotic Subjects*. New York, Hoeber, 1949.
Meyer, J. S., Barron, D. W. Apraxia of gait: a clinicophysiological study. *Brain* 83:261–284, 1960.
Meyers, R. Dandy's striatal theory of "the center of consciousness." *Archives of Neurology and Psychiatry* 65:659–671, 1951.
Michel, E. M., Troost, B. T. Palinopsia: cerebral localization with computed tomography. *Neurology* 30:887–889, 1980.
Miller, B. L., Benson, D. F., Cummings, J. L., Neshkes, R. Late-life paraphrenia: an organic delusional syndrome. *Journal of Clinical Psychiatry* 47:204–207, 1986.
Miller, G. A. The magical number seven, plus or minus two: some limits on our capacity for processing information. *Psychological Review* 63:81–97, 1956.
Miller, G. A. Some preliminaries to psycholinguistics. *American Psychologist* 20:15–20, 1965.
Miller, G. A., Galanter, E., Pribram, K. L. *Plans and the Structure of Behavior*. New York, Holt, Rhinehart and Winston, 1960.
Milner, B. Effects of different brain lesions on card sorting. *Archives of Neurology* 9:90–100, 1963.
Milner, B. Some effects of frontal lobectomy in man. In *The Frontal Granular Cortex and Behavior*. Warren, J. M., Akert, K., eds. New York, McGraw-Hill, 1964, pp. 313–334.

Milner, B. Amnesia following operation on the temporal lobes. In *Amnesia*. Whitty, C.W.M., Zangwill, O. L., eds. London, Butterworths, 1966, pp. 109–133.

Milner, B., Penfield, W. The effect of hippocampal lesions on recent memory. *Transactions of the American Neurological Association* 80:42–48, 1955.

Minsky, M. *The Society of Mind*. New York: Simon & Schuster, 1985.

Mishkin, M. Cortical visual areas and their interaction. In *The Brain and Human Behavior*. Karczman, A. G., Eccles, J. C., eds. Berlin, Springer-Verlag, 1972, pp. 187–208.

Mishkin, M. A memory system in the monkey. *Philosophical Transactions of the Royal Society of London* B298:85–95, 1982.

Mitchell, S. W. Phantom limbs. *Lippincott Magazine* 8:563–569, 1871.

Mochizuki, H., Ohtomo, R. Pure alexia in Japanese and agraphia without alexia in Kanji. *Archives of Neurology* 45:1157–1159, 1988.

Mohr, J. P. Rapid amelioration of motor aphasia. *Archives of Neurology* 28:77–82, 1973.

Mohr, J. P. Broca's area and Broca's aphasia. In *Studies in Neurolinguistics*, vol. 1. Whitaker, H., Whitaker, H. A., eds. New York, Academic, 1976, pp. 201–236.

Mohr, J. P., Leicester, J., Stoddard, L. T., Sidman, M. Right hemianopsia with memory and color deficits in circumscribed left posterior cerebral artery territory infarction. *Neurology* 21:1104–1113, 1971.

Mohr, J. P., Pessin, M. S., Finkelstein, S., Funkenstein, H. H., Duncan, G. W., Davis, K. R. Broca aphasia: pathological and clinical aspects. *Neurology* 28:311–324, 1978.

von Monakow, C., Mourque, R. *Introduction Biologique a l'etude de la neurologie et de la Psychiatrie*. Paris, Alcan, 1928.

Moniz, E. Prefrontal leucotomy in treatment of mental disorders. *American Journal of Psychiatry* 93:1379–1385, 1937.

Monrad-Krohn, G. H. Dysprosody or altered melody of language. *Brain* 70:405–415, 1947.

Montgomery, M. A., Clayton, P. J., Friedhoff, A. J. Psychiatric illness in Tourette syndrome patients and first degree relatives. In *Gilles de la Tourette Syndrome*. Friedhoff, A. J., Chase, T. N., eds. New York, Raven Press, 1982, pp. 335–339.

Mori, E., Yamadori, A. Compulsive manipulation of tools and pathological grasp phenomenon. *Clinical Neurology* 22:329–335, 1982.

Morlaas, J. *Contribution a l'Etude de l'Apraxie*. Paris, These, 1928.

Morley, C., Everett, L. D., eds. *The Shorter Bartlett's Familiar Quotations*. New York, Pocket Books, Inc., 1953.

Moruzzi, G., Magoun, H. W. Brain stem reticular formation and activation of the EEG. *Electroencephalography and Clinical Neurophysiology* 1:455–473, 1949.

Mountcastle, V. B. Modality and topographic properties of single neurons of cat's somatic sensory cortex. *Journal of Neurophysiology* 20:408–434, 1957.

Mountcastle, V. B. *Medical Psychology*, 12th ed. St. Louis, Mosby, 1968.

Mountcastle, V. B. An organizing principle for cerebral function: the unit module and the distributed system. In *The Neurosciences*. Schmitt, F. O., Worden, F. G., eds. Cambridge, MA, MIT Press, 1979, pp. 21–42.

Mountcastle, V. B. The neural mechanisms of cognitive functions can now be studied directly. *Trends in Neuroscience* 9:505–508, 1986.

Mowrer, O. H. How does the mind work? *American Psychologist* 31:843–857, 1976.

Müller, M. *The Science of Thought.* New York, Scribner, 1887.

Mungas, D. Interictal behavior abnormality in temporal lobe epilepsy. *Archives of General Psychiatry* 39:108–111, 1982.

Munk, H. *Ueber die Funtionen der Grosshirnrinde.* Berlin, Hirshwald, 1890.

Naeser, M. A., Levine, H. L., Benson, D. F., Stuss, D. T., Weir, W. S. Frontal leukotomy size and hemispheric asymmetries on computerized tomographic scans of schizophrenics with variable recovery. *Archives of Neurology* 38:30–37, 1981.

Nahor, A., Benson, D. F. A screening test for organic brain disease in emergency psychiatric evaluation. *Behavioral Psychiatry* 2:23–26, 1970.

Nauta, H.J.W. A simplified perspective on the basal ganglia and their relation to the limbic system. In *The Limbic System: Functional Organization and Clinical Disorders.* Doane, B. K., Livingston, K. E., eds. New York, Raven Press, 1986, pp. 67–77.

Nauta, W.J.H. The problem of the frontal lobe: a reinterpretation. *Journal of Psychiatric Research* 8:167–187, 1971.

Nauta, W.J.H. Neural associations of the frontal cortex. *Acta Neurobiologia Experimentalis* 32:125–140, 1972.

Nauta, W.J.H. Connections of the frontal lobe with the limbic system. In *Surgical Approaches in Psychiatry.* Laitinen, L. V., Livingston, K. E., eds. Baltimore, University Park Press, 1973, pp. 303–314.

Nauta, W.J.H., Feirtag, M. *Fundamental Neuroanatomy.* New York, W. H. Freeman & Co., 1986.

Nee, L. E., Caine, E. D., Polinsky, R. J., Eddridge, R., Ebert, M. H. Gilles de la Tourette syndrome: clinical and family studies of 50 cases. *Annals of Neurology* 7:41–49, 1980.

Needham, C. W. *Cerebral Logic: Solving the Problem of Mind and Brain.* Springfield, IL, Charles C. Thomas, 1978.

Neisser, U. The multiplicity of thought. *British Journal of Psychology* 54:1–14, 1963.

Nelson, K. Some evidence for the cognitive primacy of categorization and its functional basis. *Merrill-Palmer Quarterly of Behavioral Development* 19:21–39, 1973.

Netter, F. H. *The Ciba Collection of Medical Illustrations,* vol. 1, *The Nervous System.* Summit, NJ, CIBA, 1980.

von Neumann, J. *The Computer and the Brain.* New Haven, Yale University Press, 1958.

New Webster's Dictionary. New York, Consolidated Book Publishers, 1975.

Newell, A., Simon, H. A. *Human Problem Solving.* Englewood Cliffs, NJ, Prentice Hall, 1972.

Nielsen, J. M. *Agnosia, Apraxia, and Aphasia. Their Value in Cerebral Localization.* New York: Hafner, 1936/1948.

Nielsen, J. M. Gerstmann syndrome: finger agnosia, agraphia, confusion of right and left, and acalculia. *Archives of Neurology and Psychiatry* 39:536–560, 1938.

Nielsen, J. M., Jacobs, L. L. Bilateral lesions of the anterior cingulate gyri: report of a case. *Bulletin of the Los Angeles Neurological Societies* 16:231–234, 1951.

Nolte, J. The *Human Brain,* 2nd ed. St. Louis, Mosby, 1988.

Nozaki, K. *Kitsuné: Japan's Fox of Mystery, Romance, and Humor.* Tokyo, Hokuseido Press, 1961.
Oberg, R.G.E., Divac, I. "Cognitive" function of the neostriatum. In Divac, I., Oberg, R.G.E., eds. *The Neostriatum.* New York, Oxford University Press, 1979, pp. 291–313.
Oldendorf, W. H. *The Quest for an Image of Brain.* New York, Raven Press, 1980.
Oppenheim, H. Zur Pathologie der Grosshirngeschwulste. *Archiv für Psychiatrie* 21:560, 1889.
Orenstein, R. *The Psychology of Consciousness.* New York, W. H. Freeman, 1972.
Osgood, C. E. *Method and Theory in Experimental Psychology.* New York, Oxford University Press, 1953.
Osgood, C. E., Suci, G. J., Tannenbaum, P. *The Measurement of Meaning.* Urbana, IL, University of Illinois Press, 1957.
Oxford English Dictionary. Compact Edition. London, Oxford University Press, 1979.
Pandya, D. N., Dye, P., Butters, N. Efferent cortico-cortical projections of the prefrontal cortex in the rhesus monkey. *Brain Research* 31:35–46, 1971.
Pandya, D. N., Hallet, M., Mukherjee, S. K. Intra- and interhemispheric connections of the neocortical auditory system in the rhesus monkey. *Brain Research* 13:13–26, 1969.
Pandya, D. N., Kuypers, H.G.J.M. Cortico-cortical connections in the rhesus monkey. *Brain Research* 13:13–36, 1969.
Pandya, D. N., Seltzer, B. The topography of commissural fibers. In *Two Hemispheres, One Brain? Functions of the Corpus Callosum.* Lepore, F., Ptito, M., Jasper, H. H. (eds). New York, Alan R. Liss, 1986, pp. 47–73.
Papez, J. W. A proposed mechanism of emotion. *Archives of Neurology and Psychiatry* 38:725–743, 1937.
Parkin, A. J. Amnesic syndrome: a lesion-specific disorder? *Cortex* 20:479–508, 1984.
Patel, A. N. Syndromes of callosal infarction. *Neurology* 17:191–196, 1969.
Paterson, A., Zangwill, O. L. Disorders of visual space perception associated with lesions of the right cerebral hemisphere. *Brain* 67:331–358, 1944.
Paterson, A., Zangwill, O. L. A case of topographical disorientation associated with a unilateral cerebral lesion. *Brain* 68:188–211, 1945.
Pavlov, I. P. *Conditioned Reflexes.* G. V. Anrep, translator. London, Oxford University Press, 1927.
Pavlov, I. P. *Lectures on Conditioned Reflexes,* vol II, *Conditioned Reflexes and Psychiatry.* W. H. Gantt, translator. New York, International Publishers Co., Inc., 1941.
Pei, M. *The Story of Language.* Philadelphia, J. B. Lippincott, 1949.
Penfield, W., Jasper, H. *Epilepsy and the Functional Anatomy of the Human Brain.* Boston, Little Brown, 1954.
Penfield, W., Kristiansen, K. *Epileptic Seizure Patterns.* Springfield, IL, Charles C. Thomas, 1951.
Penfield, W., and Mathieson, G. Memory. *Archives of Neurology* 31:145–154, 1974.
Penfield, W., Perot, P. The brain record of auditory and visual experience: a final summary and discussion. *Brain* 86:595–696, 1963.

Penfield, W., Rasmussen, T. *The Cerebral Cortex of Man*. New York, MacMillan Co., 1950.
Penfield, W., Roberts, L. *Speech and Speech Mechanisms*. Princeton, NJ, Princeton University Press, 1959.
Penfield, W., Welch, K. The supplementary motor area of the cerebral cortex. *Archives of Neurology and Psychiatry* 66:289–317, 1951.
Peterson, B. W. Reticulospinal projections to spinal motor nuclei. *Annual Review of Physiology* 41:127–140, 1979.
Peterson, L. R., Peterson, M. J. Short term retention of individual verbal items. *Journal of Experimental Psychology* 58:193–198, 1959.
Petrides, M. Learning impairments following excisions of the primate frontal cortex. In *Frontal Lobe Function and Dysfunction*. Levin, H. S., Eisenberg, H. M., Benton, A. L., eds. New York, Oxford Univ. Press, 1991, pp. 256–272.
Petrides, M., Pandya, D. N. Projections to the frontal cortex from the posterior parietal region in the rhesus monkey. *Journal of Comparative Anatomy* 228:105–116, 1984.
Petrie, A. A comparison of the psychological effects of different types of operation on the frontal lobes. *Journal of Mental Science* 98:326–329, 1952.
Phelps, M. E., Huang, S. C., Hoffman, E. J., Selin, C., Sokoloff, L., Kuhl, D. E. Tomographic measurement of local cerebral glucose metabolism in humans with (F-18) 2-fluoro-2-deoxy-D-glucose: validation of method. *Annals of Neurology* 6:371–388, 1979.
Phelps, M. E., Kuhl, D. E., Mazziotta, J. C. Metabolic mapping of the brain's response to visual stimulation: Studies in humans. *Science* 211:1445–1448, 1981.
Piaget, J. *The Language and Thought of the Child*. Gabain, M., translator. London, Routledge & Kegan Paul, 1926.
Piaget, J. *The Psychology of Intelligence*. Piercy, M., Berlyne, D. E., translators. London, Routledge & Kegan Paul, 1950.
Pick, A. On reduplicative paramnesia. *Brain* 26:242–267, 1903.
Pick, A. *Aphasia*. Springfield, IL, Charles C. Thomas, 1931/1973.
Piercy, M., Smyth, V.O.G. Right hemisphere dominance for certain non-verbal intellectual skills. *Brain* 85:775–790, 1962.
Pincus, J. H. Can violence be a manifestation of epilepsy? *Neurology* 30:304–307, 1980.
Pincus, J. H., Tucker, G. *Behavioral Neurology*. New York, Oxford University Press, 1985.
Plum, F., Posner, J. B. *The Diagnosis of Stupor and Coma*, 2nd ed. Philadelphia, F. A. Davis, 1972, pp. 23–24.
Plutchik, R. *Emotion: Psychoevolutionary Synthesis*. New York, Harper & Row, 1980.
Poe, E. A. The murders in the Rue Morgue. In *The Fall of the House of Usher and Other Tales*. New York, Signet Classic, 1841/1980, pp. 49–83.
Poeck, K. Pathophysiology of emotional disorders associated with brain damage. In *Handbook of Clinical Neurology*, vol. 3. Vinken, P. J., Bruyn, G. W., eds. Amsterdam, North-Holland, 1969, pp. 343–367.
Poeck, K. *Klinische Neuropsychologie*. Stuttgart, George Thieme Verlag, 1982.
Poeck, K. Pathological laughter or crying. In *Handbook of Clinical Neurology, Vol. 45: Clinical Neuropsychology*. Vinken, P. J., Bruyn, G. W., Klawans, H. L., Frederiks, J.A.M., eds. Amsterdam, Elsevier, 1985, pp. 219–226.

Poeck, K., Kerchensteiner, M., Hartje, W. A qualitative study on language understanding in fluent and non-fluent aphasia. *Cortex* 8:299–304, 1972.

Poeck, K., Orgass, B. Gerstmann's syndrome and aphasia. *Cortex* 2:421–437, 1966.

Poeck, K., Pilleri, G. Pathologisches Lachen und Weinen. *Schweiz Archiv für Neurologie und Psychiatrie* 92:323–370, 1964.

Poetzl, O. *Die optisch-agnostischen Storungen (Die verschiedenen Formen der Seelenblindheit).* Leipzig, Franz Deuticke, 1928.

Pond, D. A. Psychiatric aspects of epilepsy. *Journal of the Indian Medical Profession* 31:144–151, 1957.

Poppelreuter, W. *Die phychischen Störungen durch Kopfschuss Bd. I: Die Storungen der niederen und höheren Sehleistunden durch Verletzungen des Occipitalhirns.* Leipzig, L. Voss, 1917.

Posner, M. I. Characteristics of visual and kinesthetic memory codes. *Journal of Experimental Psychology* 75:103–107, 1967.

Potter, H., Nauta, W.J.H. A note on the problem of olfactory associations of the orbitofrontal cortex in the monkey. *Neuroscience* 4:361–367, 1979.

Powell, E. W., Hines, G. The limbic system: an interface. *Behavioral Biology* 12:149–164, 1974.

Premack, O. Language in the chimpanzee. *Science* 172:808–822, 1971.

Pribram, K. H. The primate frontal cortex—executive of the brain. In *Psychophysiology of the Frontal Lobes*. Pribram, K. H., Luria, A. R., eds. New York, Academic Press, 1973, pp. 293–314.

Puccetti, R. The case for mental duality: evidence from split brain data and other considerations. *Behavior and Brain Science* 4:93–123, 1981.

Quinn, D. The Capgras syndrome: two cases and a review. *Canadian Journal of Psychiatry* 26:126–129, 1981.

Rappaport, D., translator. *Organization and Pathology of Thought: Selected Sources.* New York, Columbia University Press, 1951.

Rausch, H. R. Differences in cognitive function with left and right temporal lobe dysfunction. In *The Dual Brain: Hemispheric Specialization in Humans*. Benson, D. F., Zaidel, E., eds. New York, Guilford Press, 1985, pp. 247–261.

Reeves, A. G., Plum, F. Hyperphagia, rage and dementia accompanying a ventromedial hypothalamic neoplasm. *Archives of Neurology* 20:616–624, 1969.

Reeves, J. W. *Thinking About Thinking.* London, Methuen, 1965.

Regard, M., Landis, T., Hess, K. Preserved stenography reading in a patient with pure alexia. *Archives of Neurology* 42:400–402, 1985.

Reid, T. *Essays on the Intellectual Powers of Man.* Cambridge, Bartlett, 1785/1853.

Reitman, F. Orbital cortex syndrome following leucotomy. *American Journal of Psychiatry* 103:238–241, 1946.

Rickler, K. C. Episodic dyscontrol. In *Psychiatric Aspects of Neurologic Disease*, vol. 2. Benson, D. F., Blumer, D., eds. New York, Grune & Stratton, 1982, pp. 49–72.

Riddoch, G. Dissociation of visual perception due to occipital injuries with special reference to appreciation of movement. *Brain* 40:15–57, 1917.

Roberts, G. W., Ferrier, I. N., Lee, Y., Crow, T. J., Johnstone, E. C., Owens, D.G.C., Bacarese-Hamilton, A. J., McGregor, G., O'Shaughnessey, D., Polak, J. M., Bloom, S. R. Peptides, the limbic system and schizophrenia. *Brain Research* 288:199–211, 1983.

Roberts, L. Aphasia, apraxia and agnosia in abnormal states of cerebral dominance. In *Handbook of Clinical Neurology,* Vol. 4. Vinken, P. J., Bruyn, G. W., eds. Amsterdam, North-Holland, 1969, pp. 312–326.

Robinson, R. G., Benson, D. F. Depression in aphasic patients: frequency, severity, and clinical-pathological correlations. *Brain and Language* 14:282–291, 1981.

Robinson, R. G., Chait, R. M. Emotional correlates of structural brain injury with particular emphasis on post-stroke mood disorders. *CRC Critical Review of Clinical Neurobiology* 4:285–318, 1985.

Robinson, R. G., Price, D. R. Post-stroke depressive disorder: a follow-up study of 103 outpatients. *Stroke* 13:635–641, 1982.

Robinson, R. G., Szetela, B. Mood change following left hemisphere EEG in adolescent psychiatric patients with depressive or paranoid symptomatology. *Biological Psychiatry* 16:47–54, 1981.

Rochford, J., Wineapple, M., Goldstein, L. The quantitative hemisphere EEG in adolescent psychiatric patients with depressive or paranoid symptomatology. *Biological Psychiatry* 16:47–54, 1981.

Rodin, E., Schmaltz, S. The Bear-Fedio Personality Inventory and temporal lobe epilepsy. *Neurology* 34:591–596, 1984.

Roeltgen, D. P., Sevush, S., Heilman, K. M. Pure Gerstmann's syndrome from a focal lesion. *Archives of Neurology* 40:46–47, 1983.

Roland, P. E., Larsen, B., Lassen, N. A., Skinhøj, E. Supplementary motor area and other cortical areas in organization of voluntary movements in man. *Journal of Neurophysiology* 43:118–136, 1980.

Rondot, P., Tzavaras, A., Garcia, R. Sur un cas de prosopagnosie persistant depuis quinze ans. *Revue Neurologique* 117:424–428, 1967.

Rosandi, G., Rossi, G. F. On the suggested cerebral dominance for consciousness. *Brain* 90:101–112, 1967.

Rose, F. C., Symonds, C. P. Persistent memory defect following encephalitis. *Brain* 83(Part 2):195–212, 1960.

Rosenzweig, S., Mason, G. An experimental study of memory in relation to the theory of depression. *British Journal of Psychology* 24:247–265, 1934.

Ross, E. D. The aprosodias: Functional–anatomic organization of the affective components of language in the right hemisphere. *Archives of Neurology* 38:561–569, 1981.

Ross, E. D., Harney, J. H., de LaCoste-Utamsing, C. How the brain integrates affective and propositional language into a unified brain function: hypothesis based on clinicopathological correlations. *Archives of Neurology* 38:745–748, 1981.

Ross, E. D., Mesulam, M.-M. Dominant language functions of the right hemisphere? Prosody and emotional gesturing. *Archives of Neurology* 36:144–148, 1979.

Ross, E. D., Stewart, M. Akinetic mutism from hypothalamic damage: successful treatment with dopamine agonists. *Neurology* 31:1435–1439, 1981.

Rossi, G. F., Zanchetti, A. The brain stem reticular formation: anatomy and physiology. *Archives Italiennes de Biologie* 95:199–435, 1957.

Rubens, A. B. Transcortical motor aphasia. In *Studies in Neurolinguistics,* vol. 1. Whitaker, H., Whitaker, H. A., eds. New York, Academic Press, 1976, pp. 293–303.

Rubens, A. B., Benson, D. F. Associative visual agnosia. *Archives of Neurology* 24:305–315, 1971.

Rudnick, F. D. The paranoid-erotic syndromes. In *Extraordinary Disorders of Human Behavior*. Friedmann, C.T.H., Faguet, R. A., eds. New York, Plenum Press, 1982, pp. 99–119.

Ruff, R. L., Volpe, B. T. Environmental reduplication associated with right frontal and parietal lobe injury. *Journal of Neurology, Neurosurgery, and Psychiatry* 44:382–386, 1981.

Russell, W. R. Disability caused by brain wounds. *Journal of Neurology, Neurosurgery, and Psychiatry* 14:35–39, 1951.

Russell, W. R. *Brain Memory Learning—A Neurologist's View*. London, Oxford University Press, 1959.

Russell, W. R., Nathan, P. W. Traumatic amnesia. *Brain* 69:280–300, 1946.

Ryle, G. *The Concept of Mind*. New York, Barnes & Noble, 1949.

Sacks, O. *The Man Who Mistook His Wife for a Hat*. New York, Harper & Row, 1987.

Saffran, E. M., Marin, O.S.M. Immediate memory for word lists and sentences in a patient with deficient auditory short-term memory. *Brain and Language* 2:420–433, 1975.

Samuels, J. A., Benson, D. F. Some aspects of language comprehension in anterior aphasia. *Brain and Language* 8:275–286, 1979.

Sanford, A. J. *The Mind of Man*. Brighton, Sussex, England, Harvester Press, 1987.

Sapir, E. *Language*. New York, Harcourt Brace, 1921.

Sartre, J.-P. *Being and Nothingness*. New York, Citadel Press, 1965.

Sasanuma, S., Fujimura, O. *Kanji* versus *Kana* processing in alexia with transient agraphia: a case report. *Cortex* 7:1–18, 1971.

Sasanuma, S., Itoh, M., Mori, K., Kobayashi, Y. Tachistoscopic recognition of *Kana* and *Kanji* words. *Neuropsychologia* 15:547–553, 1977.

Schacter, S., Singer, J. E. Cognitive, social and physiological determinants of emotional state. *Psychological Review* 69:379–399, 1962.

Scheibel, A. B. Anatomical and physiological substrates of arousal—a view from bridge. In *Reticular Formation Revisited*. Hobson, J. A., Brazier, M. A., eds. New York, Raven Press, 1980, pp. 55–66.

Scheibel, A. B., Kovelman, J. A. Disorientation of the hippocampal pyramidal cell and its processes in the schizophrenic patient. *Biological Psychiatry* 16:101–102, 1981.

Scheibel, M. E., Scheibel, A. B. Structural organization of nonspecific thalamic nuclei and their projection toward cortex. *Brain Research* 6:60–94, 1967.

Schiff, H. B., Alexander, M. P., Naeser, M. A., Galaburda, A. M. Aphemia. *Archives of Neurology* 40:720–727, 1983.

Schilder, P. Fingeragnosie, fingerapraxie, fingeraphasie. *Nervenarzt* 4:625–629, 1931.

Schmahmann, J. D. An emerging concept: the cerebellar contribution to higher function. *Archives of Neurology* 48:1178–1187, 1991.

Schneider, C. *Psychologie der Schizophrenen*. Leipzig, Thieme, 1930.

Schneider, G. E. Two visual systems. *Science*. 163:895–902, 1969.

Schneider, J. S. Basal ganglia role in behavior: importance of sensory gating and its relevance to psychiatry. *Biological Psychiatry* 19:1693–1701, 1984.

Schrader, P. J., Robinson, M. F. An evaluation of prefrontal lobotomy through ward behavior. *Journal of Abnormal and Social Psychology* 40:61–69, 1945.

Schreiner, L., Kling, A. Behavioral changes following rhinencephalic injury in cat. *Journal of Neurophysiology* 16:643–659, 1953.

Schuell, H., Jenkins, J. J., Jiminez-Pabon, E. *Aphasia in Adults. Diagnosis, Prognosis, and Treatment.* New York, Harper & Row, 1964.

Schuster, P., Taterka, H. Beitrag zur Anatomie und Klinik der reinen Worttaubheit. *Zentralblatt für die gesamte Neurologie und Psychiatrie* 102:494–538, 1926.

Schwartz, J. M., Baxter, L. R., Jr., Mazziotta, J. C., Gerner, R. H., Phelps, M. E. The differential diagnosis of depression. *Journal of the American Medical Association* 258:1368–1374, 1987.

Scoville, W. B. Selective cortical undercutting as a means of modifying and studying frontal lobe functions in man. *Journal of Neurosurgery* 6:65–73, 1949.

Scoville, W. B., Milner, B. Loss of recent memory after bilateral hippocampal lesions. *Journal of Neurology, Neurosurgery, and Psychiatry* 20:11–21, 1957.

Searle, J. Minds, brains, and programs. *The Behavioral Brain Sciences* 3:417–457, 1980.

Searle, J. *Minds, Brains, and Science.* Cambridge, MA, Harvard University Press, 1984.

Sechenov, I. *Reflexes of the Brain.* St. Petersburg, Sushchiniski, 1863.

Segarra, J. M. Cerebral vascular disease and behavior. I. The Syndrome of the mesencephalic artery (basilar artery bifurcation). *Archives of Neurology* 22:408–418, 1970.

Segarra, J. M., Angelo, J. N. Presentation #1. In *Behavioral Change in Cerebrovascular Disease.* Benton, A. L., ed. New York, Harper & Row, 1970, pp. 3–14.

Seltzer, B., Benson, D. F. The temporal pattern of retrograde amnesia in Korsakoff's disease. *Neurology* 24:527–530, 1974.

Semmes, J. Hemispheric specialization: a possible clue to mechanism. *Neuropsychologia* 6:11–26, 1968.

Semmes, J., Weinstein, S., Ghent, L., Teuber, H. L. Correlates of impaired orientation in personal and extrapersonal space. *Brain* 86:747–772, 1963.

Serafetinides, E. A., Falconer, M. A. The effects of temporal lobectomy in epileptic patients with psychosis. *Journal of Mental Science* 108:584–593, 1962.

Serafetinides, E. A., Hoare, R. D., Driver, M. V. Intracarotid sodium amylobarbitone and cerebral dominance for speech and consciousness. *Brain* 88:107–130, 1965.

Sergent, J., Corballis, M. C. Generation of multipart images in the disconnected cerebral hemispheres. *Bulletin of the Psychonomics Society* 28:309–311, 1990.

Sergent, J., Poncet, M. From covert to overt recognition of faces in a prosopagnosia patient. *Brain* 113:989–1004, 1990.

Shallice, T. The dominant action system: an information-processing approach to consciousness. In *The Stream of Consciousness.* Pope, K. S., Singer, J. L., eds. New York, Plenum Press, 1978, pp. 117–157.

Shallice, T. Specific impairments of planning. In *The Neuropsychology of Cognitive Function.* Broadbent, D. E., Weiskrantz, L., eds. London, The Royal Society, 1982, pp. 199–209.

Shallice, T., Evans, M. E. The involvement of the frontal lobes in cognitive estimation. *Cortex* 4:294–303, 1978.

Shapiro, B. E., Alexander, M. P., Gardner, H., Mercer, B. Mechanisms of confabulation. *Neurology* 31:1070–1076, 1981.

Sherrington, C. S. *The Integrative Action of the Nervous System.* New York, Scribner, 1906.
Sherrington, C. S. *Man—On His Nature.* Cambridge, Cambridge University Press, 1940.
Sherwin, I. Seizures precipitated by the use of language: a review. *Cortex* 2:349–356, 1966.
Sherwin, I., Peron-Magnan, P., Bancaud, J., Bonis, A., Talairach, J. Prevalence of psychosis in epilepsy as a function of the laterality of the epileptogenic lesion. *Archives of Neurology* 39:621–625, 1982.
Signoret, J.-L. Memory and amnesias. In *Principles of Behavioral Neurology.* Mesulam, M.-M., ed. Philadelphia, F. A. Davis, 1985, pp. 169–192.
Skinner, B. F. *Verbal Behavior.* New York, Appleton-Century-Crofts, 1957.
Slater, E., Beard, A. W., Glithero, J. The schizophrenia-like psychoses of epilepsy. *British Journal of Psychiatry* 109:95–150, 1963.
Smith, A. Speech and other functions after left (dominant) hemispherectomy. *Journal of Neurology, Neurosurgery, and Psychiatry* 29:467–471, 1966.
Smith, A. D. Adult age differences in cued recall. *Developmental Psychology* 13:326–331, 1977.
Smith, J. S., Kiloh, L. G., Boots, J. A. Prospective evaluation of prefrontal leucotomy: results at 30 months' follow-up. In *Neurosurgical Treatment in Psychiatry, Pain, and Epilepsy.* Sweet, W. H., Obrador, S., Martin-Rodriguez, J. G., eds. Baltimore, University Park Press, 1977, pp. 217–224.
Snell, R. S. *Clinical Neuroanatomy.* Boston, Little Brown & Co., 1980.
Sokolov, A. N. *Inner Speech and Thought.* New York, Plenum, 1972.
Souques, A. Quelques cas d'anarthria de Pierre Marie. *Revue Neurologique* 2:319–368, 1928.
Sperry, R. W. Mental unity following surgical disconnection of the cerebral hemispheres. In *The Harvey Lecture Series, Vol. 2.* New York, Academic Press, 1968, pp. 293–323.
Sperry, R. W. Consciousness, personal identity, and the divided brain. In *The Dual Brain.* Benson, D. F., Zaidel, E., eds. New York, Guilford Press, 1985, pp. 11–26.
Sperry, R. W., Gazzaniga, M. S. Language following surgical disconnecting of the hemispheres. In *Brain Mechanisms Underlying Speech and Language.* Darley, F. L., ed. New York, Grune & Stratton, 1967, pp. 108–121.
Spiers, P. A. Acalculia revisited: current issues. In *Mathematic Disabilities: A Cognitive Neuropsychological Perspective.* Deloche, G., Seron, X., eds. Hillsdale, NJ, Lawrence Erlbaum Associates, 1987, pp. 1–25.
Spitzer, R. L., Wilson, P. T. Nosology and the official psychiatric nomenclature. In *Comprehensive Textbook of Psychiatry II.* Freedman, A. M., Kaplan, H. I., Sadock, B. J., eds. Baltimore, Williams & Wilkins, 1975, pp. 826–845.
Squire, L. R. The neuropsychology of human memory. *Annual Review of Neuroscience* 5:241–273, 1982.
Squire, L. R. *Memory and Brain.* New York, Oxford, 1987.
Squire, L. R., Chace, P. M. Memory function 6 to 9 months after electroconvulsive therapy. *Archives of General Psychiatry* 32:1557–1568, 1975.
Squire, L. R., Spanis, C. W. Long gradient of retrograde amnesia in mice: continuity of findings in humans. *Behavioral Neuroscience* 98:345–348, 1984.
Squire, L. R., Zola-Morgan, S. The medial temporal lobe memory system. *Science* 253:1380–1386, 1991.

Starkstein, S. E., Robinson, R. G. Neuropsychiatric aspects of cerebrovascular disease. In *The American Psychiatric Press Textbook of Neuropsychiatry*, 2nd ed. Yudofsky, S. C., Hales, R. E., eds. Washington, D.C., American Psychiatric Press, 1992, pp. 449–472.

Stedman's Medical Dictionary Illustrated. Baltimore, Waverly, 1979.

Stengel, E. Loss of spatial orientation, constructional apraxia and Gerstmann's syndrome. *Journal of Mental Science* 90:753–760, 1944.

Stern, K. Severe dementia associated with bilateral symmetrical degeneration of the thalamus. *Brain* 62:157–171, 1939.

Stevens, J. R. Psychiatric implications of psychomotor epilepsy. *Archives of General Psychiatry*. 14:461–471, 1966.

Stevens, J. R. Interictal clinical manifestations of complex partial seizures. In *Advances in Neurology*, vol. 11, *Complex Partial Seizures and Their Treatment*. Penry, J. K., Daly, D. D., eds. New York, Raven, 1975, pp. 85–112.

Strazalkowski, W. J. *The Active Character of Thinking*. London, White Eagle Press, 1982.

Strub, R. L. Acute confusional state. In *Psychiatric Aspects of Neurologic Disease*, vol. 2. Benson, D. F., Blumer, D., eds. New York, Grune & Stratton, 1982, pp. 1–23.

Stuss, D. T., Alexander, M. P., Lieberman, A., Levine, H. An extraordinary form of confabulation. *Neurology* 28:1166–1172, 1978.

Stuss, D. T., Benson, D. F. Emotional concomitants of psychosurgery. In *Neuropsychology of Human Emotion*. Heilman, K. M., Satz, P., eds. New York, Guilford Press, 1983, pp. 111–140.

Stuss, D. T., Benson, D. F. Neuropsychological studies of the frontal lobes. *Psychological Bulletin* 95:3–28, 1984.

Stuss, D. T., Benson, D. F. *The Frontal Lobes*. New York, Raven Press, 1986.

Sullivan, H. S. *Conceptions of Modern Psychiatry*. Washington, DC, William Alanson White Foundation, 1949.

Surridge, D. An investigation into some psychiatric aspects of multiple sclerosis. *British Journal of Psychiatry* 155:749–764, 1969.

Swash, M. Released involuntary laughter after temporal lobe infarction. *Journal of Neurology, Neurosurgery, and Psychiatry* 35:108–113, 1972.

Swash, M. Visual perseveration in temporal lobe epilepsy. *Journal of Neurology, Neurosurgery, and Psychiatry* 42:569–571, 1979.

Sweet, W. H., Talland, G. A., Ervin, F. R. Loss of recent memory following section of the fornix. *Transactions of the American Neurological Association* 84:76–82, 1959.

Symonds, C. Concussion and its sequelae. *Lancet* 1:1–15, 1962.

Symonds, C. Disorders of memory. *Brain* 89:625–644, 1966.

Szentagothai, J. The "module-concept" in cerebral cortex architecture. *Brain Research* 95:475–496, 1975.

Talland, G. A. *Deranged Memory—A Psychonomic Study of the Amnesic Syndrome*. New York, Academic Press, 1965.

Tanji, J., Kurata, K. Functional organization of the supplementary motor area. In *Motor Control Mechanisms in Health and Disease*. Desmedt, J. R., ed. New York, Raven, 1983, pp. 421–431.

Tatlow, W.F.T., Oulton, J. L. Phantom limbs (with observations on brachial plexus blocks). *Canadian Medical Association Journal* 73:170–177, 1955.

Taylor, M. A. Schneiderian first-rank symptoms and clinical prognostic features in schizophrenia. *Archives of General Psychiatry* 26:64–67, 1972.

Taylor, M. A. Catatonia. *Neuropsychiatry, Neuropsychology, and Behavioral Neurology* 3:48–72, 1990.
Taylor, P. The components of sickness: diseases, illnesses, and predicaments. *Lancet* 2:1008–1010, 1979.
Teasdale, G., Jennett, B. Assessment of coma and impaired consciousness: a practical scale. *Lancet* 2:81–84, 1974.
Terzian, H., Dalle Ore, G. Syndrome of Klüver and Bucy reproduced in man by bilateral removal of the temporal lobes. *Neurology* 5:373–380, 1955.
Teuber, H.-L. The riddle of frontal lobe function in man. In *The Frontal Granular Cortex and Behavior*. Warren, J. M., Akert, K., eds. New York, McGraw-Hill, 1964, pp. 410–444.
Teuber, H.-L. Battersby, W. S., Bender, M. B. Changes in visual searching performance following cerebral lesions. *American Journal of Physiology* 159:592, 1949 (Abstr).
Thompson, G. N. Cerebral area essential to consciousness. *Bulletin of the Los Angeles Neurological Society* 16:311–334, 1951.
Thoren, P., Asberg, M., Cronholm, B., Jornestedt, L., Traskman, L. Clomipramine treatment of obsessive–compulsive disorder. I. A controlled clinical trial. *Archives of General Psychiatry* 37:1281–1285, 1980.
Thurstone, L. L. Primary Mental Abilities. Chicago: University of Chicago Press, 1938.
Tilney, F. *The Brain, From Ape to Man*. New York, Hoeber, 1928.
Tilney, F., Morrison, J. F. Pseudobulbar palsy, clinically and pathologically considered, with clinical report of five cases. *Journal of Nervous and Mental Disease* 39:305–355, 1912.
Tomlinson, B. E. The pathology of dementia. In *Dementia*, 2nd ed. Wells, C. E., ed. Philadelphia, F. A. Davis, 1977, pp. 113–153.
Tonkonogy, J., Goodglass, H. Language function, foot of the third frontal gyrus and Rolandic operculum. *Archives of Neurology* 38:486–490, 1981.
Trevarthen, C. B. Hemispheric specialization. In *Handbook of Physiology, Section 1, The Nervous System, vol. III, Sensory Processes, pt. 2*. Washington, DC, American Physiological Society, 1984, pp. 1129–1190.
Trimble, M. The relationship between epilepsy and schizophrenia: a biomedical hypothesis. *Biological Psychiatry* 12:299–304, 1977.
Trimble, M. R. The interictal psychoses of epilepsy. In *Psychiatric Aspects of Neurologic Disease*, vol. 2. Benson, D. F., Blumer, D., eds. New York, Grune & Stratton, 1982, pp. 75–91.
Trimble, M. R. Personality disturbances in epilepsy. *Neurology* 33:1332–1334, 1983.
Troost, B. T. An overview of ocular motor neurophysiology. *Annals of Otology, Rhinology, and Laryngology* 90:29–36, 1981.
Tulving, E. Memory and consciousness. *Canadian Psychology* 26:1–12, 1985.
Tulving, E., Donaldson, W. *Organization of Memory*. New York, Academic Press, 1972.
Twain, M. *Mark Twain: Wit and Wisecracks*. New York, The Peter Pauper Press, 1961.
Tzavaras, A., Hécaen, H., LeBras, H. Le probleme de la specificite du deficit de la reconnaissance du visage humain lors des lesions hemispheriques unilaterales. *Neuropsychologia* 8:403–416, 1970.
Underwood, J. B. Interference and forgetting. *Psychological Review* 64:49–60, 1957.

Ungerleider, L. G., Mishkin, M. Two cortical visual systems. In *The Analysis of Visual Behavior*. Ingle, D. J., Mansfield, R.J.W., Goodale, M. A., eds. Cambridge, MIT Press, 1982, pp. 549–586.

Valenstein, E. S. *Brain Control*. New York, John Wiley & Sons, 1973.

Valenstein, E. S. Extent of psychosurgery worldwide. In *The Psychosurgery Debate*. Valenstein, E. S., ed. San Francisco, W. H. Freeman, 1980, pp. 76–86.

Valentin, G. Integritatsgefuhle der Amputaten. *Lehrbuch der Physiologie des Menschens* 2:606–609, 1844.

Vallar, G., Shallice, T. *Neuropsychological Impairments of Short Term Memories*. Cambridge, Cambridge University Press, 1990.

Van Hoesen, G. W., Pandya, D. N., Butters, N. Some connections of the entorhinal (area 28) and perirhinal (area 35) cortices of the rhesus monkey. II. Frontal lobe afferents. *Brain Research* 95:25–38, 1975.

Van Lancker, D. R., Canter, G. J. Impairment of voice and face recognition in patients with hemispheric damage. *Brain and Cognition* 1:185–195, 1982.

Veith, I. *Hysteria, The History of a Disease*. Chicago: University of Chicago Press, 1965.

Victor, M. The amnestic syndrome and its anatomical basis. *Canadial Medical Association Journal* 100:1115–1125, 1969.

Victor, M., Adams, R. D., Collins, G. H. *The Wernicke-Korsakoff Syndrome*. Philadelphia, F. A. Davis, 1971.

Victor, M., Angevine, J., Mancall, E., Fisher, C. M. Memory loss with lesions of hippocampal formation. *Archives of Neurology* 5:244–263, 1961.

Victor, M., Yakovlev, P. S. S. Korsakoff's psychic disorder in conjunction with peripheral neuritis. *Neurology* 5:394–406, 1955.

Vignolo, L. A. Auditory agnosia: A review and report of recent evidence. In *Contributions to Clinical Neuropsychology*. Benton, A. L., ed. Chicago, Aldine, 1969, pp. 172–208.

Voss, J. F. The nature of an association and its relation to thought. In *Approaches to Thought*. Voss, J. F., ed. Columbus, Ohio, Merrill, 1969, pp. 83–104.

Vygotsky, L. S. *Thought and Language*. Hanfmann, E., Vaker, G., translators. Cambridge, MIT Press, 1934/1962.

Wagenaar, E., Snow, C., Prins, R. Spontaneous speech of aphasic patients: a psycholinguistic analysis. *Brain and Language* 2:281–303, 1975.

Wall, W. D. Pain. In *Scientific Basis of Clinical Neurology*. Swash, M., Kennard, C., eds. Edinburgh, Churchill Livingstone, 1985, pp. 163–171.

Wallas, G. Stages of control. In *The Creativity Question*. Rothenberg, A., Hausman, C., eds. Durham, N.C., Duke University Press, 1976, pp. 69–73.

Walsh, F. B., Hoyt, W. F. *Clinical Neuro-ophthalmology*, 3rd ed. Baltimore, Williams & Wilkins, 1969.

Walshe, F.M.R. The brain-stem conceived as the "highest level" of function in the nervous system. *Brain* 80:510–539, 1957.

Warrington, E. K. Constructional apraxia. In *Handbook of Clinical Neurology*, vol. 4. Vinken, P. J., Bruyn, G. W., eds. Amsterdam, North-Holland, 1969, pp. 67–83.

Warrington, E. K., James, M. Disorders of visual perception in patients with localized cerebral lesions. *Neuropsychologia* 5:253–266, 1967.

Warrington, E. K., Shallice, T. Category specific semantic impairments. *Brain* 107:829–854, 1984.

Watson, J. B. *Behaviorism*. London, Kegan Paul, 1930.
Watson, R. T., Heilman, K. M. Thalamic neglect. *Neurology* 29:690–694, 1979.
Watson, R. T., Heilman, K. M., Cauthen, J. C., King, F. A. Neglect after cingulectomy. *Neurology* 23:1003–1007, 1973.
Watson, R. T., Heilman, K. M., Miller, B. D., King, F. A. Neglect after mesencephalic reticular formation lesions. *Neurology* 24:294–298, 1974.
Watson, R. T., Valenstein, E., Heilman, K. M. Thalamic neglect: Possible role of the medial thalamus and nuclear reticularis thalami in behavior. *Archives of Neurology* 38:501–506, 1981.
Watt, H. J. Experimental contribution to a theory of thinking. *Journal of Anatomy and Physiology* 40:257–266, 1905/06.
Waugh, N. C., Norman, D. A. Primary memory. *Psychological Review* 72:89–104, 1972.
Websters New Collegiate Dictionary. Springfield, MA, Merriam-Webster, 1979.
Wechsler, D. A standardized memory scale for clinical use. *The Journal of Psychology* 19:87–95, 1945.
Wechsler, D. *The Measurement and Appraisal of Adult Intelligence*. Baltimore, Williams & Wilkins, 1958.
Weinberger, D. R., Torrey, E. F., Neophytides, A. N., Wyatt, R. J. Lateral cerebral ventricular enlargement in chronic schizophrenia. *Archives of General Psychiatry* 36:735–739, 1979.
Weinstein, E. A., Kahn, R. L. Non-aphasic misnaming (paraphasia) in organic brain disease. *Archives of Neurology and Psychiatry* 67:72–79, 1952.
Weinstein, E. A., Kahn, R. L. *Denial of Illness: Symbolic and Physiologic Aspects*. Springfield, IL, Charles C. Thomas, 1955.
Weinstein, E. A., Kahn, R. L., Sugarman, L. A. Phenomenon of reduplication. *Archives of Neurology and Psychiatry* 67:808–814, 1952.
Weinstein, S. Neuropsychological studies of the phantom. In *Contributions to Clinical Neuropsychology*. Benton, A. L., ed. Chicago, Aldine, 1969, pp. 73–106.
Weinstein, S., Teuber, H. L. Effects of penetrating brain injury on intelligence test scores. *Science* 125:1036–1037, 1957.
Weisenburg, T. S., McBride, K. L. *Aphasia*. New York: Hafner Publishing Co., 1933/1964.
Weiser, H. G. Ictal "psychical phenomena" and stereoelectroencephalographic findings. In *EEG and Clinical Neurophysiology*. Lechner, E., Aranibar, A., eds. Princeton, Excerpta Medica, 1979, pp. 62–76.
Weiskrantz, L., Warrington, E. K., Sanders, M. D., Marshall, J. Visual capacity in the hemianopic field following a restricted occipital ablation. *Brain* 97:709–728, 1974.
Welch, K., Stuteville, P. Experimental production of unilateral neglect in monkeys. *Brain* 81:341–347, 1958.
Welford, A. T. Motor performance. In *Handbook of the Psychology of Aging*. Birren, J. E., Schaie, K. W., eds. New York, Van Nostrand Reinhold Co., 1977, pp. 450–596.
Welt, L. Ueber Charakterveranderungen des Menschen infolge von Lasionen des Stirnhirns. *Deutsches Archiv fuer Klinische Medicin* 42:339–390, 1888.
Wenzel, B. M., Tschirgi, R. D., Taylor, J. L. Effects of early postnatal hemidecortication on spatial discrimination in cats. *Experimental Neurology* 6:322–339, 1962.
Wepman, J. M., Jones, L. V. Five aphasias: a commentary on aphasia as a regres-

sive linguistic problem. In *ARNMD*, vol. 42, *Disorders of Communication*. Rioch, D. M., Weinstein, E., eds. Baltimore: Williams & Wilkins, 1964, pp. 190–203.

Wernicke, C. *Das Aphasische Symptomenkomplex*. Breslau: Cohn & Weigart, 1874.

Wernicke, C. *Lehrbuch der Gehirnkrankheiten, Vol. 1. Tragweite der Aphasie fur das Verstandniss der Tindenfunctionen*. Kassel, Theodor Fischer, 1881.

Wexler, B. E. Cerebral laterality and psychiatry: a review of the literature. *American Journal of Psychiatry* 137:279–291, 1980.

White, J. C., Sweet, W. H. *Pain—Its Mechanisms and Neurosurgical Control*. Springfield, IL: Charles C. Thomas, 1955.

Whiteley, A. M., Warrington, E. K. Prosopagnosia: a clinical, psychological, and anatomical study of three patients. *Journal of Neurology, Neurosurgery, and Psychiatry* 40:395–403, 1977.

Whitty, C.W.M., Lewin, W. A Korsakoff syndrome in the post-cingulectomy confusional state. *Brain* 83:648–653, 1960.

Wiener, P. P., ed. *Dictionary of the History of Ideas*. New York, Charles Scribner & Sons, 1973.

Wigan, A. L. *The Duality of the Mind*. London, Longman, 1844.

Wilde, O. The Importance of Being Earnest. In *The Literature of England*, 3rd ed., vol. 2. Woods, G. B., Watt, H. A., Anderson, G. K., eds. Chicago, Scott, Foresman, 1895/1941, pp. 970–1002.

Williams, D. The structure of emotions reflected in epileptic experience. *Brain* 79:29–67, 1956.

Wilson, R. S., Kasniak, A. W., Klawans, H. L., Garren, D. G. High speed memory scanning in parkinsonism. *Cortex* 16:67–72, 1980.

Wilson, S.A.K. A contribution to the study of apraxia with a review of the literature. *Brain* 41:164–216, 1908.

Wilson, S.A.K. *Aphasia*. London, Kegan Paul, 1926.

Winner, E., Gardner, H. The comprehension of metaphor in brain-damaged patients. *Brain* 100:717–729, 1977.

von Wolff, C. *Psychologia Rationalis*. Frankfurt, Officiana Libraria Regeriana, 1734.

Wolpe, J. *The Practice of Behavior Therapy*. New York: Pergamon Press, 1969.

Woodworth, R. S., Schlosberg, H. *Experimental Psychology*, rev. ed. New York, Holt, 1954.

World Health Organization. *Manual of the International Classification of Diseases, Injuries, and Causes of Death*, 9th Revision (ICD-9). Geneva, World Health Organization, 1977.

Wundt, W. *Principles of Physiological Psychology*, vol. 1. Tichener, E. B., translator. Leipzig, Englemann, 1873–74 (New York, Macmillan, 1904).

Yakolev, P. I. Motility, behavior, and the brain. *Journal of Nervous and Mental Disease* 107:313–335, 1948.

Yakovlev, P. I., Lecours, A. R. The myelogenetic cycles of regional maturation of the brain. In *Regional Development of the Brain in Early Life*. Minkowski, A., ed. Oxford, Blackwell, 1967, pp. 3–23.

Yamadori, A. Ideogram reading in alexia. *Brain* 98:231–238, 1975.

Yamadori, A. Right unilateral dyscopia of letters in alexia without agraphia. *Neurology* 30:991–994, 1980.

Yingling, C. D., Skinner, J. E. Regulation of unit activity in nucleus reticularis thalami by the mesencephalic reticular formation and the frontal granular

cortex. *Electroencephalography and Clinical Neurophysiology* 39:635–642, 1975.
Young, J. A. *Philosophy and the Brain.* Oxford, Oxford University Press, 1987.
Young, R. M. *Mind, Brain, and Adaptation in the Nineteenth Century.* New York, Oxford, 1970/1990.
Zaidel, E. Auditory vocabulary of the right hemisphere after brain bisection or hemidecortication. *Cortex* 12:191–211, 1976.
Zaidel, E. Lexical organization in the right hemisphere. In *Cerebral Correlates of Conscious Experience.* Buser, P. H., Rougeul-Buser, A., eds. Amsterdam, Elsevier, 1978, pp. 177–197.
Zaidel, E. Language in the right hemisphere. In *Dual Brain: Hemispheric Specialization in Humans.* Benson, D. F., Zaidel, E., eds. New York, Guilford Press, 1985, pp. 205–231.
Zangwill, O. L. *Cerebral Dominance and Its Relation to Psychological Function.* Springfield, IL, Charles C. Thomas, 1960.
Zangwill, O. L. Neuropsychological models of memory. In *The Pathology of Memory.* Talland, G. A., Waugh, N. C., eds. New York, Academic Press, 1969, pp. 161–166.
Zangwill, O. L. Consciousness and the cerebral hemispheres. In *Hemisphere Function in the Human Brain.* Dimond, S., Beaumont, J., eds. London, Paul Elek, 1974, pp. 264–278.
Zarcone, V. Narcolepsy. *New England Journal of Medicine* 288:1156–1166, 1973.
Zihl, J., von Cramon, D., Mai, N. Selective disturbance of movement vision after bilateral brain damage. *Brain* 106:313–340, 1983.
Zola-Morgan, S., Squire, L. R., Amaral, D. Human amnesia and the medial temporal region: enduring memory impairment following a bilateral lesion limited to the CA 1 field of the hippocampus. *Journal of Neuroscience* 6:2950–2967, 1986.
Zurif, E. B., Caramazza, A., Myerson, R. Grammatical judgements of agrammatic aphasics. *Neuropsychologia* 10:405–417, 1972.

Index

Abulia, 84
Acalculia
  clinical examples, 199–202f
  definition, 199
  variations, 202
Acetylcholine, 242
Acquiring process, in memory, 178–179
Acute confusion
  causes, 78t
  clinical characteristics, 78, 79
  clinical examples, 78–79, 181–183
  neuroanatomical substrate, 192–193
Adrenergic system, 92f
Affect
  definition, 101
  discordance with mood, 101
  varieties, 115t
Affective disorders
  clinical examples, 106–111
  focal damage to cerebral hemispheres and, 115
  thought disorders and, 228
Affective facade, 101
Age–associated memory impairment, 190
Aging
  neurotransmitters and, 242
  senescence and, 190
Agnosia, 121
Agraphia, 146, 148, 168, 174
Akinesia, 84
Akinetic mutism
  causes, 81–82
  characteristics, 82t
  clinical example, 80–82
  locus of damage, 82t
Alcoholism, Korsakoff's disease and, 183, 184f
Alertness
  degrees of, 75
  impaired, 75
  staging, 75
  stimulus–response paradigm, 75

Alexia
  with agraphia, 165–166. *See* Central alexia
  without agraphia, 125, 153–154. *See* Posterior alexia
  and color agnosia, 123
  definition, 146
  in Japanese patients, 169
  types, 168t. *See also specific types of alexia*
Alien hand syndrome, 58–60f, 73
Alzheimer's disease
  clinical examples, 203–204, 237
  dementia of, 171, 228–229
  ideational apraxia and, 63
  neuroanatomical substrate, 206–207
  neurotransmitter systems and, 242
  subiculum in, 196
Amelodia, 162–164f
Amnesia
  clinical definition, 186t
  etiologies, 187t
  from head trauma, 183–184
  true, 193
Amnesic aphasia, 151–152f
Amnesic stroke, 185, 188
Amorphosynthesis, 40, 93
Anarithmetria, 201–203, 206
Angular gyrus
  in animal species, 18–19f
  cross–modal associations and, 19, 137, 206
Anomia, variations, 171–173f
Anomic aphasia, 151–152f
Anosognosia
  attention disorders and, 87–88
  clinical examples, 86–87
  in hemiplegia, 109
Anoxic amnesia, 188
Anterior alexia
  with Broca's aphasia, 173
  clinical examples, 166, 167
  locus of pathology, 168t, 174f
  neighborhood characteristics, 168t
  written language and, 167, 168t

Anton's syndrome
  amnesic stroke and, 185, 188
  anosognosia of, 88
  clinical example, 87–88
Anxiety disorders, serotonin and, 242
Aphasia
  amnesic, 151–152f
  behavioral complications, 232–234
  classification, 161t
  clinical examples, 155–161
  definition, 146
  frontal language disorders, 162t
  heteromodal association cortex damage and, 252
  neurological studies, early, 11
  subcortical lesions and, 162
Aphasic acalculia, clinical examples, 199–201f
Aphasic agraphia, 174
Aphemia, 150–151f, 162
Aphemia plus, 156–157f
Apperception, 30, 31
Apperceptive agnosia, 126
Apperceptive visual agnosia, 121, 122–123
Apraxia, 56, 57
Aprosodia, 106–107
Aristotle, 14–15
Arousal
  phasic aspects of, 97
  stages, 97
Articulation, 176
Articulatory initiation disturbance, 171
Artificial intelligence, 13–14
Associationism, 14–18
Associative agnosia, 126
Associative visual agnosia, 121
Astereognosis, 40
Attention
  deficit, hierarchical stages, 86t
  dichotomy, 76
  directed, 259
  neural basis, 96f
  neuroanatomical aspects, 93
  neuroanatomical network, 90t
  phasic aspect, 97
  phasic disorder, 92
  tonic aspects, 97
Auditory agnosia, 36
Auditory disturbances, case reports, 33–36f

Auditory sensory system, 45f
Auras, epileptic, 106
Automatic system, neural processing steps, 72
Awakeness
  alterations, 75, 192
  in arousal, 97
Awareness, 74

Bain, Alexander, 15
Basal ganglia
  in cognitive function, 51
  in motor activities, 56–57, 66–67f
Basal–limbic dysfunction, 118
Basolateral limbic circuit, 221f
Behaviorism, 16
Benign senescent forgetfulness, 190
Berkeley, George, 15
Bifrontal traumatic brain damage, 204–205
Big Broca aphasia, 156–157
Bilateral upper motor neuron disease, 111
Blindness, 120
Brain. *See also* Left hemisphere; Right hemisphere
  alteration of function, 10
  communication flow, 144f
  damage, behavioral abnormalities and, 12
  focal damage, language loss and, 142
  function, thinking and, 3–4
  operations for intractable pain, 37–38
  psychoarchitectural map, 23f
Brain/mind combinations, 20t
Brain scan. *See* Radionuclide brain scan
British empiricists, 15, 49
Broca, Paul, 11
Broca's aphasia
  anterior aphasia and, 108
  articulatory initiation disturbance, 171
  classification, 160, 161t
  clinical example, 155–156f
  depressive reaction, 232, 233
  frontal alexia and, 173
  left hemisphere pathology and, 142
  with literal alexia, 166
Broca's area, damage, 107

Brodmann areas
  4. See Precentral gyrus (Brodmann area 4)
  6, 68
  8. See Frontal eye fields (Brodmann area 8)
  17, 136, 137, 248
  37, lesion of, 152f
  eye movements and, 134
  in heteromodal association cortex, 250–251
  sensory input and, 248, 250
  in unimodal association cortex, 250
  in visual–spatial function, 137, 248

Calcarine cortex (Brodmann area 17), 136, 137, 248
Calculation ability, studying, 202
Calculation impairment. See Acalculia
Callosal disconnection anomia, 172
Callosal separation syndrome, 40–41
Capgras syndrome, 218–220f
Cataplexy, 77
Catastrophic reaction, 101, 109
Catatonia
  abnormal dopamine activity and, 242
  definition, 82
Catatonic schizophrenia, clinical example, 229–230
Category-specific anomia, 172
Category-specific naming problems, 172–173
Cellular neuroanatomy, 21–25
Central alexia
  clinical example, 165–167
  locus of pathology, 168t, 174f
  neighborhood characteristics, 168t
  reading and, 173
  written language and, 168t
Central nervous system
  damage, pain and, 38–39
  somesthetic stimuli pathways, 44f
Cerebellum
  cognitive function and, 51
  dysfunction, 53t
Cerebral disconnection syndrome, 60–61f
Cerebral tone
  alterations, neurotransmitters and, 76–77f
  tonic aspect of arousal and, 97

Cerebrovascular accident, depression, 233–234
Character disorders, 228
Cholinergic system, 91, 92f
Chomsky, Noam, 17, 142
Chronic pain, personality disorder, 38, 234–235
Circumstantiality, 104
Clouding of consciousness, 88, 182
Cognition
  definition, 5–6, 198–199
  disorders, 111–114
    clinical examples, 199–206
    neuroanatomical substrate, 206–207
  neural basis, 207
  varieties of activities, 198–199
  verbal dimensions, 207
  visual–spatial information and, 207
  vs. thinking, 5
Cognitive control. See Executive control
Color agnosia, 123
Color appreciation, 137
Color naming, 125
Columns or modules, 45
Coma vigil, 81
Command system, 72–73
Communication
  disorders, 141–143
    clinical examples, 148–169f
    varieties, 143–148
  flow in brain, 144f
  neural basis, 175–176f
Competition, in thought processing control, 257
Comprehension, of spoken language, 170–171f
Computation, 206
Computed tomography
  of Broca's aphasia, 155f
  of Broca's area lucency, 150f
  of conduction aphasia, 157–158f
  of hemorrhagic infarctions in bilateral medial thalamic structures, 90f
  left hemisphere intracerebral hemorrhage, 160f
  in neurological practice, 11
  of occipital lobe, in palinopsia, 130f
  of right medial occipital infarction, 128f

Concept formation, 207
Conditioned reflex, 16
Conditioning, learning and, 16
Conduction aphasia, 157–158f, 172, 200
Confabulation
  frontal dysfunction and, 187
  in Korsakoff's disease, 186
Confusional state, acute. See Acute confusion
Consciousness, 21
Consolidation, 179
Constructional tasks, 133
Control mechanisms, 256–258f
Corpus callosum, 20, 165
Cortex
  areas of, 18–19, 22–23f
  functional classification, 24f
  myelinogenesis and, 22f, 23–24
  neural processing divisions, 248–249f. See also specific divisions
Cortical anarthria, 151
Cortical blindness, 87
Cortical deafness, case report, 34, 35f
Cortical dementia, 191. See also Alzheimer's disease
  vs. subcortical, 237–239t
Cortical eye fields, 135f
Cortical functions, hierarchy, 251–253t
Cortical homunculus, 47f
Cortical–limbic regions, 222
Cortical–spinal dysfunction, 53t
Covert seizure discharge, 131
Cross–modal association. See also Heteromodal association
  definition, 32
Cross–modal associations
  angular gyrus and, 19, 137, 206
  importance, 17–18
  language functions and, 176
  memory and, 252
  neural circuits, 226, 260
Cross–model cortex. See Heteromodal association cortex
CT. See Computed tomography

Deafness, cortical, 33–34, 35f
Deep dyslexia, 166–167, 168t, 169, 173–174

Degenerative dementia, 170–171
Degradation, in thought processing control, 256–257
Delirium. See Acute confusion
Delusions, 229
Dementia
  clinical examples, 237–238
  cortical vs. subcortical, 237–239t
  progressive, with thalamic degeneration, 89–91f
  retrieval problems, 191
  thought disorders of, 228–229
  types, 191
Denial, of hemiplegia, 88
Depression
  after cerebrovascular accident, 107–108, 233–234
  during aphasia rehabilitation, 232, 233
  thought disorders and, 228
Descartes, René, 6–7
Diagram making, 142
Diencephalon–upper brain stem junction, 91
Directed thought, 258–260
Disconnection anomia, 172
Disconnection theory, 142
Discrimination, 48
  definition, 31–32
  in sensory processing, 32t
  visual, 120–121
Dopamine, abnormal activity, 242
Dorsal raphe nuclei, 91
Drive
  basic mental control functions and, 210
  definition, 97, 101
  disorders, 111–114
  neural basis, 223–224
Dual mind notion, 20
Dynamic aphasia, 159
Dysgraphia, 79
Dyslexia, deep, 166–167, 168t, 169, 173–174

EEG (electroencephalography), 11
Emotion
  definition, 102
  dichotomies, circular representation, 100f

Emotion *(cont'd)*
  disorders
    clinical examples, 102–114
    neuroanatomical substrate, 114–116*t*
    energizing force of behavior, 115
    hemispheric variations, 240–241*f*
    importance, 99
    neural basis, 116–118*f*
    normal response modifications, 117–118
    varieties, 101–102
Encephalitis, learning disorder of, 185
Endophasia, 143–144
Environmental agnosia, 127–128
Epilepsy
  emotional experiences, 106
  interictal state, behavioral abnormalities, 109–110
  pathological laughter and, 106
Episodic dyscontrol, 113–114
Etorhinal area, learning and, 195–196
Ettlinger, George, 18
Executive control
  description, 210
  disorder, memory and, 216
  neural basis, 224
  prefrontal cortex and, 226
Expressive aphasia, 155–156*f*
Extrapyramidal motor functions, 51, 53
Eye movement system, 134–135

Facial recognition tests, 127
Fantastic confabulation, 216–217*f*, 219, 220
Ferrier, David, 8
Finger tapping act, basal ganglia and, 56–57
Fluency–nonfluency, repetition and, 169–170
Fluent aphasia
  characteristics, 148*t*
  hemispheric region, 147*f*
Fluent verbal output, 169
Foreign accent syndrome, 151
Forgetfulness, 190
Formulation process, 176
Fornix, 187, 194
Frontal alexia. *See* Anterior alexia
Frontal association cortex, 136

Frontal ataxia or apraxia, 58
Frontal behavior, 113
Frontal communication activities, 163*t*
Frontal control systems, in thought disorders, 242–243
Frontal eye fields (Brodmann area 8), 68–69, 95–96, 134
Frontal language disorders, 162*t*
Frontal lobe
  damage
    behavior alterations, 113
    drive and, 223–224
    infarction, 163–165*f*
    retrieval problems, 191–192
  destructive procedures for, 117
  subdivisions, 220–221
Frontal-lobishness, 113, 209–210*t*
Frontal personality syndrome, 113
Frontal system, medial, 115
Functional systems. *See also specific systems*
  fixed operations, 254
  independence of, 254
  integration, 254–255
  interactions, 255
  multiple and simultaneous, 256
  successive, 255–256
  types, 25–26*t*
Functionalism
  cellular neuroanatomy, 21–25*f*
  comparative neuroanatomy, 18–19
  definition, 14
  functional systems, 25–26*t*
  hemispheric specialization, 20–21*t*
Future memory
  description, 210
  neural basis, 224–225

Gage, Phineas, 209, 211–212*f*
Gall, Franz Joseph, 6*f*, 7–8
Galton, Sir Francis, 15–16
Gating systems, in thought processing control, 257–258*f*
Gaze paresis, 84
Gerstmann syndrome, 199–203*f*, 206
Geschwind syndrome, 104–105*t*, 236–237
Gestural language, 145
Glucose metabolism alterations, in depression, 108–109

Hallucinations, 192, 220
Hartley, David, 8, 15
Head trauma, amnesia and, 183–184, 187
Hemianopia, 120, 135
Hemiplegia, denial, 86–87
Hemispatial neglect, 84–85
Hemispheric specialization, 20–21t
Hemispheric systems, thought disorders and, 240–241f
Heschl's gyrus
  focal lesion, 34–36
  pure word deafness and, 154
  sensory input and, 248, 250
Heteromodal association. *See also* Cross–modal association
  cortical functions, essential, 121
  definition, 32
  description, 48
  in language processing, 176
  in sensory processing, 32t
  in visual imaging, 138f, 139
Heteromodal association cortex
  areas, 250–251
  classification, 24–25f
  cognitive networks, 252
  memory and, 195
  neural networks, 221, 252
  pathology, 252
Heteromodal processing, 139–140
Higher cortical function
  hierarchy, 253t
  neuroanatomical foundation, 248–251f
Higher mental control
  disorders, clinical examples, 211–223f
  functions, *See specific higher mental control functions*
  neural basis, 223–226f
  neuroanatomical substrate, 220–223f
  vs. cognition, 208
Higher mental control functions, 208–226f
Hippocampal–limbic system, 193f
Hobbes, Thomas, 15
Holding process, in memory, 178
Homonymous hemianopia, 153, 173
Hume, David, 15
Humphrey, George, 10
Humors, typology of, 99

Huntington's disease, 189, 191, 237–238
Hydrocephalus, obstructive, 57–58f
Hyperactivity, 223
Hypergraphia, 104
Hypokinesia, 84
Hypothalamus, gliosis of mamillary bodies, in Korsakoff's disease, 186–187

Ideational apraxia, 62–64
Ideomotor apraxia
  in anterior callosal separation syndrome, 40–41
  clinical examples, 61–64, 73
  disconnection explanation, 63f
  neuroanatomical sites, 62
Idiotypic cortex, 24
Imaging methods, 11
Imitative behavior, frontal damage and, 216
Immediate recall
  description, 179
  disorders
    clinical examples, 181–183
    neuroanatomical substrate, 192–193
  neural basis, 195
Impulsivity, 233
Inattention, 84
Indifference, 101
Inferior longitudinal fasciculus, 137
Inferotemporal cortex, 137
Inflection, 145
Information processing, 13–14t
Inintention, 84
Inner speech, 143–144
Instinct, 102
Integration, of functional systems, 254–255
Intelligence, prefrontal function and, 208–209
Intelligences, 25. *See also* Functional systems
Intention, 97
  neuroanatomical network, 90t
Intentional movements, motor activation programs, 95f
Interictal personality disorder, 236–237
Interlaminar nuclei, in sensory gating, 257–258f

Intermodal association, 17–18, 195
Interparietal area. See Angular gyrus
Intractable depression, 117
Inverted U concept, of mental tone, 76–77f

James–Lange theory, 99
Juxtastriate cortex, 136

Kant, Emmanuel, 9
Klüver–Bucy syndrome, 102–103, 104t, 114
Koestler, Arthur, 15
Korsakoff's disease
  clinical example, 183, 184f
  site of pathology, 186–187
  Wernicke's encephalopathy and, 186
Kosten's syndrome, 38

Lacunes, 183
Language
  definition, 143
  disorders, 109, 120
  fundamental functions, 146–148t
  hemispheric participation, 145t
  loss, left hemisphere and, 142
  processing steps, 175–176f
  spoken
    comprehension, 147–148, 170–171f
    repetition of, 147, 149f
  thought and, 9–10
  varieties, 145–146
  whole–brain approach, 142
Learning
  characteristics, 180–181
  conditioning and, 16
  definition, 179–180
  disorders
    clinical examples, 183–188f
    neuroanatomical substrate, 193–194f
  neural basis, 195–196
Left hemisphere
  in animal species, 19f
  areas of damage, in anterior, central and posterior alexia, 174f
  Brodmann area 37 lesion, 152f
  comprehension tasks and, 171f
  language areas, 147f
  language functions, 145t

  lesion locations in acalculia, 202f
  motor areas, 67f
  naming, pertinent areas for, 172
Left posterior cerebral artery infarction, 153–154f
Lethargy/drowsiness, 192
Leucotomy
  behavioral alterations, 209
  postoperative damage, 111–113, 205–206f
Lexicon, 241
Limbic rage syndrome, 113–114
Limbic system
  learning and, 196
  supramodal association and, 253
  thought disorders and, 239–240
Linguistics
  comparative, 146
  theories, 142
Little Broca aphasia, 156–157
Locke, John, 9–10, 15
Locked–in syndrome, 81
Locus coeruleus, 91
Long–term memory, 181. See also Retrieval
Lower motor neuron
  anatomy, 52f
  paralysis, characteristics, 51, 52t

Magnetic gait, 57
Magnetic resonance imaging (MRI)
  in neurological studies, 11
  of posterior cortical atrophy, 132f
Mechanical agraphia, 174
Medial limbic circuit, 221f
Medial temporal region, 193
Melody, 145
Memory,
  aging and, 190
  disorders
    clinical examples, 181–192
    neuroanatomical substrate, 192–194f
    unilateral lesions and, 193
    varieties, 178–179
  functions, 179–181
  individuality and, 177
  neural basis, 195–197
  neurophysiological processes, 178–179
  psychological processes, 178–179
  studies, types of, 178
  temporal lobe and, 177–178

Mental attributes, as brain area products, 141–142
Mental control
  anatomic areas, 90t, 91
  disorders
    clinical examples, 77–91f
    neuroanatomical substrate, 91–96f
  levels, 96–97. See also Arousal; Attention
  neural basis, 96–98f
  varieties, 74–77. See also specific varieties of mental control
Mental tasks, 3
Mental tone, 76–77f
Mesencephalic reticular formation, 91, 94f, 95f
Mesencephalic/diencephalic nuclei, 194
Mesencephalon
  cholinergic system, 91
  reticular formation, 91, 93f
Midline diencephalic region, 193
Midline system, 93
Mill
  James, 15
  John Stuart, 15
Mind/brain dichotomy, 6–9
Minnesota Multiphasic Personality Inventory, 100
Modality-specific anomia, 173
Module, 25
Mood
  discordance with affect, 101
  disorders, clinical examples, 102–106
  neurochemical changes and, 114
Mood-consistent affect, 115
Motivation, 102. See Drive
Motor Activity
  neural basis, 70–73t
  varieties, 71t
Motor aphasia, 155–156f
Motor apraxia. See Ideomotor apraxia
Motor aprosodia (amelodia), 162–164f
Motor association cortex, 23
Motor cortex, 22, 67–70f
Motor disorders
  clinical examples, 57–64
  neuroanatomical substrate, 64–70f
Motor function
  cortical homunculus and, 47f
  pyramidal vs. extrapyramidal, 51, 53

tripartite anatomical differentiation, 53
tripartite scheme of, 55–56f
varieties of, 51–57f
Motor planning, stages, 56
Motor representation, 72–73
Motor system
  of behavioral expression, 54f, 55
  of effective behavior, 54f, 55
  as multi-loop system, 50
  responses
    activities in, 70–71
    functional components, 69–70f
    integrative, 51
    reflexive, 51
    steps in, 56t
    types, 51
  of visceral activities, 53, 54f
MRI (magnetic resonance imaging), 11
Multimodal cortex. See Heteromodal association cortex
Mutism, akinetic. See Akinetic mutism
Myelinogenesis, cortical areas and, 22f, 23–24

Naming
  acquired impairment. See Anomia
  disorders, 148
  functional system interactions, 255
Narcolepsy, clinical example, 77–78
Narcotic analgesics, 39
Neglect
  anosognosic phenomena and, 88
  hemispatial, 84–85
  right hemisphere predominance, 85–86
  sensory, 84
  unilateral, 84, 92
Neomammalian (effector) brain, 55f
Neuroanatomy
  cellular, 21–25
  comparative, 18–19
Neurobehavior, 4
Neurological function, basic, 29
Neurological studies, 11
Neuroophthalmology, 120
Neuropsychology, 12
Neurotransmitter systems, in thought disorders, 242

Neurotransmitters. *See also specific neurotransmitters*
  altered sleep stages and, 75
  asymmetry, 108–109
  cerebral tone alterations, 76f
Non–REM sleep, 91, 97
Nonfluent aphasia
  characteristics, 148t
  hemispheric region, 147f
Nonfluent verbal output, 169
Nonverbal auditory agnosia, 36
Norepinephrine
  altered sleep stages and, 75
  decreased output, 242
Nucleus reticularis, 94f, 97

Obsessive–compulsive disorder, 117, 228
  with Tourette's syndrome, 235–236
Obstructive hydrocephalus, 57–58f
Occipital alexia. *See* Posterior alexia without agraphia. *See* Posterior alexia
Optic dysmetria, 132
Oriental languages, reading, neural basis of, 169f

Pain
  definition, 38
  gating mechanisms, 97, 257–258f
  intractable, relief by brain operations, 37–38
  treatment approaches, 39
Pain asymbolia, 36–37
Paleomammalian–limbic brain, 55f
Palinopsia, 130–131f, 140
Paragraphia, 200
Paranoia, 233
Paraphasia, 200
Paraphasic anomia, 171–172
Paraphasic substitution, 200
Parietal alexia. *See* Central alexia
Parietal lobe, angular gyrus, 18–19
Parietal-occipital cortex (Brodmann area 19), 95, 136
Parkinson's disease
  abnormal dopamine activity and, 242
  dementia of, 191
Paroxysmal behavioral disorders, narcolepsy and, 77
Pathological crying, 105, 111
Pathological laughter, 105–106, 111

Pavlov, Ivan, 16
Perception, 30, 31
  disordered, 170
  in language processing, 175f
  neuroanatomical correlates, 170
Percepts, 32, 49
  interaction, 255
  multiple and simultaneous processing, 256
Peripheral nerve destruction, 39
Perseveration, 200
Personality
  alteration, following brain damage, 117
  definition, 102
Personality disorder(s)
  with chronic pain, 234–235
  in frontal damage, 212–214
  types, 99
PET (positron emission tomography), 11, 108
Phantom limb phenomenon, 41–43f
Phrenology, mental faculties of, 7–8t
Piaget, Jean, 10
Pick, Arnold, 10
Polymodal cortex. *See* Heteromodal association cortex
Polysomnography, of narcolepsy, 77–78
Positron emission tomography (PET), 11, 108
Post–traumatic amnesia (PTA), 187
Posterior alexia, 153–54, 167, 168t, 173, 174f
Posterior cerebral artery occlusion, 185
Posterior cortical atrophy, 131–132f
Posterior hemispheric localization, 207
Posterior–lateral prefrontal cortex, 222
Postural control, 72
Precentral gyrus (Brodmann area 4), 67–68f, 250
Prefrontal cortex
  in animal species, 18–19f
  connections to subcortical motor centers, 222–223
  control functions, 226f
  damage, 206
    behavioral disorders of, 211–220f
    manifestations, 209–210t
  intelligence and, 208–209
  limbic system connections, 222f
  neural circuits, 222–223f

Prefrontal surgery, behavior and, 111–113, 209
Premotor cortex (Brodmann area 6), 68
Preverbiculum, 143–144
Primary analyzers, 136
Primary cortex, 248, 250, 251, 253t
  subcortical connections, 253
Primary memory, 179
Primary motor cortex, 67–68f
Primary sensory cortex, 22
Primary visual receptive system, 46f
Priming, retrieval and, 197
Problem solving, 207
Progressive supranuclear palsy, 191
Prosody, 145, 165
Prosopagnosia, 11, 126–127
Pseudo–depressed frontal personality syndrome, 113
Pseudo–psychopathic personality syndrome, 113
Pseudo–retarded frontal personality syndrome, 113
Pseudobulbar affect, 110–111
Psychic blindness, 103
Psychoanalytic theory, 101
Psychogenic amnesia, 188
Psychological tests, 207
Psychomotor retardation, 223
Psychosis, in sleep deprivation, 78
Psychotic breakdown, 111
Psychotropic medications, 230
PTA (post–traumatic amnesia), 187
Pure amnesia, 186
Pure word deafness
  diagnosis, 152–153
  disordered reception and, 170
  neuropathological patterns, 154
Pure word dumbness, 150–151f
Pyramidal motor functions, 51, 53

Quadrantopia, 120

Radionuclide brain scan
  of cortical deafness, 35f
  left posterior cerebral artery infarction, 153f
  of unilateral inattention/inintention, 83f

Reading
  neuroanatomical correlates, 173–174f
  in Oriental languages, 169f
  testing, 148
Recent memory, 179–181
Reception
  definition, 31, 120
  disordered, 170. See also Pure word deafness
  in language processing, 175f
  neuroanatomical correlates, 170
  in sensory processing, 32t
  of visual information, 137
Receptive aphasia. See Wernicke's aphasia
Recognition
  definition, 139
  neuroanatomical correlates, 170–171
Reduplicative paramnesia, 217–218, 219, 220
Reflex epilepsy, with schizophrenia–like disorders, 230–232
Reflex system, 71–72
Reflexes, 16, 93
Rehearsal, 255
Release phenomenon, 131
REM–off cells, 91
REM–sleep, 91, 97
Remote memory, 181. See also Retrieval
Repetition, fluency–nonfluency and, 169–170
Reptilian brain, 55f
Reticular activating system, 91–92, 93f, 192
Reticular system, 97
Retrieval
  description, 181
  disorders, 216
    clinical examples, 189–192
  in memory, 179
  neural basis, 196–197
  neuroanatomical substrate, 194
  priming and, 197
Retrograde amnesia, 187, 189–190
Rhythm, 145
Right hemisphere
  in communication, 165
  language characteristics, 165t
  language functions, 145t
  predominance, in neglect, 85–86

Rolando, fissure of, 169
Rote memory, 199

Scanning process, in memory, 179
Scanning speech, 149–150
Schema, 25. *See also* Functional systems
Schizophrenia
    abnormal dopamine activity and, 242
    catatonia and, 82
    clinical examples, 229
    negative symptoms, 228
    positive symptoms, 228
Schizophrenia–like disorders, with reflex epilepsy, 230–232
Scotomata, 120
Sechenov, I.M., 16
Secondary analyzers, 136
Secondary memory, 179–181
Selective attention, 76
Self–analysis. *See* Self–awareness
Self–awareness
    definition, 211
    neural basis, 225–226*f*
Self–consciousness. *See* Self–awareness
Semantic anomia, 172
Semantic language, 146
Semantic paralexia, of deep dyslexia, 167, 169
Semantic recognition, neuroanatomical correlates, 170–171
Senescence, 190
Sensation
    conscious recognition of, 32
    neural basis, 48–49
    varieties of, 30–32
Sensorimotor reactions, 29
Sensory aphasia. *See* Wernicke's aphasia
Sensory association cortex, 23
Sensory attention pathways, 93, 94*f*
Sensory disorders. *See also specific sensory disorders*
    clinical examples, 33–43*f*
    neuroanatomical substrate, 43–48
Sensory excitation, 72, 73
Sensory functions, 30, 47*f*
Sensory gating, 257–258*f*
Sensory input system, 92
Sensory neglect, 84
Sensory processing steps, 32*t*

Sensory reception, 31
Sequencing
    description, 209–210
    neural basis, 224
Serotonergic system, 92*f*
Serotonin
    altered sleep stages and, 75
    disturbances, 242
Serotoninergic cells, 91
Short–term memory, 179–181. *See also* Learning
Simultanagnosia, 132
Skinner, B.F., 16–17
Sleep
    altered thought processing, 75
    deprivation, 78
    disorders, 77–78, 242
    neuroanatomy, 91
    stages, 75
Sleep time, optimal, 75
Sleep/wakefulness cycle, 91
SMA (supplementary motor area), 69
Social speech, 144
Sociopathic personality, 228
Somatic function, 30
Somesthesis
    disturbances, 36–43*f*
    subdivisions, 30
Somesthetic stimuli pathways, 44*f*
Somnolent akinetic mutism, 81
SPECT, 11
Speech
    definition, 143
    disturbances
        with language disorders, 151
        pure, sites of, 151
    forms, 144
    inner, 143–144
    motor aspect of, 51
    scanning, 149–150
Split–brain patients, 133–134
    right hemisphere language capacity, 165*t*
Spoken language. *See* Language, spoken
Spontaneous confabulation, 216–217*f*, 219, 220
Spontaneous speech, 146–147*f*
Stereognosis, 30
Storing process, in memory, 179
Strangelove effect, 58–60*f*
Stress/homeostasis theory, 99

Striato–pallidal–nigral system
  dysfunction, 53t
  motor programs, 56
Subangular alexia, 173
Subcortical dementia, 191, 237–239t
Subcortical limbic structures, 222
Subcortical system, with prominent frontal influence, 253–254t
Subcortical (thalamic) aphasia, 159–160f
Subliminal awareness, 140
Succession, of functional systems, 255–256
Supplementary motor area (SMA), 69
Supramodal association cortex, 251, 253
Syntactic functions, disordered, 171
Syntax, 146, 176

Tactile function, 30
Temporal grading, 209–210
Temporal gyrus, 18–19
Temporal lobe
  damage, 108
    in posterior aphasia, 233
  hyperconnection, 237
  personality disorders, 102–105t
Temporal–parietal lesions, neglect and, 84
Tertiary association cortex, 23
Tertiary memory, 181. *See also* Retrieval
Thalamic damage, bilateral, with inintention, 89–91f
Thalamic nuclei, in sensory gating, 257–258f
Thalamus, 43
Thinking, 3, 4, 260
  brain function and, 3–4
  definition, 3, 4–5
  philosophical views, 13
  theoretical views, 13
  vs. cognition, 5
Third alexia. *See* Anterior alexia
Thought
  abnormal, 10
  definition, 143
  directed, 258–260
  language and, 9–10

Thought content
  alteration, 259–260
  definition, 5, 260
Thought disorders, 227–244. *See also* Schizophrenia
  clinical examples, 229–239t
  neural basis, 243–244
  neuroanatomical substrate, 239–243t
  terminology, 227
  varieties, 228–229
Thought processing
  control mechanisms, 256–258
  definition, 5
  functional systems, governing characteristics, 253–256
  functional systems and, 25–26
  multiple levels, 260
  neural model, 247–248
Timbre, 145
Toland, John, 8
Tonic arousal system, 93, 94f
Topographagnosia, 128–130f
Tourette's syndrome, with obsessive–compulsive traits, 235–236
Toxic encephalopathy. *See* Acute confusion
Transcortical motor aphasia, 158–159, 162
Transcortical sensory aphasia, 159, 170
Transient electrical nerve stimulation (TENS), 39
Transmodal association, 17–18
Transmodal cortex. *See* Heteromodal association cortex

Unawareness, of attentional deficit, 88
Unconcern, in attentional disorder, 88
Unilateral attention, anatomical base, 95
Unilateral brain damage, emotional disorders, 100–101
Unilateral dominance theory, 88
Unilateral inattention, 76, 82–83f, 92
Unilateral inintention, 82–83f, 84
Unilateral neglect, 84, 92
Unilateral revisualization disturbance, 85f
Unimodal association, 48
  definition, 32
  description, 121
  in language processing, 175f

in sensory processing, 32t
visual–spatial function and,
137–138f
Unimodal association cortex, 251–252
areas, 250
classification, 24f
memory storage and, 139, 195
primary visual analyzer, 136
reciprocal connections, 221
Upper motor neuron, 51, 52f
anatomy, 52f
paralysis, characteristics, 51, 52t

Verbal aphasia, 152
Verbal auditory agnosia, 36
Verbal dysdecorum, 113, 163–165f
Verbal regulation, in thought disorders, 241–242
Vigilant akinetic mutism, 81
Visceral–endocrine peripheral nervous system, 222
Visual agnosia, 123–126f
Visual allesthesia, 130
Visual discrimination
definition, 120–121
types, 137
unimodal association and, 137–138f
Visual field disturbance, in amnesic stroke, 188
Visual gnosis
definition, 120
disorders, 122–125f, 134t
studies, 121–122
Visual imagery
neuroanatomical substrate, 169–174
in thinking, 119
Visual–Metaphor Test, 205
Visual neglect, 85

Visual percepts, 136
interaction, 255
Visual processing
disorders
clinical examples, 122–134
higher, 134t
neuroanatomical substrate, 134–137f
steps, 140
Visual reception, 120
Visual sensations, 31
Visual–spatial acalculia, 202
Visual–spatial agnosia, 139
Visual–spatial competency, 216
Visual–spatial discrimination disturbance, 121
Visual–spatial function
neural basis, 137–140f
varieties, 120–122
Visual stimulation, 140
Visual–Verbal Test, 205–206
Vygotsky, Lev, 10

Watson, John, 9, 16
Wechsler Adult Intelligence Scale, 205
Wernicke's aphasia, 108, 157, 170, 233
Wernicke's encephalopathy, 186
White matter tracts, in visual processing, 136
Wilson's disease, 191
Wisconsin Card Sort Test, 206, 215
Word production anomia, 171
Word recognition anomia, 172
Word selection anomia, 152, 172
Writing
competency, 148
disorders, categories of, 174
Written speech, 144

NO LONGER THE PROPERTY
OF THE
UNIVERSITY OF R.I. LIBRARY